Clinical Applications
for
Motor Control

Clinical Applications
for
Motor Control

Edited by

Patricia C. Montgomery, PhD, PT
Therapeutic Intervention Programs, Inc.
Hopkins, Minnesota

Barbara H. Connolly, EdD, PT, FAPTA
University of Tennessee Health Science Center
Memphis, Tennessee

An innovative information, education, and management company
6900 Grove Road • Thorofare, NJ 08086

BS

Clinical applications for motor control/(edited by) Patricia Montgomery, Barbara Connolly.
   p,; cm.
Includes bibliographical references and index.
  ISBN 1-55642-545-7 (alk. paper)
  1. Physical therapy--Case studies. 2. Neuromuscular diseases--Pathophysiology. 3. Movement disorders--Pathophysiology. 4. Motor ability. 5. Motor learning.
  [DNLM: 1. Movement Disorders--rehabilitation--Case Report. 2. Motor Skills--physiology--Case Report. 3. Physical Therapy Techniques--Case Report. 4. Psychomotor Performance--Case Report. WL 390 C641 2002] I. Montgomery, Patricia. II. Connolly, Barbara H.
  RM701 .C58 2002
  615.8'2--dc21

                                                    2002010007

Printed in the United States of America.

Published by: SLACK Incorporated
             6900 Grove Road
             Thorofare, NJ 08086 USA
             Telephone: 856-848-1000
             Fax: 856-853-5991
             www.slackbooks.com

Contact SLACK Incorporated for more information about other books in this field or about the availability of our books from distributors outside the United States.

For permission to reprint material in another publication, contact SLACK Incorporated. Authorization to photocopy items for internal, personal, or academic use is granted by SLACK Incorporated provided that the appropriate fee is paid directly to Copyright Clearance Center. Prior to photocopying items, please contact the Copyright Clearance Center at 222 Rosewood Drive, Danvers, MA 01923 USA; phone: 978-750-8400; website: www.copyright.com; email: info@copyright.com.

Last digit is print number: 10 9 8 7 6 5 4 3 2 1

10/29/03

CONTENTS

ACKNOWLEDGMENTS

We would like to acknowledge the artwork of Sandy Lowrance that was initially prepared for the first edition of this text (***Motor Control and Physical Therapy: Theoretical Framework and Practical Application***) and has been reprinted in this revision titled ***Clinical Applications for Motor Control***. Our appreciation also goes to the authors of the individual chapters for being so responsible and efficient, and to our families for their support during the process of writing and editing.

ABOUT THE EDITORS

Patricia C. Montgomery, PhD, PT received her BS degree in physical therapy from the University of Oklahoma, Norman, Okla, her MA degree in educational psychology, and her PhD in child psychology from the University of Minnesota, Minneapolis. Dr. Montgomery has a private practice in pediatrics in the Minneapolis-St. Paul area and has taught in physical therapy programs at several academic institutions. She is currently an associate professor at the University of Tennessee Health Science Center and also provides continuing education courses for physical therapy clinicians.

Barbara H. Connolly, EdD, PT, FAPTA received her BS degree in physical therapy from the University of Florida, Gainesville. She received an MEd in special education and an EdD in curriculum and instruction from Memphis State University, Tenn. She is professor and chairman of the department of physical therapy at the University of Tennessee Health Science Center. She holds an academic appointment in physical therapy at the University of Indianapolis and serves as a guest lecturer at numerous other programs in physical therapy. Additionally, Dr. Connolly remains active in the clinic through the University of Tennessee faculty practice.

CONTRIBUTING AUTHORS

Joanell A. Bohmert, PT, MS, received her BS degree and advanced MS degree in physical therapy from the University of Minnesota, Minneapolis. She is a full-time clinician with the Anoka-Hennepin school district with a focus on pediatrics and neurology. Ms. Bohmert was actively involved in the development and revision of the *Guide to Physical Therapist Practice* as a member of the project advisory group and liaison to the musculoskeletal panel for Part Two; member of the task force on development of Part Three; a project editor for the second edition, Parts One and Two; and is currently a member of the American Physical Therapy Association board of directors oversight committee for the second edition. She has lectured extensively on the *Guide* and is an APTA Trainer for the *Guide*.

Nancy N. Byl, PhD, PT, FAPTA, is currently professor and chair of the department of physical therapy and rehabilitation science at the University of California, San Francisco. Dr. Byl received her BS degree in physical therapy and an MPH in public health from the University of California, San Francisco. She received her PhD in special education from the University of California, Berkeley and San Francisco State University. In 2000, she was awarded a Catherine Worthingham Fellowship from the American Physical Therapy Association. Dr. Byl has engaged in research and published extensively in the areas of motor control and neuroplasticity.

Lisa M. Cipriany-Dacko, PT, MA, received BS and MA degrees in physical therapy from Boston University, Mass. She also received an MA degree in motor learning from Columbia University, NY. She is currently an assistant professor and academic coordinator of clinical education at Arcadia University (formerly Beaver College) in Glenside, Pa. She has published numerous articles on physical therapy and elder individuals.

Carol A. Giuliani, PhD, PT, received a BS degree in physical therapy from California State University at Long Beach, and MS and PhD degrees in kinesiology, with an emphasis in the neural control of movement, from the University of California at Los Angeles. Dr. Giuliani currently is a professor in the division of physical therapy at the University of North Carolina at Chapel Hill.

Patricia Leahy, PT, MS, NCS (deceased), received a BS degree in physical therapy from the University of Pittsburgh and an MS degree in physical therapy from Temple University, Philadelphia, Pa. She was certified as a neurologic clinical specialist by the American Board of Physical Therapy Specialties. At the time of her death, Ms. Leahy was an assistant professor in the physical therapy department of the Philadelphia College of Pharmacy and Science. She was active in the neurology section of the American Physical Therapy Association, and a memorial scholarship in her name was established to honor her dedication to the profession.

Kathye E. Light, PhD, PT, received her BS degree in physical therapy from the University of Missouri, Columbia, her MS degree in physical therapy from the Medical College of Virginia, Virginia Commonwealth University, and her PhD in kinesiological motor control from the University of Texas, Austin. She is presently an associate professor of physical therapy at the University of Florida. Dr. Light's research interests include motor control and learning issues related to neurologic rehabilitation and adult aging.

Roberta A. Newton, PhD, PT received a BS degree in physical therapy and a PhD in neurophysiology from the Medical College of Virginia/Virginia Commonwealth University. Dr. Newton is a professor and director of Temple University's Institution on Aging. Dr. Newton conducts research on balance control, falls, and fall prevention/reduction in older adults.

Carol A. Oatis, PhD, PT has a BS degree in physical therapy from Marquette University, Milwaukee, Wis and a PhD in anatomy with an emphasis on biomechanics from the University of Pennsylvania, Philadelphia. She is an associate professor in physical therapy at Arcadia University (formerly Beaver College) in Glenside, Pa, where she teaches applied anatomy and biomechanics, as well as clinical decision-making. Her present research interests include motion analysis of locomotion, particularly modeling knee joint behavior during locomotion in individuals with osteoarthritis.

Mary M. Rodgers, PhD, PT received BS and MS degrees in physical therapy and biomechanics from the University of North Carolina at Chapel Hill, and a PhD in biomechanics from Pennsylvania State University, State College. Dr. Rodgers is a research health scientist with the Department of Veterans Affairs and holds academic appointments in the Departments of Rehabilitation Medicine and Orthopaedic Surgery at Wright State University School of Medicine, Dayton, Ohio.

Mary Ann Seeger, PT, MS received her BS degree in physical therapy from the University of Colorado, Boulder and her MS degree in physical therapy from the University of Southern California. Ms. Seeger is employed in a private practice in Portland, Oregon. Ms. Seeger also holds an appointment as an instructor at the University of Tennessee Health Science Center. Her many roles include being a clinician with practice focused on adults with balance and vestibular disorders, a consultant to other clinicians in the areas of balance and vestibular disorders, and a teacher at numerous post-professional and graduate seminars around the country.

Ann F. VanSant, PhD, PT received a BS degree in physical therapy from Russell Sage College, Troy, NY, her master's degree from Virginia Commonwealth University, and her doctorate from the University of Wisconsin, Madison. Her teaching and research are related to life span development of motor abilities. She is currently editor of *Pediatric Physical Therapy*, the journal of the pediatric section of the American Physical Therapy Association, and is a professor in the Department of Physical Therapy, College of Allied Health Professions, Temple University, Philadelphia, Pa.

Marilyn Woods, PT, has a BS degree from Nebraska Wesleyan University, Lincoln and a certificate in physical therapy from Mayo Clinic School of Physical Therapy. She is a member of the APTA-trained faculty for the *Guide to Physical Therapist Practice*. She has given numerous workshops on the *Guide* to clinicians and has been active in the

Minnesota chapter APTA quality assurance program for more than 20 years. Ms. Woods spent many years as a generalist in a small rural hospital in northern Minnesota. Currently, she is a supervisor of home care rehabilitation at Park Nicollet Health System, Methodist Hospital in St. Louis Park, Minn.

Mitzi B. Zeno, PT, MS, NCS received a BS degree in biology from Graceland College, a BS degree in physical therapy from the University of Central Arkansas, and an MS degree in physical therapy from Texas Woman's University, Dallas. Ms. Zeno is an assistant professor in the Department of Physical Therapy at the University of Tennessee Health Science Center. She teaches in the areas of neurologic physical therapy to entry-level and post-professional students in the physical therapy programs. Her research interests include the assessment of motor control in adults and children with neurologic disorders.

Audrey Zucker-Levin, PT, MS, GCS, received her BS and MS degrees in physical therapy from Long Island University. She is currently a PhD candidate in pathokinesiology at New York University. Ms. Zucker-Levin is an assistant professor in the Department of Physical Therapy at the University of Tennessee Health Science Center. She teaches in the areas of kinesiology/pathokinesiology, neurobiology, and prosthetics to entry-level and post-professional students in the physical therapy programs. Ms. Zucker-Levin was previously employed at the Johns Hopkins Geriatrics Center in Baltimore, Md, and continues to practice clinically through the University of Tennessee faculty practice. Her research interests are in the areas of geriatrics and prosthetics.

INTRODUCTION

In the 10 years since the publication of the first edition, empirical evidence in the areas of neurophysiology, biomechanics, motor control, motor learning, motor development, and cognitive training has continued to expand. Physical therapists increasingly are becoming an entry point into the health care system and are responsible for diagnosing movement disorders. As a result, physical therapists must remain current in their knowledge of the research literature and possible applications to patient care. In addition, the *Guide to Physical Therapist Practice* has evolved as the framework for examination, evaluation, and intervention by physical therapists. *Clinical Applications for Motor Control* attempts to provide "state-of-the-art" information that allows physical therapist students and practitioners to apply current concepts in a problem-solving approach within the framework of the *Guide*. Evaluation and intervention strategies should be modified by practitioners as new empirical evidence is obtained. *Clinical Applications for Motor Control*, therefore, is an evolving document that will change in future editions to reflect evidence-based practice.

CHAPTER 1

A Framework for Examination, Evaluation, and Intervention

Barbara H. Connolly, EdD, PT, FAPTA
Patricia C. Montgomery, PhD, PT

Our framework for examination, evaluation, and intervention must be one that allows us as dynamic health care professionals to change as new information becomes available. Advances in research in the areas of neurophysiology, biomechanics, motor control, motor learning, motor development, and cognitive training provide us with new and more effective methods to evaluate and treat patients with movement disorders. The purpose of this book is to provide physical therapy students and practitioners with state-of-the-art information in the above-mentioned areas. New information in the areas of neuroplasticity and balance should be of particular interest to those practitioners who are providing care to both the pediatric and adult populations.

A case study format is used to emphasize and illustrate the importance of applying research information in the clinical setting. Students and clinicians need to be diagnosticians of movement disorders and able to apply this state-of-the-art information to patients. The *Guide to Physical Therapist Practice* has stimulated the entire profession of physical therapy to become more active in diagnosis, prognosis, and the establishment of functional outcomes. The case study format used in this text allows students, who have little experience in applying theoretical information to practical problems, to use a problem-solving approach and to use the *Guide to Physical Therapist Practice*.

Figure 1-1. An open system devoid of feedback. Information travels in only one direction. Neurons 1 and 2 conduct impulses toward neuron 3, which in turn directs its activity toward the muscle.

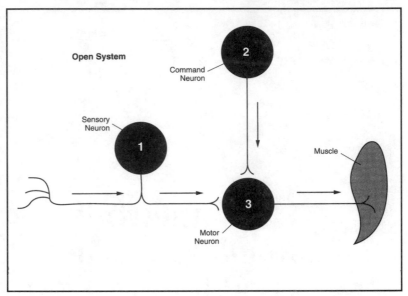

HISTORICAL PERSPECTIVES

For the past 30 years, the approaches to patients with neurologically based movement disorders have changed from reflexive or hierarchical models of motor control to more contemporary models of motor control. Most of the early approaches were based on a hierarchical model of motor control in which the reflex served as the basic functional unit of movement. In these models, the cortex was viewed as the highest functioning component of the system and spinal level reflexes as the lowest. Newer models, in particular the *distributed control model*, propose a different neural organization of motor control. In this model, the controller varies depending on the task. No longer is the cortex considered the boss.

Two general models of neural organization that are used to describe motor function are the *open system* and the *closed system*. The open system model is characterized by a single transfer of information without feedback loops (Figure 1-1). This model is used in the traditional reflexive hierarchical theory of motor control. However, the closed system model has multiple feedback loops and supports the concept of distributed control (Figure 1-2). Additionally, in the closed model, the nervous system is viewed as an active agent with structures that enable the initiation and generation of movement, not merely an agent that reacts to incoming stimuli. In the early hierarchical theories of motor control, more focus was placed on the open system, and the child was viewed as a reactive rather than a proactive individual as advocated in the distributed control model.

In the field of motor learning, *closed loop* and *open loop* theories are proposed to account for the processes of learning and performing motor tasks. Closed loop theory stresses the use of feedback, particularly when learning new tasks. The use of feedback during new tasks is important as the individual uses *internal trial and error* as opposed to primarily *external trial and error* in making judgments about the correctness of the motor performance. Interestingly, during the 2000 World Olympics, a gold medalist diver discussed the importance of *imagery* (or internal trial and error) as an important

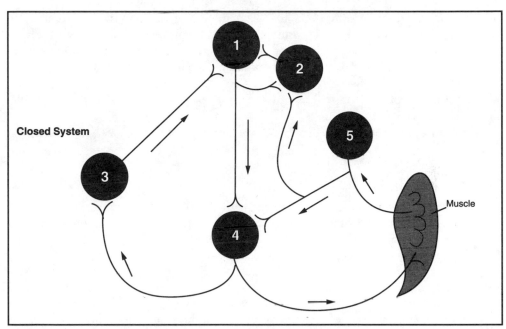

Figure 1-2. A closed loop system with multiple feedback loops. Although neuron 1 appears to be at the top of the hierarchy, and thus in command of the system, it is apparent on closer analysis that there is no hierarchy in this organizational arrangement of neurons. By inspecting neurons 1 to 4, it is easy to see that each of these elements could conceivably be under control of at least one other neuron: neuron 1 receives information from neurons 2 and 3, neuron 2 receives information from neurons 1 and 5, and so on. Only neuron 5 appears to be outside the sphere of influence of other neurons. Neuron 5 is indirectly affected by the activity in neuron 4.

aspect of her training for the Olympics. She had been injured and was unable to physically practice her diving and thus had to mentally practice. This mental practice occurred without physical practice until shortly before the Olympic competition, and yet the diver was able to perfect her dive to the point of winning a gold medal. Open loop theory accounts for skills that are well-established, performed rapidly, or where feedback is not used due to the speed needed to accomplish the task (ie, ballistic type movements). As we work with patients with neurological impairments, we strive to attain use of open loop systems, but we need to use closed loop systems during the early intervention period.

REVIEW OF TRADITIONAL NEUROPHYSIOLOGIC APPROACHES

Physical therapists use combinations of techniques from a variety of theoretical frameworks in the evaluation and treatment of patients with movement disorders. A majority of the traditional reflexive/hierarchical neurophysiologic approaches relied on the examination of reflexive behavior (ie, flexor withdrawal, asymmetrical tonic neck reflex, Moro response, body righting, labyrinthine righting, and equilibrium reactions) as a basis of treatment. This early emphasis on reflexes led therapists to conceptualize the central nervous system (CNS) in a stimulus-response type paradigm or as a passive agent in movement. Treatment often was based on inhibition of abnormal postural reflex activity and facilitation of normal postural control and movement. These early approaches were developed when much less was known about mechanisms that control movement and did not address parameters of movement such as initiation, rate, and synergistic organization. In this text, we will focus on current theories of motor control that identify the multiple systems that are involved in a complex dynamic interaction resulting in motor behavior.

The most commonly used neurophysiologic approaches are reviewed superficially in the following pages.

Ayres—Sensory Integration

As a young occupational therapist in the early 1950s, A. Jean Ayres, PhD, realized that functional limitations of many adults with brain injuries were due to sensory or perceptual factors rather than motor problems. She reasoned that understanding how the brain processes sensation, especially vestibular and somatosensory input, would provide the basis for treatment of perceptual dysfunction. *Sensory Integration* (SI), the neurobehavioral theory developed by Dr. Ayres, stressed the CNS's ability to organize and interpret sensory information. In Ayres' original theory, higher level processes of perception and cognition were considered dependent on brainstem and midbrain processing of sensory input (hierarchical). SI theory was developed to explain an observed relationship between deficits in sensory processing and deficits in academic or neuromotor learning. The basic assumptions put forward by Ayres included the following:

1. Plasticity exists within the CNS
2. SI processes occur in a developmental sequence
3. The brain functions as an integrated whole, but is comprised of systems that are hierarchically organized
4. Eliciting an adaptive behavior promotes SI and, in turn, the ability to produce an adaptive behavior reflects SI
5. People have an inner drive to develop SI through participation in sensorimotor activities[1]

Currently, the SI approach places a greater emphasis on a systems view of the nervous system. However, this view retains Ayres' concept of an interactive holistic hierarchy. In current SI theory, the assumption is made that the person and the nervous system are *open systems*. The open system is viewed as one in which the person and the nervous system are capable of self-regulating and self-organizing through a spiral process of self-actualization.[1] Important aspects of the new model are the inclusion of behavioral, as well as neurobiologic, components and the expanded role of the environment on motor behaviors.

Ayres devised tests to identify and measure symptoms of sensory dysfunction and began publishing her findings in the mid 1960s. She continued to develop standardized tests until the time of her death in 1988. The last test developed by Dr. Ayres was the Sensory Integration and Praxis Tests. Through the use of these tests, supplemented by clinical observations, children are identified as having sensory integrative disorders in the following:

1. Postural-ocular movement
2. Tactile discrimination

3. Sensory modulation

4. Bilateral integration and sequencing

5. Somatodyspraxia

Motor dysfunction in sensory integrative theory is addressed primarily from the aspect of motor planning or praxis, and SI was not developed to address neuromotor dysfunction as exists in the child with cerebral palsy. Although assessment and treatment principles initially addressed the child with learning disabilities, SI has been incorporated into treatment for patients with varying brain pathology. Motor behavior during treatment is used to evaluate changes in organization and interpretation of sensory input. Ayres proposed that somatosensory and vestibular functions are ontogenetically and phylogenetically early and are the underpinnings of normal development. Sensory feedback and repetition are important principles of motor learning incorporated into SI theory.

Treatment is administered to meet the sensory needs of the individual. The sensory environment and sensory requirements of tasks are changed depending on the individual's response to treatment. The *adaptive response* refers to active participation in treatment, so sensory information must be organized by the individual in order to complete a task, solve a problem, or plan a movement. Behavioral goals that, as much as possible, are determined by the patient are stressed. SI is practiced mainly by occupational therapists, but physical therapists also have incorporated SI into treatment regimens for patients with neurologic impairments. Training beyond entry-level preparation is available and consists of professional development courses in theory, test mechanics, and interpretation.

Bobath—Neurodevelopmental Treatment

Neurodevelopmental treatment (NDT) is an approach developed by Dr. Karel Bobath, an English physician, and his wife, Berta Bobath, a physiotherapist. Evaluation and treatment principles for neuromotor dysfunction were originally proposed in the late 1940s and were based on research done in the 1920s and 1930s with animals and humans. Emphasis has evolved from assessing localized spasticity to evaluating patterns of movement. Dysfunction is envisioned as the result of loss of control from damaged higher CNS centers. The CNS lesions are thought to result in a release of abnormal reflex activity from higher control. Currently, the NDT approach has incorporated new theories of motor control and has begun to address posture and its control as resulting from a cooperative interaction of the sensorimotor system with other systems, including the musculoskeletal system, cardiopulmonary system, and other regulatory and command systems, as well as the environment.[2] New assumptions have been incorporated into NDT theory based on current models of motor control. The new assumptions are:

1. Postural control uses both feedback and feed-forward mechanisms of execution

2. Postural control appears to be learned and modified through experience

3. Postural activity is initiated at the base of support

4. The development of postural control is expressed by an ability to assume positions in which the center of mass is progressively higher off the base of support and in which the size of the base of support is reduced

5. The development of postural control is an essential component of skill acquisition[2]

NDT was developed for children with cerebral palsy and adults with acquired hemiplegia, although this approach has been applied to patients with many types of neural dysfunction involving the motor system. In the NDT approach to treatment of children, normal development and quality of movement are addressed. The Bobaths stressed the importance of early intervention in children before abnormal or primitive movement patterns become habitual, leading to muscle asymmetries, contractures, and deformities. Currently, NDT has begun to use the *disablement model* in the planning and implementation of NDT treatment. In using this model, less focus is placed on quality of movement, and more focus is placed on the identification of impairments in relationship to functional goals. Additionally, NDT theory now stresses the necessity for the therapist to identify how, by improving the quality of movement, a change of function will occur if indeed quality of movement is a treatment goal. Treatment principles in NDT include normalizing abnormal muscle tone (spasticity, flaccidity, rigidity, and spasms), inhibiting or integrating primitive postural patterns, and facilitating normal postural reactions. This is done primarily through direct handling of the patient through key points (usually proximal) of control, although positioning and family/caregiver education also is stressed. In addition to numerous publications, basic training in NDT is taught in a continuing education format simultaneously to occupational therapists, physical therapists, and speech pathologists. The Bobaths considered all of these professionals to be concerned with motor aspects of behavior. Instructors are certified by a professional organization, and basic 8-week pediatric courses, 2- to 3-week courses in treatment of adults with hemiplegia, and advanced courses in treatment of infants are offered.

Brunnstrom—Movement Therapy in Hemiplegia

The Brunnstrom approach developed by Signe Brunnstrom, a physical therapist, is based on clinical information and neurophysiologic principles that were prevalent during the early 1960s. Brunnstrom identified numerous common characteristics seen in patients with hemiplegia. These common characteristics included the presence of basic limb synergies in both the upper and lower extremities and the order of recovery stages from the time of the initial insult. She stated that, although patients with hemiplegia have common characteristics, individual differences occur since no two patients are exactly alike. In synergistic patterns, these differences are related mainly to the relative strength of the synergy components and not the nature of the synergy.[3,4]

Using the Brunnstrom approach, the patient is assessed for the following:
- The presence of flaccidity (Stage 1)
- Emergence of basic limb synergies (Stage 2)
- Voluntary performance of part or all of the basic limb synergies (Stage 3)
- Mixing and matching of the basic limb synergies (Stage 4)
- Relative independence of basic extremity synergies (Stage 5)
- Isolated, coordinated joint movement (Stage 6)

Additionally, evaluations of sensation (tactile and passive motion sense), pain, passive range of motion, trunk balance, hand function, facial function, presence of selected postural reflexes, and stance/gait are vital to the overall evaluation of the patient.

Therapeutic procedures are aimed at promoting voluntary control of the basic limb synergies by the patient through the use of sensory input (tactile, proprioceptive, visual, and auditory) and positive reinforcement. Selected postural reflexes, such as the asymmetric tonic neck, tonic lumbar, and tonic labyrinthine reflexes, are used to facilitate voluntary movement. Brunnstrom stressed that training sessions must be planned so that only those tasks that the patient can master or almost master are demanded. Once the patient is able to move voluntarily through the synergies, the patient is encouraged to learn a number of movement combinations that deviate from the basic synergies and which are more functional. In particular, hand activities are stressed as the patient is able to move out of the basic synergy patterns in the involved upper extremity.

Brunnstrom advocated that preparation for walking be emphasized early in the treatment approach but that extensive walking be postponed so that a poor gait pattern could be avoided. The preparation for walking included training in trunk balance, modification of motor responses in the legs, and training of alternate responses of antagonistic muscles. In the training for standing and walking, Brunnstrom advocated the use of sensory input and behavioral modification by providing the patient with knowledge of result of his efforts.

Carr and Shepherd—Motor Relearning Approach

The motor relearning approach, developed by Janet Carr and Roberta Shepherd in the 1970s, focuses on an understanding of normal movement and how movement is learned or relearned.[5] Carr and Shepherd stated that an adult who has experienced a neurologic insult may no longer know how to move and may have to relearn those movements.[6] They further stated that those factors that are relevant to the *learning* of a motor skill are also relevant to the *relearning* of the skill. The major factors in the learning or relearning process as identified by Carr and Shepherd include:

- Identification of a goal
- Inhibition of unnecessary activity
- Ability to cope with the effects of gravity and therefore to make balance adjustments while shifting weight
- Appropriate body alignment
- Practice (physical and mental)
- Motivation
- Feedback and knowledge of results

Carr and Shepherd stated that the therapist should be aware of the effects of these factors in learning a skill; the therapist should assess the impact of problems on the patient with neurologic deficits. The importance of one of these factors, *knowledge of results*, is illustrated in Figure 1-3.

In the motor relearning approach, observation is a major part of the evaluation. Accordingly, the therapist who understands the subtleties and variations of normal movement should be able to evaluate with accuracy the patient's problems with movement. Through this critical observation, the therapist should be able to judge the most essential missing or abnormal components of movement and therefore provide interventions to address primary or secondary problems. The examination includes assessment of tone through movement, handling, and the effect of tonic reflexes. Additionally, the therapist examines overall movement and function, hand function, balance (both static and dynamic), and sensation. Although the assessments suggested in the approach are subjective, the authors stated that these observations were reliable and provided qual-

Figure 1-3. Average root-mean squared (or RMS) error for the two acquisition knowledge of results (KR) relative frequency conditions for day 1 (blocks 1-8), day 2 (blocks 9-16), immediate, and delayed no-KR retention tests. Results show that practice with lower relative frequencies of KR may be beneficial to

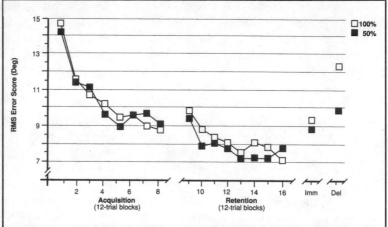

long-term retention and learning (reprinted with permission by the American Psychological Association. Winstein C, Schmidt RA. Reduced frequency of knowledge of results enhances motor skill learning. *J Exp Psych: Learning, Memory, and Cognition.* 1990;16:4).

itative information about the patient's function.[5] Other objective quantitative measures could be used as needed. Videotaping the patient is encouraged as a means of documenting function and improvement.

The techniques used in this approach represent a combination of other approaches. However, the authors insist that there can be no routine treatment for patients according to their medical diagnosis and that the developmental sequence should not be adhered to in adults. Many of the Bobath treatment techniques are suggested for use, such as holding and placing, reflex inhibiting movement patterns, weight bearing/approximation/compression, balance activities on a therapy ball, inhibitive casts, and walking facilitation. Many of the hand activities are based on the Bobath approach as well. The Rood techniques of brushing, application of ice, pounding, tapping, as well as vibration are incorporated into treatment. Carr and Shepherd encourage the use of electromyogram (EMG) biofeedback as a therapeutic technique to either decrease hypertonus during movement or to aid in the contraction of specific muscles. The use of a mirror for visual feedback is encouraged as a means of self-correction and self-awareness.

Johnstone—Treatment of Cerebrovascular Accident

Margaret Johnstone is a Scottish physiotherapist who has worked with patients with neurologic deficits since the time she treated patients with gunshot wounds of the brain in the mid 1940s. The main objective of her treatment approach is to attack spasticity in the patient with a cerebrovascular accident (CVA) 24 hours a day.[7] Treatment is based on reflex inhibition with special attention to inhibiting the tonic neck reflexes through use of air splints and positioning. The optimal position for the affected upper extremity in the air splint (40 mmHg pressure when fully inflated by mouth) is with shoulder external rotation; elbow, wrist, and finger extension; forearm supination; and thumb abduction. The goal is to maintain full wrist extension, thus avoiding the typical wrist and finger flexion postures of the patient with a CVA, and to maintain a pain-free shoulder.

During early stages of recovery, the patient is positioned sidelying on the unaffected side with the affected arm in the air splint protracted and supported by a pillow. Attention also is paid to positioning the affected leg in protraction with hip internal rotation and hip, ankle, and knee flexion. The patient can lie on the affected side if the limbs are positioned properly. Main problems are considered to be an imbalance of muscle tone and the presence of unwanted, disabling postures from loss of CNS control from higher centers. Based on a hierarchical, reflex model with sensory as well as motor emphasis, Johnstone's approach also relies on a normal, developmental model following sequences of movements, proximal to distal. The air splint is designed to apply even, deep pressure to the soft tissues to address sensory dysfunction. Johnstone outlined principles of early bed and transfer mobility, as well as early mat exercises. She also described more advanced exercises as the patient improves, with emphasis continuing on the use of air splints and positioning.

Kabat, Knott, Voss—Proprioceptive Neuromuscular Facilitation

Herman Kabat, MD, has been credited, along with his coworker, Margaret Knott, physical therapist, for developing the approach initially termed *proprioceptive facilitation.* Knott and Dorothy Voss, another physical therapist, later used the term *proprioceptive neuromuscular facilitation* or *PNF.*[8] PNF was developed initially for use with children with cerebral palsy but soon was applied to patients with other types of neurologic disorders. Today, PNF is used extensively with patients with orthopedic as well as neurologic problems.[9]

Guidelines for this theory were obtained from studies of animal behavior and learning, as well as human development. A developmental framework is evident in such principles as cervico-caudal and proximal to distal progressions and fetal reflexive motor behavior. This suggests that recapitulation of motor sequences is important. Sensory elements are incorporated. For example, reversals of movement used in PNF are an orderly sequencing of tactile, auditory, and visual cues. Manual contacts and tone of voice are used to modulate the patient's efforts to move.

Along with principles of motor development, principles of motor learning using involuntary and voluntary effort with repetition and use of specific patterns are stressed. PNF uses resistance and stretch to facilitate specific motor patterns, and rotation is a key element in many of these patterns. Specific patterns are used with reversing movements to establish an interaction between agonists and antagonists in an attempt to correct imbalances among muscle groups. Diagonal rather than straight plane movements are used primarily and are identified by specific titles, such as D1 and D2. Reflexes are stimulated to initiate movement and to promote postural control. These patterns are known as *irradiation patterns.* Coordination within and between patterns of a segment and between segments is stressed. Maximal resistance is used to promote irradiation and the patient's voluntary effort is used whenever possible. Adjunctive physical agents such as heat and cold are employed when appropriate.

General treatment in PNF includes the use of recapitulation of total patterns of developing motor behavior, spiral and diagonal patterns of movement, coupling voluntary movement with postural and righting reflexes, appropriate sensory cues and techniques for facilitating movement and postural responses, maximal resistance for maximal excitation and inhibition, and repetitive activity for conditioning and training. Specific placements of the therapist's hands are an important aspect of the PNF approach as it was originally developed.

Rood—Rood Approach to Neuromuscular Dysfunction

An approach to treatment of neurologic dysfunction was proposed in the 1950s by Margaret S. Rood, a physical therapist.[10] The approach of Rood to neurologic dysfunction represented her philosophy of treatment, which was concerned with the interaction of somatic, autonomic, and psychologic factors and their interactions with motor activities. This approach was one of the first that considered motor functions to be inseparable from sensory mechanisms. Therefore, sensory factors and their relationship to motor functions assumed a major role in the analysis of dysfunction and in the application of treatment. Specifically, Rood used sensory stimuli by stroking or brushing at a given speed and for a given duration for activation of a phasic muscle response. She applied cold for visceral stimulation and somatic relaxation and applied pressure and stretch for postural muscle activation. Over the years, the types of stimuli used have been modified by both Rood and other practitioners, and brushing is no longer used in treatment.[11]

In the Rood approach, muscle groups are analyzed according to the types of work they perform and their responses to specific stimuli. Light work refers to movement with reciprocal inhibition of antagonists. This may occur in voluntary movement or autonomic nervous system action. Heavy work is defined as the holding or co-contraction of muscles that are antagonists in normal movement and that are used to provide a stable support of a joint in a fixed position. Some muscles perform both light and heavy work functions. Using these concepts of light and heavy work, Rood outlined the normal developmental sequence by using the following order of activation of muscles groups:

1. Reciprocal innervation—reflex activation for movement patterns using reciprocal innervation of proximal joints in the developmental sequence until voluntary movement without the reflex is achieved
2. Coinnervation—co-contraction of antagonists and agonists working together to stabilize the body beginning at the head and neck and working downward
3. Heavy work—movement superimposed on co-contraction
4. Skill—skilled work with emphasis on distal portions of the body that requires control from the highest cortical level

In addition to using the concepts of light and heavy work in the developmental sequence, the Rood approach identified two major sequences in motor development that are distinctly different, but inseparable due to their interaction. The two sequences are those of skeletal functions (Figure 1-4) and vital functions. The skeletal functions include activities of the head, neck, trunk, and extremities while the vital functions include vegetative, respiratory, and speech activities.

The developmental sequence, both skeletal and vital, can be used to analyze the stages during which acquisition of the four levels of control (reciprocal innervation, coinnervation, heavy work, and skill) occurs. Additionally, stimulation of the sensory receptors is done in the sequence of normal development from the most primitive reflexes to the skill level.

The purpose of treatment is to restore that component in the sequence in the manner in which would be normally acquired. Therefore, the Rood approach to treatment is proposed to be applicable to any type of neurologic dysfunction at any age.

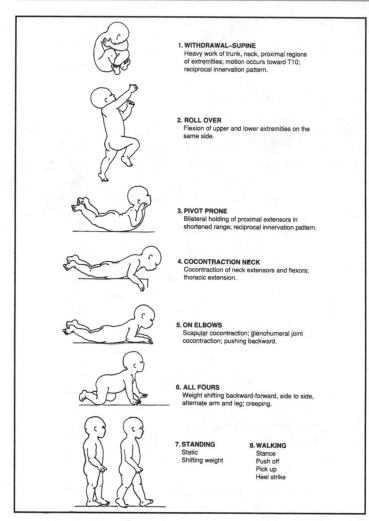

1. WITHDRAWAL–SUPINE
Heavy work of trunk, neck, proximal regions of extremities; motion occurs toward T10; reciprocal innervation pattern.

2. ROLL OVER
Flexion of upper and lower extremities on the same side.

3. PIVOT PRONE
Bilateral holding of proximal extensors in shortened range; reciprocal innervation pattern.

4. COCONTRACTION NECK
Cocontraction of neck extensors and flexors; thoracic extension.

5. ON ELBOWS
Scapular cocontraction; glenohumeral joint cocontraction; pushing backward.

6. ALL FOURS
Weight shifting backward-forward, side to side, alternate arm and leg; creeping.

7. STANDING
Static
Shifting weight

8. WALKING
Stance
Push off
Pick up
Heel strike

Figure 1-4. The skeletal function sequence according to Rood (adapted from Rood, M. The use of sensory receptors to activate, facilitate, and inhibit motor response, autonomic and somatic in developmental sequence. In: Sately C, ed. *Approaches to Treatment of Patients with Neuromuscular Dysfunction.* Dubuque, Iowa: William C. Brown; 1962:26-37).

CONTEMPORARY THEORETICAL FRAMEWORKS

Contemporary systems theories, such as ***dynamical action theory***, consider numerous systems or factors that contribute to the learning or relearning of motor skills. Traditional neurophysiologic theories from the 1950s and 1960s were based on a narrow developmental, hierarchical model. The use of this traditional model for physical therapy intervention has not been fully supported or substantiated through empirical studies. Research with animals and humans disseminated in recent years regarding motor control, motor development, and motor learning has prompted physical therapists to revise theoretical frameworks for evaluating and managing patients with movement disorders. Traditional theoretical frameworks that are used in clinical environments are continually being modified to incorporate principles supported by empirical studies and to integrate principles of systems theories. Clinicians, therefore, must remain current in their knowledge of basic and applied research and not rely on anecdotal information to determine intervention strategies and treatment techniques.

Variables Affecting Outcomes

A complete patient history should include those factors that may impact the motor behaviors of the developing child or of the adult who has pathology involving the nervous system. Physical therapists may have examined several of these factors in the past, but may not have fully appreciated the possible impact on functional skill acquisition. Systems theories have prompted physical therapists to examine a greater variety of variables that may influence a patient's ability to achieve functional outcomes following physical therapy intervention.

A factor that most physical therapists take into consideration is the patient's age. In general, the recovery process will be different in the child versus the adult. Additionally, information regarding acquisition of developmental milestones will be more important in the diagnosis, prognosis, and management of the child. In the adult patient, information relative to current living situations and prior community and work activities will be more applicable as the therapist plans an appropriate intervention program.

Cultural beliefs and traditions need to be recognized and incorporated into all aspects of patient management. For example, in some cultures, the therapist must address the male head of the family rather than the mother or female spouse when giving instructions for a home program. In other cultures, in which there is a matriarchal system, the grandmother or oldest living female in the family must be consulted even before an examination takes place.

A general health history for the patient provides information about systems or environments that might impact current management. An example of the interaction between health history and the environment would be to determine the relationship between an elderly patient with a history of frequent falls and the living environment. The patient might experience fewer falls if the living space has installation of brighter lighting and a nonslippery floor surface. Another example would be the child with a history of failure to thrive and repeated hospitalizations. As the child experiences fewer hospitalizations, the rate of progress may change.

Physical therapists need to know if the patient receives medication and what possible effects the medication may have on motor behaviors. Common examples are antiseizure medications, which may influence the alertness and arousal of the patient. If the antiseizure medication is increased during the course of therapeutic interventions, a loss of motor function may occur due to effects on the alertness and arousal state of the patient. Medications given to patients with Parkinson's disease have well-recognized "on" and "off" periods of effectiveness that have a direct correlation with the patient's ability to move. Some medications, such as those used in chemotherapy, may decrease the patient's overall strength and endurance for physical activity.

Although current anthropometric measurements are important during an examination of a patient, information about past anthropometrics also may be vital to the evaluation process. Musculoskeletal impairments may have been present prior to the current neurologic condition as a result of previous excessive stress or weight bearing on joints. This may occur, for example, in the patient who has a past history of obesity.

Movement is performed within the context of an individual's unique musculoskeletal system and neuromuscular status in relation to the task to be accomplished and the environment in which the task is attempted. A child who is short in stature may not demonstrate a reciprocal lower extremity pattern in ascending and descending stairs. The child may choose to use a "step to" pattern because of the relationship of the height of the step and the length of the extremity. This child may score below age level on a standardized test item when in fact a reciprocal pattern would be seen if a smaller step height were used. Increases or decreases in height (as in childhood and adolescence or in aging) may contribute to the degree of coordination of a motor skill or whether it can be accomplished at all. Likewise, the child with short fingers may choose to use the thumb and middle finger for a pincer grasp instead of the using the thumb and index finger.

Understanding how anthropometric factors may impact the prognosis for the individual patient is critical in overall management. An example of this would be a child with myelomeningocele. The decision to remain a household ambulator with orthotics and a walker or to use a wheelchair will be related to height and weight in relation to the energy expenditure required for mobility. The recovery of an adult who has had a CVA may be more difficult if the patient has excessive weight due to the increased energy expenditure required for movement and the completion of activities of daily living (ADLs).

Evidence-Based Practice

Information regarding physical therapy treatment strategies and specific hands-on techniques has been disseminated through various methods. In the absence of empirical studies, anecdotal information provided through expert opinion has been a common method of sharing information regarding the management of patients with pathology involving the nervous system. In order to become more effective and efficient in the provision of physical therapy services, the necessity of using empirical evidence to guide practice has become evident, and reliance on anecdotal information should be minimized. The reader is referred to texts that specifically focus on experimental designs and generalizability of results, topics that are not intended to be the focus of this chapter.

Harris[12] stated that the following questions should be asked when critiquing clinical treatment techniques and determining if the technique meets minimum scientific criteria:

- Are the theories underlying the treatment approach supported by valid anatomic and physiologic evidence?
- Is the treatment approach designed for a specific type of patient population?
- Are potential side effects of the treatment presented?
- Are studies from peer-reviewed journals provided that support the treatment's efficacy?
- Do the peer-reviewed studies include well-designed, randomized, controlled clinical trials or well-designed single-subject experimental studies?

Therefore, when determining a treatment strategy, three basic questions should be addressed:

1. Has the intervention been documented to be effective on an anatomic or physiologic level?
2. Do we have empirical information regarding the most efficient way to provide the intervention?
3. Does the intervention make a difference (ie, the "so what?" question)?

One example would be physical therapy intervention that is designed to elongate the hamstring muscles. The first question is addressed by empirical evidence that suggests prolonged stretching of muscle fibers results in increased range of motion and flexibility. DeDeyne discussed the cellular and adaptive mechanisms of muscle fibers that may be the scientific basis for stretching.[13]

Figure 1-5. Straight leg raise before stimulation.

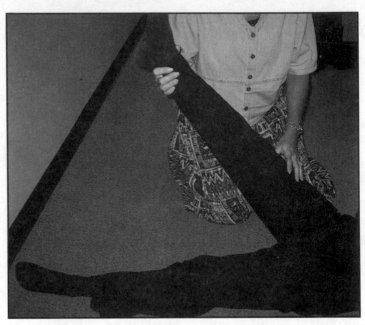

In regard to the second question, there have been studies that attempted to address the most efficient way to provide the intervention. Bandy and associates demonstrated that a single 30-second stretch of the hamstrings done daily was as effective as protocols that required more frequent or longer stretching.[14] This research was done with non-disabled adult subjects, however, so direct extrapolation to patients with pathology to the nervous system is not possible. For example, Steffen and Mollinger were unable to show any change in knee flexion contractures in nursing home residents following a 6-month intervention using a prolonged static stretch with a splint, 3 hours a day, 5 days per week.[15] Holt et al[16] demonstrated that resistance to stretch of the hamstring muscles could be measured in a reproducible manner from day to day in children with severe multiple disabilities. Resistance to stretch then was measured before and after 6 weeks of daily activities, including 60 seconds of passive static stretching (5 days per week). Resistance to stretch of the hamstrings was unchanged following the 6-week intervention period. It is obvious that more studies of stretching protocols as applied to patients with specific clinical characteristics need to be completed to guide our intervention.

If we are comfortable with the empirical evidence regarding the effectiveness of a technique such as stretching and can document that there has been elongation of the hamstrings with an increase in range of motion and flexibility (eg, increase in straight leg raising) in an individual, we must ask the third question—"So what?" Does it make a difference in the patient's functional abilities or contribute to the care administered by caregivers (Figures 1-5 and 1-6)? If a patient's hamstrings are elongated, but there is no change in functional abilities, then the cost effectiveness and appropriateness of the intervention can be questioned. The "so what?" question is at the basis of determining the extent to which lessening impairments contributes to improved functional outcomes and lessening of disability.

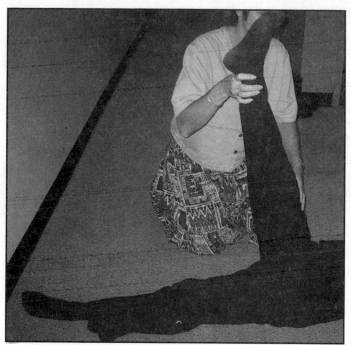

Figure 1-6. Straight leg raise after stimulation.

FUNCTIONAL OUTCOMES

Determination of effective outcomes must occur as we change our theoretical models. Outcomes should be related to age-appropriate functionality. The use of functional behavioral outcomes that are well-defined and that can be observed and measured must be used. In the absence of empirical evidence regarding an intervention, documenting that the patient has achieved specific objectives contributes to the validity of the intervention until empirical evidence can be accumulated.

Establishing Functional Outcomes

In the past, some physical therapy outcomes were based on traditional neurophysiologic facilitation techniques and could not be documented objectively (eg, decreasing muscle tone, decreasing the influence of primitive reflexes, or improving sensory processing). Regardless of the theoretical framework being used, it is preferable to describe impairments in relation to the functional problems hypothesized to be associated with them. Changes in the status of some impairment, such as weakness, are easy to quantify. An example would be the patient achieving increased repetitions of specific exercises. The objective documentation of increased strength is not particularly valuable, unless it relates to improved function (ie, the "so what?" question). In this instance, two-part outcomes are indicated: one related to strength and a second to improved function in which weakness is hypothesized to play a role. If physical therapy intervention improves strength, endurance, flexibility, or some other variable, but does not improve the individual's ability to function, it can be argued that the intervention is of little value to the patient. In a time of high health care costs and limitations placed on physical therapy services, only services that produce functional improvement or maintain levels of function should be provided.

Several examples of functional limitation(s), impairment(s), treatment goal(s), and functional outcome(s) for patients with disorders of or injury to the nervous system are provided to assist the physical therapy student who has had little experience in patient management. A logical approach is to start by defining the patient's functional problems and hypothesizing which impairment(s) may be contributing factors. Goals of physical therapy intervention and the functional outcomes that will measure change(s) in behavior can then be determined. The following section shows examples of this.

CASE STUDY
Twenty-Four Examples

Example 1
- Functional Limitation(s): a shuffling gait and complaints of fatigue, inability to lift body weight up on toes to reach objects overhead
- Impairment(s): decreased strength of gastrocnemius muscles bilaterally
- Treatment Goal(s): to increase strength of calf muscles by achieving a tiptoe position 10 times
- Functional Outcome(s): following intervention, the patient will be able to achieve a tiptoe position to reach objects overhead. The patient will demonstrate improved push-off during gait (using chalk on the ball of the foot to document changes in the gait pattern) and have fewer complaints of fatigue with ambulation

Example 2
- Functional Limitation(s): inability to use an ankle strategy during balancing in stance (unable to remain standing in one place) and decreased toe clearance during the swing phase of gait with a tendency to trip
- Impairment(s): decreased strength of ankle dorsiflexors
- Treatment Goal(s): to increase strength of ankle dorsiflexor muscles by performing three sets of repetitions of resistive ankle dorsiflexion with red elastic band
- Functional Outcome(s): following intervention, the patient will clear the toe during gait 100% of the time. The patient will be able to maintain balance in standing for 3 minutes without bending at the hips or moving the feet

Example 3
- Functional Limitation(s): difficulty rising from sitting at a bench to standing and inability to walk up stairs
- Impairment(s): diminished strength in hip and knee extensors
- Treatment Goal(s): increase strength in hip and knee extensors
- Functional Outcome(s): following intervention, the patient will be able to rise from sitting at a bench to standing independently three times and walk up 10 stairs holding a rail

Example 4

- Functional Limitation(s): limited household ambulation with complaint of fatigue
- Impairment(s): decreased endurance
- Treatment Goal(s): increase endurance for ambulation
- Functional Outcome(s): following intervention, the patient will be able to walk 100 yards using a cane and complete daily household routines without reporting fatigue

Example 5

- Functional Limitation(s): poor toe clearance during gait with tendency to trip
- Impairment(s): decreased passive range of motion (PROM) in ankle dorsiflexion
- Treatment Goal(s): increase PROM into ankle dorsiflexion by 10 degrees
- Functional Outcome(s): following intervention, the patient will clear the toe during gait 100% of the time

Example 6

- Functional Limitation(s): difficulty using upper extremities for ADLs
- Impairment(s): decreased active range of motion (AROM) of one shoulder into forward flexion
- Treatment Goal(s): increase AROM of shoulder
- Functional Outcome(s): following intervention, the patient will be able to comb his hair with the affected arm and put on and take off a stocking hat using both hands

Example 7

- Functional Limitation(s): limited reciprocal arm swing during gait with stiffness in the trunk and difficulty maintaining balance on uneven terrain
- Impairment(s): decreased trunk mobility
- Treatment Goal(s): increase trunk mobility/flexibility
- Functional Outcome(s): following intervention, the patient will be able to rotate his trunk while sitting to obtain an object placed behind him and demonstrate a reciprocal arm swing during gait 50% of the time. He will be able to walk outside on grass and gravel and maintain his balance

Example 8

- Functional Limitation(s): inability to remember verbal instructions, limiting ability to participate in therapy sessions and daily routines
- Impairment(s): poor short-term memory
- Treatment Goal(s): improve short-term memory
- Functional Outcome(s): following intervention, the patient will perform a three-step command of motor tasks, two of three trials, and will remember the sequence needed for putting on his socks and shoes

Example 9

- Functional Limitation(s): difficulty orienting within environments and remembering how to locate different areas within the hospital
- Impairment(s): poor spatial orientation ability and memory for places
- Treatment Goal(s): improve spatial orientation and memory for places
- Functional Outcome(s): following intervention, the patient will be able to find his way from his room to the physical therapy department and to the hospital cafeteria independently

Example 10

- Functional Limitation(s): cannot identify objects by touch with right hand and must rely on vision or use of other hand, limiting bilateral use of the hands for functional activities
- Impairment(s): poor tactile sensation and processing of tactile information on one side of the body
- Treatment Goal(s): improve tactile processing and awareness of tactile input by having patient match circle, square, and triangle explored tactually with involved hand to same three-dimensional objects explored with the opposite hand
- Functional Outcome(s): following intervention, the patient will be able to find familiar objects in a dresser drawer using either hand, two of three trials

Example 11

- Functional Limitation(s): avoids using involved hand to perform bilateral tasks
- Impairment(s): hypersensitivity to touch in one hand
- Treatment Goal(s): improve tolerance to tactile input and functional use of extremity by tolerating various textures and using hand to find objects hidden in various materials (eg, sand, gravel)
- Functional Outcome(s): following intervention, the patient will use the involved hand to do bilateral ADL tasks such as washing and drying dishes

Example 12

- Functional Limitation(s): disregards one side of the body, has difficulty with ADLs that require two hands, and is prone to injury of the extremities on the involved side
- Impairment(s): decreased sensory awareness on one side of the body
- Treatment Goal(s): improve sensory awareness of involved side
- Functional Outcome(s): following intervention, the patient will shave both sides of his face with only one verbal reminder and will check the position of his involved arm and leg periodically for safety

Example 13

- Functional Limitation(s): loses balance in situations where a number of people are moving simultaneously
- Impairment(s): uses vision rather than multiple sensory inputs which impairs balance when standing in environments with multiple moving visual stimuli

- Treatment Goal(s): decrease reliance on vision for balance
- Functional Outcome(s): following intervention, the patient will maintain balance using a cane when walking through a crowded shopping mall

Example 14

- Functional Limitation(s): leans to one side and occasionally falls out of chair unless restrained by a seat belt
- Impairment(s): decreased sitting balance
- Treatment Goal(s): improve proprioceptive awareness and perception of the vertical
- Functional Outcome(s): following intervention, the patient will maintain a symmetrical sitting posture for 5 minutes with no more than three verbal or tactile reminders

Example 15

- Functional Limitation(s): disregards the right side of visual space and does not orient to objects to the right side of the body
- Impairment(s): right visual field deficit
- Treatment Goal(s): improve visual scanning and perception
- Functional Outcome(s): following intervention, the patient will orient spontaneously to a television set or person on his right side, two of three trials

Example 16

- Functional Limitation(s): initiates movement too slowly to perform some functional tasks effectively and safely
- Impairment(s): difficulty in initiating movement (akinesia)
- Treatment Goal(s): improve speed of initiation of movement
- Functional Outcome(s): following intervention, the patient will be able to move from sitting in a chair to answer a telephone within six rings, and will be able to move in and out of an elevator safely

Example 17

- Functional Limitation(s): moves too slowly to perform some functional tasks effectively and safely
- Impairment(s): performs movements slowly and cannot vary speed of movement
- Treatment Goal(s): improve speed of movement
- Functional Outcome(s): following intervention, the patient will be able to walk safely across a street in the time allowed by a green light; and will be able to move on and off an escalator safely

Example 18

- Functional Limitation(s): has a tendency to fall when attempting to stand or walk independently
- Impairment(s): poor balance in standing
- Treatment Goal(s): improve balance in standing and walking

- Functional Outcome(s): following intervention, the patient will maintain independent standing balance for 5 minutes, initiate a step to regain balance when losing balance in upright, and will be able to walk 100 feet on even surfaces

Example 19

- Functional Limitation(s): difficulty maintaining standing balance when handling objects with the upper extremities
- Impairment(s): poor synergistic organization of posture and active movement
- Treatment Goal(s): improve synergistic organization of posture and active movement
- Functional Outcome(s): following intervention, the patient will be able to lift 1-, 3-, and 5-pound weights off a table without falling forward

Example 20

- Functional Limitation(s): cannot combine shoulder flexion with elbow extension to reach for objects above the head.
- Impairment(s): poor synergistic organization of upper extremities
- Treatment Goal(s): improve upper extremity coordination
- Functional Outcome(s): following intervention, the patient will be able to reach overhead to obtain objects from a shelf, three of five trials.

Example 21

- Functional Limitation(s): inability to rise from sitting to standing in a chair without arms
- Impairment(s): poor synergistic organization for postural control
- Treatment Goal(s): improve synergistic organization of movement and sequencing of weight shifts
- Functional Outcome(s): following intervention, the patient will be able to rise from sitting to standing from a chair without arms, one of three attempts

Example 22

- Functional Limitation(s): inability to perform wheelchair transfers independently
- Impairment(s): poor motor planning
- Treatment Goal(s): improve motor planning
- Functional Outcome(s): following intervention, the patient will transfer independently and safely from a wheelchair to a bed or chair 100% of the time

Example 23

- Functional Limitation(s): difficulty with toe clearance during ambulation with tendency to trip
- Impairment(s): lack of knee flexion and ankle dorsiflexion during ambulation
- Treatment Goal(s): improve gait pattern or synergistic movements of lower extremities during gait
- Functional Outcome(s): following intervention, the patient will walk 100 yards, clearing his toes safely

Example 24

- Functional Limitation(s): limited ability to ambulate in community settings
- Impairment(s): poor reciprocation of lower extremities during ambulation with decreased stride length and decreased speed and endurance
- Treatment Goal(s): improve gait pattern and endurance
- Functional Outcome(s): following intervention, the patient will demonstrate improved stride length (measured with chalk footprints on a gait grid [Figure 1-7]) and will be able to walk 50 feet further at a faster rate (timed with stop watch) than noted at initiation of treatment (see Figure 1-3). The patient will be able to participate in a 30-minute shopping excursion without fatigue

SUMMARY—PATIENT MANAGEMENT

It should be noted that, in some instances, several factors are hypothesized to contribute to the same functional limitation. For example, either weakness in hip and knee extensors or poor synergistic organization of movement, or both, could contribute to difficulty in rising from sitting on a chair without arms to standing. The advantage of focusing on functional outcomes is that, if the patient does not improve following treatment to increase strength of hip and knee extensors, then other factors can be considered and emphasized in treatment. If intervention outcomes focused only on impairments, the relationship to functional skills would be unclear.

Often, several treatment goals are worked on simultaneously. An example is intervention to address poor toe clearance during gait, which may be due to weak ankle dorsiflexors or plantarflexors, limited range of motion into dorsiflexion, or poor synergistic organization of movement. Following intervention, if the patient has normal AROM and adequate strength at the ankle, yet drags the toe during gait, poor synergistic organization may be hypothesized to be the most plausible factor contributing to the functional limitation.

A controversial issue among physical therapists is how much to emphasize quality of movement as a treatment goal in patients with damage to the nervous system. Quality movement usually is considered to be the ideal or typical pattern of movement observed in nondisabled children and adults. In some instances, normal patterns of movement are not attainable due to anthropometric factors or degree of pathology in the neuromuscular, musculoskeletal, and/or cardiopulmonary systems. Latash and Anson proposed that changes in any of these systems due to pathology may change the priorities of the nervous system and compensatory patterns of movement displayed by patients may, in come cases, be optimal.[17] Rather than categorizing movements as normal or abnormal, movements could be considered typical or less typical and functional or nonfunctional. Trying to obtain normal movements may be self-defeating for the patient, the patient's family, and the physical therapist. Identifying maladaptive movement strategies that may lead to secondary problems, however, is important. An attempt should be made to assist the patient in using adaptive movement strategies that also will be functional.

In our opinion, rather than concentrating on quality or normal movement, the physical therapist should concentrate on improving function. Perhaps the movement pattern that is the most functional and results in the greatest independence should be considered the best pattern. Emphasis on function is evident in the current health care system, as

Figure 1-7. Assessment using a gait grid.

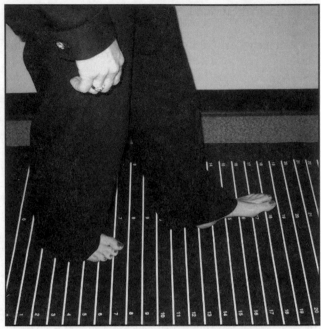

documentation of improved functional abilities following physical therapy intervention usually is required by third-party payers. Determining meaningful functional outcomes also is essential for the patient and the physical therapist in order to measure efficacy of intervention and patient satisfaction.

SUMMARY

Motor control, motor learning, and motor development are areas of interest to physical therapists working with patients of various ages with disorders of the nervous system. Contributing authors have attempted to incorporate the most recent empirical evidence from these fields of study into a theoretical framework that is integrated with the *Guide to Physical Therapist Practice*. Specific examination and evaluation procedures, intervention strategies and techniques, and functional outcomes are presented in a problem-solving approach. Contributing authors have presented several different motor control models and systems theories. Knowledge of contemporary theories and practical applications to patient management will prepare the physical therapist to be the primary diagnostician of movement disorders.

REFERENCES

1. Fisher AG, Murray EA, Bundy AC. *Sensory Integration: Theory and Practice*. Philadelphia, Pa: FA Davis Co; 1991:3-26.
2. Cupps B. *Postural Control: A Current View*. NDTA Network; Laguna Beach, Calif; 1997:1-7.

3. Brunnstrom S. *Movement Therapy in Hemiplegia: A Neurophysiological Approach.* Hagerstown, Md: Harper and Row, Publishers, Inc; 1970.

4. Sawner KA, LaVigne JM. *Brunnstrom's Movement Therapy in Hemiplegia: A Neurophysiological Approach.* Philadelphia, Pa: JB Lippincott; 1992.

5. Carr JH, Shepherd RB. *A Motor Relearning Program for Stroke.* London: Aspen Systems, Corp; 1983.

6. Carr JH, Shepherd RB. *Physiotherapy in Disorders of the Brain.* London: William Heinemann Medical Books Ltd; 1980.

7. Johnstone M. *Restoration of Motor Function in the Stroke Patient: A Physiotherapist's Approach.* 3rd ed. New York, NY: Churchill Livingstone; 1987.

8. Voss DE. Proprioceptive neuromuscular facilitation. *American Journal of Physical Medicine.* 1967;46:838–898.

9. Voss DE, Ionta MK, Myers BJ. *Proprioceptive Neuromuscular Facilitation: Patterns and Techniques.* 3rd ed. Philadelphia, Pa: Harper and Row; 1985.

10. Rood MS. Neurophysiologic reactions: a basis for PT. *PT Review.* 1954;34:444.

11. Stockmeyer SA. An interpretation of the approach of Rood to the treatment of neuromuscular dysfunction. *American Journal of Physical Medicine.* 1967;46:789-815.

12. Harris S. How should treatment be critiqued for scientific merit? *Phys Ther.* 1996;76:175-181.

13. DeDeyne PG. Application of passive stretch and its implications for muscle fibers. *Phys Ther.* 2001;81:819-827.

14. Bandy WD, Irion J, Briggler M. The effect of time and frequency of static stretching on flexibility of the hamstring muscles. *Phys Ther.* 1997;10:1090-1096.

15. Steffen TM, Mollinger LA. Low-load prolonged stretch in the treatment of knee flexion contractures in nursing home residents. *Phys Ther.* 1995;75:886-895.

16. Holt S, Baagoe S, Lillelund F, et al. Passive resistance of hamstring muscles in children with severe multiple disabilities. *Dev Med Child Neurol.* 2000;42:541-544.

17. Latash ML, Anson JG. What are "normal movements" in atypical populations? *Behavioral & Brain Sciences.* 1996;19:55-106.

Motor Control, Motor Learning, and Motor Development

Ann F. VanSant, PhD, PT

INTRODUCTION

As physical therapists, we are interested in foundation sciences related to human movement. Our understanding of motor behavior serves as a basis for our work with individuals whose functional limitations arise from impairments of motor control. Among kinesiologists there are a variety of perspectives and approaches to the study of human movement. For example, biomechanists offer the theory and models of physical mechanics. These theories and models are frequently used by physical therapists to analyze and solve our patients' movement problems. However, the biomechanical perspective represents just one approach that can be used to study human movement. Motor control, motor learning, and motor development represent three other areas of kinesiology that have much to offer physical therapy. Each of these specialized areas offers a unique perspective that can add to our abilities as physical therapists to analyze and solve patients' movement problems.

DEFINITIONS OF MOTOR CONTROL, LEARNING, AND DEVELOPMENT

According to Brooks, a neurophysiologist, "Motor control is the study of posture and movements that are controlled by central commands and spinal reflexes, and also to the functions of mind and body that govern posture and movement."[1] Schmidt and Lee, as psychologists and kinesiologists, define motor learning as a set of processes associated with practice or experience that leads to relatively permanent changes in the capability for producing skilled action.[2] And finally, the study of motor development, according to Roberton, a physical educator, is the study of life span change in motor behavior.[3]

Motor control, learning, and development represent three distinct approaches to understanding motor behavior. Yet, scientists who study these three areas have shared ideas and themes in the past and continue to do so. Each discipline is ultimately directed toward understanding motor behavior. For motor control, the question is "How is the control of motor behavior organized?" For motor learning, the question is "How is motor behavior acquired through practice or experience?" And, for motor development, the question is "How does motor behavior change with age?" The "How?" in each of these questions refers to the search for understanding of the processes that underlie observable motor behavior.

Although motor control, learning, and development researchers have a common interest in processes that underlie motor behavior, one of the differences among them is the time scale over which the processes are studied. Motor control scientists are interested in processes lasting milliseconds or, at the most, seconds. Motor learning scientists are interested generally in processes that occur across hours, days, and weeks, although for highly practiced skills the processes of learning may extend across months or years. Those who study motor development generally are interested in processes of change that involve time periods ranging from months to decades. The relative span of time that attracts interest has to do with the rate of change in the motor behavior being studied (Table 2-1).

Obviously the specialized areas of motor control, learning, and development share the focus of motor behavior. Those interested in motor control seek to understand how motor behavior is controlled and organized. Those interested in motor learning study how motor behaviors are acquired through practice and experience. Those interested in motor development examine age-related processes of change in specific age groups or across the whole human life span. The perspectives of each of these disciplines within the study of motor behavior influence and enrich the others and offer to physical therapists alternate perspectives to help solve problems of human movement dysfunction.

Motor Control—An Overview

The specialized area of motor control as we know it today grew out of the subdisciplines of neurophysiology and cognitive psychology. Early in this century, physiologists studied both motor behavior and the neural processes underlying that behavior. Since that time, and until very recently, neurophysiologists tended to concentrate exclusively on understanding microscopic internal neural processes that coordinated and controlled motor behavior of animals. Their studies were carried out in laboratories with anesthetized animals. More recently, technological advances have enabled neuroscientists to study more general processes involved in the control of natural movements of awake animals and in human subjects performing motor skills.

TABLE 2-1

Motor Control, Learning, and Development: A Comparision

Motor Control	Control and organization of processes underlying motor behavior	Milliseconds
Motor Learning	Acquisition of skill through practice and experience	Hours, days, weeks
Motor Development	Age-related processes of change in motor behavior	Months, years, decades

Over the last 30 years, cognitive psychologists brought to the study of motor control concepts derived from cybernetics and information processing. *Feedback*, one of these concepts, arose from cybernetic theory and has become a routine element of motor control models. Over time, neural functions were modeled as computer functions and processes such as motor programs and memory served major roles.

Physical therapists have a long-standing tradition of studying the neurosciences in order to understand how the nervous system is organized and how it controls motor behavior. The classical neurophysiologic approaches to patient care, which originated in the work of Knott and Voss,[4] Rood,[5] the Bobaths,[6] Brunnstrom,[7] and Fay,[8] represented a distinct shift away from relying on biomechanical concepts alone to solve patient problems, to the use of a motor control model (see Chapter 1). The motor control model dominant at the time consisted of a control hierarchy, with reflexes serving as the foundation for volitional control of movements. This model is still commonly understood and often used to explain the abnormal motor behavior of individuals with impairments of the central nervous system (CNS). Simply put, individuals with brain dysfunction demonstrate reflexive motor behaviors that are no longer under volitional control. The reflexes arise from the intact lower levels of the motor control hierarchy. Physical therapists[4-7] used the hierarchical model to suggest that rebuilding control after brain injury could be accomplished by activating the higher levels of control by using sensory stimulation and requests for volitional action.

When the original neurophysiologic approaches to physical therapy were developed, neurophysiologists were actively studying the electrical activity of single neurons and complex sensory receptors such as the muscle spindle.[9,10] It was the study of the muscle spindle and the gamma motor system that provided a generation of physical therapists with understanding of the concept of feedback as an integral part of motor control, whereas the physiology of the muscle spindle strongly influenced the therapeutic practices advanced by Rood,[11] as well as Knott and Voss[12] through proprioceptive neuromuscular facilitation (PNF). Brunnstrom[7] and the Bobaths[13,14] were less influenced by microscopic elements of motor control, focusing instead on observable elements of motor behavior theorized to represent reflexes mediated at the spinal, brainstem, and midbrain levels of the motor control hierarchy.

Figure 2-1. A traditional model.

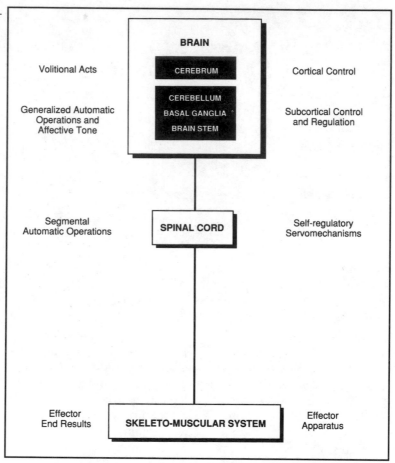

As technology advanced, the simultaneous monitoring of electrical activity at multiple sites within the CNS became possible. This advance led to increasingly complex models of motor control developed to explain relationships among various elements of the nervous system.[1,15] With this came a deeper appreciation of the complexity of the nervous system and hesitancy to assign specific functions to specific structures within the CNS (Figures 2-1 and 2-2). Neuroscientists began to adopt a notion of shared function that recognizes the contributions of multiple structures to the production of functional behaviors. This was an important trend that affects our current understanding of motor control. Gradually, network models that demonstrate this interconnectivity and interdependence of neural elements began to appear in the neuroscience literature. An example of this trend is evident in models of neural control of locomotion, in which neural networks are used to portray oscillatory processes that control the alternating phases of gait.[16] The impetus for the adoption of network theory was not only the increasing appreciation of the complexity of neural processes, but also the increasing availability of computers to assist in the modeling of networks as control elements.

Current Issues in the Study of Motor Control

A general change has taken place in the way theorists view issues related to the control of motor behavior.[17,18] This change in large part is the result of the publication of

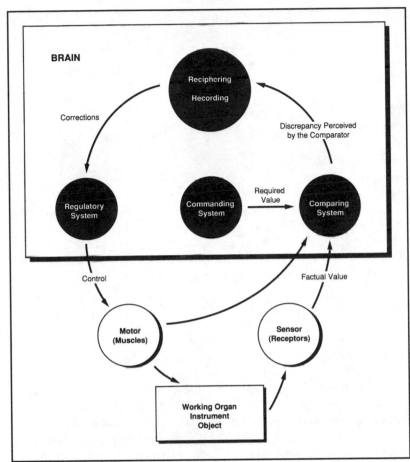

Figure 2-2. A contemporary model taken from Bernstein's work.

the work of Bernstein,[19] a Russian physiologist. Bernstein's writings captured increasing attention among motor control theorists. Bernstein is most well-known for his "degrees of freedom" problem: How does the brain control so many different joints and muscles of the body? The statement of the degrees of freedom problem brought renewed focus on the physical aspects of the body, particularly the musculoskeletal system and its role in motor control. Previously, theorists focused almost exclusively on the role of the nervous system in controlling movements.

The way in which the CNS solves the degrees of freedom problem is proposed to be through muscle synergies or coordinate structures.[20] The brain simplifies the task of controlling numerous muscles by constraining them to function collectively.[21]

Two lines of thought have emerged to explain these muscle linkages or synergies. One emphasizes motor programs; the other emphasizes that muscle synergies are not predetermined like a computer program, rather they arise as a result of complex interactions among the individual and the environments in which the person functions. Motor programs include information that specifies fixed relationships among muscles.[1,2,22,23] Programs are stored in memory and recalled to guide action. An alternate explanation is that the CNS creates solutions to the demands for action at the time they are needed. The muscle linkages emerge from the CNS, taking into account the physical structure of the body and the context in which the action must be performed.

The concept of a synergy, or muscles working in collective groups, is not a new concept to physical therapists. However, the processes that underlie the appearance of muscle linkages are new concepts. Traditionally, synergies were viewed as the behavioral manifestation of hard wired reflexes, present at birth. Synergies are viewed as either motor programs or as emergent properties of the body systems within the context of a meaningful environment.[24] The nervous system, the musculoskeletal system, and the cardiopulmonary system all contribute to the production of movement. No longer is the nervous system considered the sole source of motor control.

Synergies as Motor Programs

A motor program simplifies the degrees of freedom problem by providing a single unit rather than many units to control. Some contemporary models of motor control constitute hierarchies that incorporate motor programs. In these models, the motor program is selected through higher level control processes but carried out by lower levels. This arrangement frees up the higher levels to engage in processes of planning actions. Those who research motor control theory from the perspective of motor programs are interested in determining what elements of the motor program are fixed and what elements can be controlled.[1,2]

Currently, a motor program is characterized by an invariant order in which fundamental elements come into action. Thus, if one were considering a motor program for an overarm throwing of a ball, the order in which the muscles contract would be fixed. The relative duration of the various muscular contractions would be fixed, as would the relative force levels among muscles acting in the program. What can vary in the program, and therefore would need to be controlled, are the absolute level of force and the overall duration of the program. In the overarm throwing task, this means the throw may be light or forceful or the throw may be carried out slowly or quickly.

The speed and force that can be generated within a specific program are, however, limited. For example, if speed is increased in an underarm throwing pattern, the relative timing of various muscles can change and a new program is used as the individual begins to use a windmill pattern as a windup for the throw. A similar change from one pattern to another can be seen when walking speed increases to a point where a switch to a running pattern occurs. These examples can be explained as shifts from one program to another.

One model that has evolved to explain control within the programming concept is the mass spring model of control. Support for the mass spring model has been provided by Fel'dman, a Russian motor control theorist.[25] He proposed that we control the final position of a limb by specifying the relative stiffness of opposing muscles. Movements end at the point where agonist and antagonist stiffness is balanced across the limb. Noncontractile elastic properties of muscle are a part of the model, and antagonistic muscles are viewed as two opposing springs. Polit and Bizzi, two neuroscientists, found that monkeys, after having learned to perform simple one-joint movements involving pointing to targets, were able to point correctly with vision occluded and following deafferentation of the limb, regardless of the starting position.[26] It appeared that the monkeys had stored information about muscle tensions at the end position of pointing at the target. This research is supportive of the theory that the motor control system solves the degrees of freedom problem by treating the musculoskeletal system as though it were a mass spring system.

The mass spring model offers a relatively simple explanation of discrete movements to an endpoint. It has been extended to relatively elaborate tasks, such as handwriting.

Hollerbach[27] created a system of four springs arranged at right angles to each other, with each attached to the same mass or weight. This is like a four-muscle system attached around a limb segment. If the mass is displaced in any direction, the system oscillates until an equilibrium point is reached. This more complex model of springs in oscillation can produce action similar to handwriting. If the displacement of such a four-spring system happens to occur in a diagonal direction, the mass oscillates in a circular pattern. By varying the stiffness of the springs, the circular pattern can be altered to make elliptical loops. Attach a pen to the system and the product is much like the letters of cursive writing. Slight alterations to the elliptical loops produce a variety of recognizable letters. Thus, the mass spring model can be extended to explain complex tasks.

Emergent Properties of the Nervous System

The notion of emergent properties of a neural network is an outgrowth of application of network models to issues of motor control, particularly to the control of locomotion.[28] By specifically placing elements depicting neurons in a series, patterns of neural function can be modeled. If one element in the chain is activated, the others will be activated in a fixed order, mimicking one of the fundamental properties of a synergy or coordinate structure: the elements are constrained to produce a fixed pattern of activity.

Not only can fixed patterns of activity result from the function of a network, but sets of neurons can be arranged in a circular pattern so that cyclic function results. Cyclic function, as a pattern of activation and rest, becomes an emergent property of the network. By constraining the relationship between the elements of the system, a new property emerges that is not an inherent property of any element of the system: that is, no element of the system possesses the property of cyclic activity, but when arranged in a network, cyclic activity can result.

Emergent network properties have disadvantages, as well as advantages. One particular disadvantage is the tendency for circularly arranged networks to produce resonating oscillatory behavior. This means that they may get progressively carried away during repetitive functions. Damping mechanisms are needed in network models to control the oscillations. Damps ultimately return oscillators to a point of static equilibrium when the energy of the system has dissipated.

While oscillatory function is quite common in biological systems,[20] biological oscillations typically do not resonate uncontrollably. Living organisms have the ability to sustain stable levels of oscillatory function. Thus, the network model cannot be used to explain some fundamental properties of living systems. The problem with network modeling is that it is based in the physics of closed systems in which fuel or energy is not exchanged with the surrounding environment. Ultimately, closed physical systems are not well suited to modeling the functions of living systems.[29] Biological oscillations appear to be more accurately portrayed by nonlinear or limit cycle oscillators, typical of open physical systems.

The modeling of open systems is a relatively new area of physics. Yet, the constructs of the newer models of motor control are grounded in principles related to the thermodynamics of open systems (not to be confused with open loop control of movement) and principles of nonlinear limit cycle oscillators. One important characteristic of limit cycle oscillators is the property of entrainment of one oscillating function to another, such that they share a common periodicity. Entrainment has been used to explain interlimb coordination during locomotion.[29] Entrainment underlies the temporally pat-

Figure 2-3. This diagram demonstrates the periodic oscillation of the pectoral and dorsal fin of a fish. The relationship between the fins becomes coordinated at the X marked on the diagram. Prior to that time, the dorsal fin oscillated at a faster rate than the pectoral fin. The process of entrainment of one oscillating fin to the other resulted in a shared frequency. In this case, the dorsal fin has become entrained to the slower rhythm of the pectoral fin, and the movements of the fins are "coordinated" (adapted from Gallistel CR. *The Organization of Action: A New Synthesis.* Hillsdale, NJ: Lawrence Erlbaum Associates Publishers; 1980).

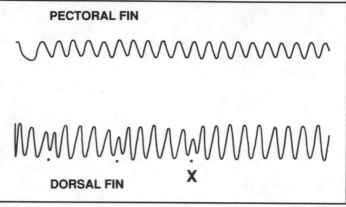

terned relationship between the limbs during their individual cyclic gait patterns. Figure 2-3 illustrates the concept of entrainment.

At first glance, the use of oscillators to model motor control appears to be limited to repetitive cyclic tasks, such as various gait patterns. Yet, oscillators also may be used to model discrete noncyclic behaviors with specific start- and endpoints.

The science of open systems that is leading to formulation of such control models is not just useful to us as therapists. The properties of nonlinear systems are being used to model a host of natural phenomenon, from shoreline formations and tornado development to the formation of biological structures such as leaves and honeycombs.[30] Why is this new theory preferable to the traditional models? Simply put, complex natural patterns can be reduced to a few simple principles. These principles, when applied in the context of the physical world, lead to new understanding of a vast array of complex natural forms and patterns. Human movement is an example of an array of complex natural forms and patterns.

One aspect of the newer control models is particularly rich for physical therapists. This is the notion that synergies emerge and are constrained by the physical characteristics of the human body and characteristics of the specific environmental context in which actions are performed.[31] As an example, imagine a child in a huge rocking chair (Figure 2-4A). If she were to get out of the rocker, there are several strategies she might use. She could slide off the front of the chair, extending her legs and trunk while holding fast to the armrests. Or, she could turn to lie prone on the chair and get off backwards by lowering her legs to the floor (Figure 2-4B). One action pattern that she cannot perform from this chair is the common sit-to-stand action pattern that involves flexing forward over feet contacting the floor, followed by extension to attain standing. This is because the chair is too big or she is too small to be able to sit and have her feet on the floor. But, the child can perform other actions that larger people cannot. She can curl up on her side on the seat of the chair and probably can slide out under the side arms (Figure 2-4C). Thus, the size of her body and the size of the rocking chair mutually constrain the actions possible.

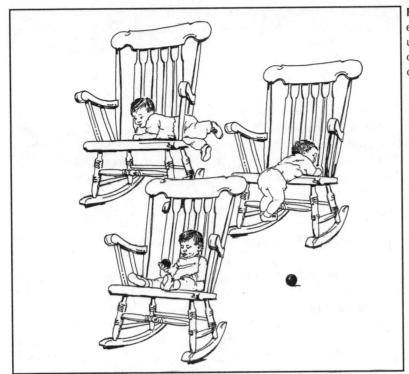

Figure 2-4. Different action patterns used to remove oneself from a chair.

In the examples of throwing and locomotion patterns that were used previously to illustrate different motor programs, when the speed of the individual increased to a critical level, there was an abrupt qualitative shift from one pattern to another. In the programming concept, this shift is explained as a switch from one program to another. Newer theory, based on principles of open systems, would explain this switch as a function of scaling up a variable until a qualitatively different organizational pattern emerges from the system. Qualitative change from one action pattern to another is an emergent property. The laws and principles under which such qualitative change may occur are corollaries of theory of open systems. This newer theoretical framework is termed dynamical action theory.[31]

Motor Control Theory Applied to Physical Therapy

The theoretical perspective one adopts affects what aspects of patient function are evaluated and the procedures used to solve clinical problems.[32,33] The classical neurophysiologic approaches to patient care were formulated from the perspective of a motor control hierarchy resting on progressively more complex levels of reflex organization. Therapists evaluated the presence of specific reflexes and reactions, presumed to be controlled at various levels of the CNS, and determined the level of neural function. Therapists facilitated and inhibited reflexes to promote advancement to a higher level of control, ultimately for the purpose of improving the patient's functional competence in daily life.

Functional motor behaviors are of critical importance in the evaluation of patients regardless of the theoretical model adopted to explain motor control. It is important, however, to remember that functional behavior implies that the patient acts in the context of a meaningful environment. Therefore, two basic elements that need to be assessed are functional motor behaviors and the environmental conditions under which they are performed.

A fundamental construct within the newer models of control rest on the notion of coordinate structures, synergy patterns, or muscle linkages. I suggest that the behavioral expression of these linkages within functional tasks should constitute a primary focus of physical therapy examinations. Specifically, the following question can serve as a starting point for the therapist applying motor control theory in clinical practice: "What postural and movement patterns are part of patients' behavioral repertoire?" I would further suggest that impairments in motor control would evidence as a limited repertoire of movement patterns and difficulty when switching from one pattern to another.

The movement patterns used to perform fundamental tasks of daily life have begun to be identified[34-38] as have standing postural synergies.[39] However, the descriptions of qualitatively different patterns used to perform the fundamental of tasks of daily life are far from complete.

Another key aspect of contemporary patient evaluation is an analysis of environmental contexts in which motor behaviors are displayed. The environmental conditions under which our patients function can be systematically explored.[40,41] Environments can be considered either stable or variable. Stable environments simplify demands for motor control. Stable environments are predictable and allow individuals to perform at a self-determined speed. Parallel bars are an example of a stable environment for walking. Stable environments, however, are not all the same. Home and hospital rooms can be stable, in that the elements in the room are fixed and unchanging, yet they differ from one another. We need to concern ourselves with the features of the environments in which our patients ultimately will be required to function. Walking surfaces and the heights of chairs and beds are examples of the variable features of stable environments.

Variable environments require a greater degree of motor control than do stable environments. This is because the individual must adjust movements to the changing demands of the environment. A busy city street is a good example of a variable environment, as it has a large degree of unpredictability. Yet, even variable environments can have some degree of predictability. We rely on this predictability to ensure our safety. For example, stoplights provide predictable patterns of traffic flow. But there are instances when we must be able to slow, speed up, or stop our movements in order to meet the demands of the environment. Our patients often are not given opportunities to experience variable and unpredictable environments as part of a full course of rehabilitation. Rather, we tend to teach skills in the stable environments of hospitals, rehabilitation centers, and homes. As a result, we are unsure, as our patients often are, of their ability to function across the full range of circumstances that are commonly encountered in daily life.

By viewing the individual and the environment as an interacting unit in the formation of movement patterns, the potential for structuring the environment to bring out specific patterns also becomes apparent as a therapeutic principle. Therapists are familiar with structuring patients' environments to promote general forms of motor behavior. Common examples are arranging the room of a patient with hemiplegia to encourage turning toward the involved side of the body or positioning a toy so a child will orient and reach to touch it. But we have not fully exploited the idea of the physical environment as a constraining variable that would lead to specific motor patterns.

Conversely, we need to examine the environment to determine what ?
ble given the relative size of the patient and objects in the environmer

Several years ago, I was treating a young man recovering from head in.,
sistently postured with his right arm in elbow flexion and had developed a contractu.
of approximately 30 degrees. While splinting and casting had been used to prevent further contracture, active extension of this elbow, necessary to maintain functional range
of motion, seldom was performed. Traditional techniques of handling and facilitating
elbow extension, while effective, were hampered by his limited attention span and motivation to participate in therapy. Repeatedly asking the patient for elbow straightening or
pushing him off balance to evoke protective extension were boring after multiple training sessions. Yet, the young man proved to be quite interested in trying out his abilities
in a familiar and meaningful skill. I turned a sliding board into a striking board by having him hold it in a manner similar to the way in which one would hold a baseball bat.
A tennis ball was tossed to him, and he swung the sliding board with appropriate timing and directional control to hit the ball. His elbow extended quite naturally, achieving
in a matter of seconds what had been an underlying goal of therapy for several months.
He performed a task in which he had to straighten his elbow in the context of a meaningful environment. In this example, the environmental conditions were such that the
patient had to time his movement to coincide with the arrival of the tennis ball. Had he
not been successful, this task could have been simplified by having him use the board to
strike a stationary ball, such as in a golf swing or batting in T-ball.

In summary, newer theories of motor control lead to different examination, evaluation, and intervention strategies. The types of information gathered during examination
are not the same as those we would gather using our traditional examinations. They go
beyond the common view of the environment as the source of reflex stimuli. Rather, the
environment is seen as both a constrainer and promoter of meaningful behavior. Motor
patterns now are viewed as more than reflexive responses. They are the elements of
behaviors that arise as an emergent property of a highly complex system that is tuned to
function in meaningful environments.

MOTOR LEARNING—AN OVERVIEW

The specialized area of motor learning grew out of the subdiscipline of psychology
concerned with processes of learning.[42] In the early part of this century, experimental
studies explored three main learning issues: massing versus distributing the practice of
tasks, instruction in the whole versus the parts of tasks, and the transfer of learning from
one task to another.

By the middle of this century, motor learning had been established as a specialized
area of study with problems that differed from those studied by researchers interested in
verbal learning. Since that time, cybernetics and information processing science have
exerted a major influence on the study of motor learning, as they did on the study of
neurophysiology. The contribution of these new sciences to the study of learning
includes recognition of the influence of feedback on the motor learning process. Both
motor learning theorists and neuroscientists have applied information theory to their
areas of study.[1,2] This commonality and technologic advances have allowed neuroscientists to study human subjects. Additionally, neuroscientists and motor control scientists
from a psychological background share ideas in interdisciplinary research focused on
how skills are acquired and controlled.

Physical therapists, who work with individuals with neurologic impairments, are becoming increasingly familiar with motor learning literature. Recently, our association with medical sciences, often at the expense of behavioral sciences, tended to direct attention away from principles of learning, although there was explicit recognition of the role of learning in the restitution of functional skills.[43,44] Treatment rather than teaching tended to embody the traditional way of thinking about physical therapy interventions. Regaining motor skills following CNS damage was based predominately on repetitively evoking reflexes to facilitate postures and movements. Practice involved repetition of reflexively facilitated behaviors. Rehabilitative practices involved teaching motor skills, including the breaking down of functional activities into component parts for ease of learning[45] and periods of practice. Much of what therapists learned about teaching motor skills was acquired through practical experiences, rather than through reading literature related to the science of motor learning.

When Adams[46] published a theory of motor learning, much attention and research was generated to investigate his theory. Adams' closed loop theory was based on learners receiving both ongoing intrinsic feedback arising from the proprioceptive system, as well as extrinsic feedback generated as a consequence of one's actions. The closed loop theory also included two different forms of memory as critical components. Later, Schmidt[47] proposed an open loop theory that incorporated two memory structures termed the motor schema and the motor program. Schmidt's theory is particularly relevant for skills that are performed either so rapidly or automatically that intrinsic proprioceptive feedback critical to Adams' closed loop theory is not used for deliberate control processes.

Over the past 25 years, the theories of motor learning advanced by Adams and Schmidt have led those studying motor behavior to consider theories of motor control. Specifically, the debate of whether movements were controlled centrally or peripherally was a spark that kindled interest in contemporary motor control issues.[2] This debate generated increased understanding of how different types of movements are controlled, and subsequently how different types of movements might be learned. Feedback is essential for learning, but may not be necessary for the performance of well-learned tasks.

Current Issues in the Study of Motor Learning

Four contemporary issues are presented to demonstrate the importance of motor learning research to physical therapists. These include the difference between motor performance and motor learning, the appropriate use of feedback, the impact of practice schedules, and the transfer of learning across tasks and conditions of practice.

Performance and Learning

An issue of importance to physical therapy is the differentiation between performance and learning. Performance can be observed, learning cannot. Motor learning is an internal process associated with practice or experience that produces a relatively permanent change in the capability for motor skill.[2] Although we help our patients learn motor skills, generally, as therapists we are more familiar with variables that affect performance than variables that affect learning. Some of the familiar performance variables known to evoke temporary effects are fatigue, head turning that evokes a reflexive response, or an audience watching the patient perform. Learning variables, in contrast, continue to influence performance after they are removed.

Feedback

Extrinsic feedback represents information concerning performance supplied to the learner. Feedback is necessary for learning. The relative frequency with which feedback is supplied to the learner is an area of research that is germane to physical therapists. Current research suggests that contrary to what might be predicted, a relatively low frequency of providing feedback enhances learning.[2,48] This is true despite the fact that performance might suffer during periods of low frequency feedback. Additionally, Winstein has shown that the fading of feedback, or progressively decreasing the rate with which feedback is given, appears to be most effective in promoting learning.[49,50]

The fading of feedback is contrary to customary practice in physical therapy in which more feedback often is considered better, particularly if performance is not up to standard. It has been suggested that the reason individuals learn better with less feedback is they do not become as dependent on feedback, rather they engage in processes that enable learning, such as reviewing their last performance of the task, and determining for themselves what should be done to improve the next performance of the task. If learning involves an improved capacity to perform a skill, opportunities to self-assess and then take corrective action are integral components of success in acquiring skills.

Practice Schedules

Among motor learning researchers, the terms blocked practice and random practice are used to denote two different practice schedules. Blocked practice refers to consistent practice of one task. Random practice means varying practice among a group of distinctly different tasks. It appears that varying practice among different tasks is more effective in promoting learning than concentrating on a single task.[51] Schmidt and Lee suggested that the recall of tasks inherent in random practice seems to assist with processes that ensure learning.[2]

Transfer of Learning

A final issue that arises from the motor learning research literature that is of great importance to physical therapists concerns the transfer of learning. There are two distinct types of transfer, from one task to another and from one learning condition to another. Many of our traditional neurophysiologic approaches emphasized the practice of early-appearing developmental tasks which were thought to positively affect the ability to perform later-appearing higher order tasks. For example, performance of prone extension patterns was considered fundamental and a prerequisite to the normal performance of standing. General motor abilities such as stability or extensor antigravity control, which developed in prone extension, were hypothesized to be essential to normal performance of standing. Yet, research into the existence of general motor abilities that might underlie the transfer of skill from one task to another has indicated that such transfer is very small, if it exists at all.[2]

Motor Learning Theory Applied to Physical Therapy

Because physical therapists are increasingly becoming aware of the research findings of motor learning, there is an increasing trend for therapists to view their role with patients as a teacher of motor skills. This perspective is apparent in the publications of Carr and Shepherd,[52,53] Winstein,[48-50] and Shumway-Cook and Woollacott.[54] With the acceptance of the role of teacher comes a concern for the basic principles of motor learning and a reexamination of the traditional guiding hypotheses of physical therapy.

A common experience of therapists is that some traditional treatment procedures such as facilitation and inhibition of reflexes affect performance at the time they are applied, but have no lasting effect. The differentiation between treatment procedures that affect learning and those that affect performance should lead to more considered and appropriate use of intervention procedures and more effective outcomes.

Understanding that feedback is necessary for learning provides a different perspective on therapy sessions. In the past, feedback appears to have held a motivational role in therapy, being used as an incentive for continued participation in practice sessions. While the idea of withdrawing hands on facilitation to promote increased volitional participation is a traditional practice, the idea of withdrawing feedback to enhance learning is not. Winstein's finding,[49,50] that the fading of feedback enhances learning, is important for the way we work with our patients during practice sessions. In general, we need to allow patients the opportunity to judge and correct their own performance. Accurate and timely feedback given in a frequency designed specifically to promote learning should become standard practice.

Issues related to the transfer of learning are very relevant to therapists. In traditional approaches, much time is devoted to practicing lower order tasks that are considered to positively affect performance of developmentally later-appearing tasks. Motor behavior research suggests that to the extent that the tasks are different, this practice is ineffective. Transfer between tasks appears to be dependent on the similarity between the tasks. Further, the similarity seems to rest within the elements that define motor programs. When motor programs differ, transfer of training from one task to another is quite small. Thus, the relative timing and phasing of muscle activity within a motor program is quite specific. Practice of one motor pattern is unlikely to transfer to performance of a different pattern.

How does what we know about transfer of training affect our practice as therapists? There are times in therapy when performance of the task is the primary objective, and little concern is directed toward which movement patterns are used to accomplish the task. There are other instances when patients demonstrate a stereotypic set of postural or movement patterns, and the objective of treatment may be directed toward the patient being capable of performing a very specific movement pattern. In this latter example, it is important to state clearly which pattern is the objective of treatment. And, practice must be structured to allow the patient to acquire that specific pattern.

In summary, the research findings of motor learning provide useful information for the therapist who accepts the role of a teacher of motor skills. The way we structure practice, provide feedback, and even the way our treatment objectives are stated can be influenced positively by knowledge gained through motor learning research.

MOTOR DEVELOPMENT—AN OVERVIEW

The roots of motor development as a specialized area of study can be found in the work done early in the past century by developmental psychologists and physicians. These individuals described the sequential acquisition of motor skills in infants and young children. Studies were conducted that examined the relative contributions of maturational and environmental factors to the process of age-related change in behavior. The pioneers of motor development were influenced by the motor control and learning theories of their times. For example, McGraw studied the neuromuscular development of infants to look for the onset of cortically mediated volitional control over subcortical reflexive behaviors.[55] She further studied the relative roles of maturational and experiential factors on the motor skill development of a set of twins.[56,57]

The field of motor development has been defined as an area separate from developmental psychology since World War II when psychologists abandoned the study of motor development, preferring to focus on the development of cognitive skills.[58] Professionals in physical education, medicine, and health disciplines including physical therapy became more involved in defining and studying the problems associated with age-related changes in motor behavior.[59-61] Generally, this second generation of motor development researchers was interested in development of infants and children, although some adopted a broader perspective involving life span changes in motor behavior.

Traditional theories of motor development paralleled traditional concepts of motor control.[61] In fact, the classic hierarchical model of CNS organization, originally proposed as a model of neural evolution,[62] laid the groundwork for developmental theory. Processes of hierarchical integration and progressive differentiation incorporated in Jackson's notion of neural evolution are evident in the work of McGraw.[55] These processes were proposed as fundamental to changes in organismic developmental theories.[63]

For about 25 years following World War II, motor development researchers tended to focus on describing the product of motor development. These products included performance measures on standardized tests of skill performance, including features such as how far and how fast children of different ages were able to throw a ball and run.[59] Studies during this period carefully described the movement patterns used by children to perform a variety of motor skills.[64] In the 1970s, the influence of information processing models of motor control began to be seen in the study of the development of motor skills.[65,66] The information processing approach to motor development incorporates a variety of memory structures that are similar to schema and motor programs. Because feedback is an integral part of these models, they are equally well suited for and applied to the study of both motor control and learning processes.

Recently, a resurgence of interest in motor development appeared within psychology. This seems in large part to be due to the influence of dynamical action theory applied by Kugler, Kelso, and Turvey[67] and Thelen.[68] Their work seems to have given impetus to application of the systems theoretical perspective to infant motor development.[69-71]

Current Issues in the Study of Motor Development

The issues in motor development that impact the practice of physical therapy include the concept of motor development as a lifelong process, a greater understanding of developmental sequences, new information concerning prenatal development of movement abilities, and the use of systems theory, particularly dynamical action theory, as a tool for research and expansion of our understanding of motor development.

Motor Development as a Lifelong Process

The concept of life span development had its beginnings among developmental psychologists who continued to study their young subjects well into adulthood.[72] The life span concept appeared in the motor development literature in the late 60s, and now there are an increasing number of contemporary texts that adopt what is called a life span approach to motor development.[73-76] Roberton[3] has rightfully pointed out, however, that few of these texts included chapters that cover a single topic across the life span. Rather, chapters tend to be devoted to different phases of the life span. To a large extent, this would seem to result from the paucity of research conducted from a life span perspective. It is easier to gather studies of different phases or age groups and report on them as representative of a particular period within the life span. It is more difficult to integrate the findings of studies of a single function that are carried out under a variety of conditions with representation of age groups.

We are beginning to accumulate a body of literature generated using a life span developmental perspective that describes age differences in motor performance of functional tasks. The tasks of rising to standing from the floor,[77-82] rolling from supine to prone,[83-85] rising from a chair,[86] and rising from bed[87,88] have been studied in a variety of age groups. Because the conditions under which the subjects perform have been kept consistent across the age groups, reasonable comparisons can be made across a wide portion of the life span. We have charted the incidence of different movement patterns used to perform these tasks from early childhood through later adulthood.[89,90] The results of these studies indicate that age differences in movement patterns can be expected across the life span. We have discovered that variability in performance differs with age and with activity level. Currently, the relationship between body dimensions and motor performance in these tasks is under investigation. This line of inquiry is particularly well suited to life span study. Physical growth is a well-accepted correlate of childhood motor development. Body dimensions and movement patterns used to perform functional righting tasks demonstrate a variable relationship across the life span.[91] The increase in weight that commonly occurs during the middle adult years alters the shape of the body and may well influence the form of functional movement patterns long after the physical growth associated with early years is finished.

The patterns of change in movements used to perform functional tasks do not entirely support the traditional concept of developmental progression during childhood to maturity in young adulthood, followed by regression during the middle and later adult years. The variable patterns of movement suggest that patterns of change in motor behavior may be more complex than the simple progression and regression hypotheses would suggest.[61] Much is to be learned from a life span perspective toward motor development. This information will impact our expectations for individuals of different ages who require physical therapy services.

Developmental Sequences

Developmental sequences take many forms. There are sequences of tasks, such as those described by Gesell and Amatruda[92] and Shirley.[93] These sequences outline the order in which a variety of developmental skills are acquired, such as rolling before sitting, sitting before creeping, and so forth. There also are developmental sequences of body action within performance of a single skill or task. Developmental sequences of body movements within tasks were described by McGraw.[55] She described how the form of body movement changes with age and outlined developmental sequences for several tasks of interest to physical therapists, including rolling, sitting, prone progression, rising to standing, and walking (Figure 2-5). Finally, there are developmental sequences of movement patterns for body regions.[78,84,86,87]

Neurophysiologic approaches to patient care incorporate developmental principles as guides for the progression of patients from states of physical dependency. The predomi-

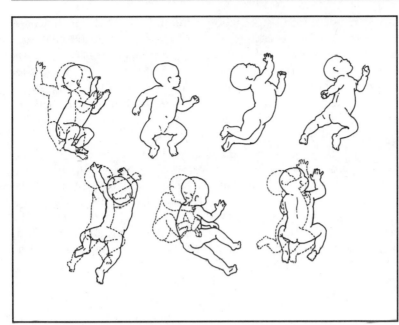

Figure 2-5. Rolling sequence from supine to prone (adapted from McGraw MB. *The Neuromuscular Maturation of the Human Infant.* New York, NY: Hafner Publishing Co; 1945).

nant pattern of progression was termed the developmental sequence,[12] or the skeletal function sequence,[94] and comprised a sequence of motor skills predominantly selected and adapted from the work of McGraw[55] and Gesell.[95] Unfortunately, the ordering of developmental accomplishments was interpreted as though it were the only order for attainment of skills and led to prescriptive use of developmental sequences in physical therapy. Early-appearing developmental patterns were construed as essential preparatory steps for later-appearing functions. According to Knott and Voss "...a recapitulation of the developmental sequence is a means to the end—the ability to care for one's body, to walk, and to engage in productive work."[12] It is worth noting, however, that Knott and Voss recognized that recapitulation of developmental tasks was not the only means to functional competence.

Careful reading of the original descriptions of developmental accomplishments[93,95-97] reveals that the order in which they are accomplished varies from person to person. This finding raises serious doubts about the prerequisite nature of early-appearing tasks for later-appearing functions. If one person is able to skip a developmental step, then obviously that step is not universally essential for later functional accomplishments. The extent to which early tasks lay a foundation for later skills is a matter of conjecture. Further, if motor learning research can be used to shed light on this debate, one would have to question how performance of early-appearing skills could influence essentially different skills appearing later in development.

Prenatal Development of Movement Abilities

Ultrasonography has allowed a new perspective on fetal development. Rich descriptions of the many varied activities of the human fetus have been made possible by ultrasonography.[98] Most notably, the concept of an active infant has surfaced.[99-101] This new concept challenges the older idea that the infant is predominantly passive and dominated by reflexive behaviors evoked by environmental stimuli. As a result, the spontaneous movements of the young infant are no longer ignored and have become the subject of careful study.[102,103] The rhythmical patterns of infancy have been interpreted as suggesting the existence of motor programs[102] and central pattern generators.[103] It is not coincidental that the interpretation of these spontaneous movements has rested on concepts common to motor learning and motor control. As in the past, when reflexes were used to explain behavior, now more contemporary concepts of programs and pattern generators are being used to explain infant behavior.

Systems Theory

Systems theories also are influencing our understanding of motor development.[67,104-106] This influence began gradually but has taken on intensity over the past few years. In 1964, Anokhin, a Russian neuroscientist, characterized neural development as a process of systemogenesis[107] through which different regions of the brain develop at different rates in anticipation of the demand for vital functions. Thus, sets of brain structures collectively function to meet the specific circumstances of the individual in an ecologically appropriate context. Importantly, the ecologically appropriate context for infant development involves an interaction with a mother or caregiver. The functions of both mother and infant are matched to ensure survival and proper development.

This idea of elements collectively functioning to meet the needs of the individual in concert with environmental demands is seen in Milani-Comparetti's interpretation of fetal movements.[99] He characterized the emerging behavioral repertoire of the fetus as directed toward the process of being born and surviving during the early postnatal period. Thrusting and locomotor movements of the fetus were adapted to the process of birth, in which both infant and mother actively participated. Breathing and sucking patterns were developed prenatally to ensure extrauterine survival. Thus, behavioral systems were envisioned as ecologically appropriate to the context in which the fetus or infant would function.

Two contemporary systems theories are currently being used to explain a variety of developmental processes in infancy and childhood. These two theories are termed perception-action theory and dynamical action theory. Perception action theory has roots in the work of the Gibsons.[108,109] Perceptual systems are considered critical for any action system. Specifically, motor development is viewed as much a function of perceptual system change as it is a function of change in motor systems.

Dynamical action theory, another example of systems theory, has been increasingly applied to explain motor development.[67-71,101,104,105,110-113] A set of propositions central to this theory were clearly delineated by Heriza.[71,114] They include the assumption that behavior represents a compression of the degrees of freedom inherent in the complexity of a developing individual. Behavior also is viewed as an emergent property of a self-organizing system. Behavior is constructed in the context of a specific task. Many subsystems of the body and environment contribute to the production of behaviors. There are preferred patterns of behaviors that are termed attractor patterns. Development can be considered to be a series of new behaviors appearing as a series of shifts between attractor patterns. What pushes the system to reorganize and produce a new pattern is termed a control parameter. Control parameters act as catalysts for change. Examples of developmental control parameters may be found in the physical characteristics of the body that change with growth, for example, the length of a limb or the weight of a body part. Control parameters may also be found in other body systems and in the physical and social environments in which individuals must function. Control parameters gradually change until a point is reached where previous behavioral patterns are unstable and the shift to a new behavioral form occurs. The idea of gradually increasing the scale of a parameter to influence motor behavior was introduced in our discussion of dynamic systems of motor control: change in locomotor patterns can be achieved by increasing the speed of locomotion, causing the system to reorganize behavior from a walk to a run. Similarly, if we reconsider the child in the rocking chair (see Figures 2-4), we begin to appreciate the role of physical growth in the emergence of new motor patterns and the potential application of dynamical action theory to advance our understanding of developmental issues. As one grows, some patterns become impossible, while others are enabled by the changing size of the individual and the changing physical and social environments in which one functions. No longer can motor development be viewed solely as a process of maturation of the CNS. Clearly the physical parameters of the body and its relationship to the physical environment contribute to the emergence of new patterns of motor behavior during development.

MOTOR DEVELOPMENT THEORY
APPLIED TO PHYSICAL THERAPY

The issues of life span change in motor behavior, developmental sequences, fetal motor behavior, and constructs of dynamical action theory are impacting physical therapy. Because of a new understanding of development as a lifelong process, the concept of age-related change in motor behavior of individuals across the life span is beginning to be more widely appreciated. This broader perspective influences which motor skills and constituent motor patterns are taught to patients. A concern for the range of age-appropriate skills and movement patterns influences therapeutic programs for individuals of all ages.

Careful review of information concerning developmental sequences suggests that they be used less prescriptively. Because there is little information concerning the relationship between early- and later-appearing behaviors, the use of an early-appearing behavior, such as prone extension or creeping, to prepare for a developmentally later-appearing function, such as walking, is not well founded (Figure 2-6). As a result, therapists should carefully consider the manner in which they help patients acquire functional skills. Strict adherence to a developmental sequence as a pattern of progression no longer appears valid or appropriate. Sequences that describe the skills expected at a particular age do, however, outline the functional accomplishments that are expected of infants and children. Some of these tasks, specifically rolling, sitting, rising from supine or sitting to standing, and walking continue as integral elements of physical independence across a wide period of the life span. Each of these skills should be carefully considered when helping patients attain or regain physical independence.

The new knowledge of developmental sequences of body action and movement patterns is beginning to be applied in physical therapy. At present, the most common interpretation of this information is that age-appropriate body actions and movement patterns should be used when instructing patients in performance of functional skills.[78,82,86,87]

Studies of fetal movement have influenced our perception of infants as active agents in their environments. Such active infant concepts are impacting the behaviors we seek

Figure 2-6. Trunk extension in upright may have different requirements of motor control than extension in prone.

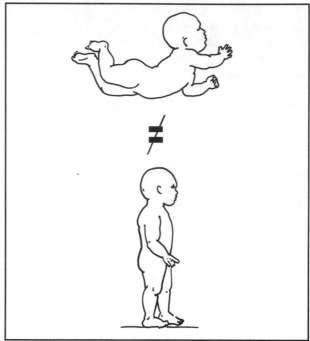

to evaluate. The evaluation of self-control, as used in the Brazelton neonatal assessment[115]; the Test of Infant Motor Performance, which includes spontaneous movements[116]; and the assessment of general movements in infants[117] are all examples of increasing acceptance of an active organism concept in contrast to traditional assessments that only focused on infant reflexes.

The extension of this active organism concept to our interventions requires recognition that individuals who come to treatment have a role to play in changing their behavior. We need to continue to adopt a model of intervention in which the patient is given active roles in producing action, evaluating feedback, and generating corrective action rather than considering the individual a passive recipient of our procedures.

The impact of developmental systems theories, particularly dynamical action theory, on physical therapy is just beginning to be realized. There is now greater concern for the physical constraints or determinants of motor pattern changes, such as those brought about by physical growth. The short stature of many disabled children may well be a contributing factor in determining which movement patterns are used to perform functional tasks, as is the extra body weight that inactive patients carry. No longer is the CNS considered the sole determinant of developing movements. The question of whether movement patterns emerge or if they are learned as a part of the developmental process continues to be a fertile area for debate and research. Such controversy can only lead to a greater understanding of motor control, learning, and development.

SUMMARY

Motor control, motor learning, and motor development represent three different perspectives of motor behavior. The interdisciplinary sharing of ideas and themes in the past continues to be evident today. Motor control theories are used to explain how the control of motor behavior is organized. Currently, the concept of muscle synergies or coordinate structures has a central role to play in the organization of motor control. The impact of these newer control theories on motor development and learning is strong. The focus on coordinate structures and systems models of organization in each of these three disciplines is evident. Coordinate structures are envisioned by some as motor programs stored in memory and by others as emergent properties of the system.

Identification of those variables in a motor program that can be controlled and those that are fixed has implications for the motor learning theorist. By knowing what is controlled, the motor learning researcher's question "How is motor behavior acquired through practice or experience?" begins to be answered.

For the motor development theorist, the question "How does motor behavior change across long periods of time?" is strongly influenced by current concepts of motor control. Systems theory, which had its beginnings as a theory of control, is providing a new understanding of the dynamic relationships in developing individuals among the environment and perceptual, musculoskeletal, and nervous systems. Because all of these systems change across the human life span, there are multiple possibilities for explaining life span motor development even in individuals thought to be exhibiting stable behavior. As physical therapists, our understanding of motor behavior is expanded and our approaches to patient care made more versatile by knowledge of theories of motor control, learning, and development.

REFERENCES

1. Brooks VB. *The Neural Basis of Motor Control.* New York, NY: Oxford University Press; 1986:5,129-150.

2. Schmidt RA, Lee TD. *Motor Control and Learning: A Behavioral Emphasis.* 3rd ed. Champaign, Ill: Human Kinetics; 1999.

3. Roberton MA. Motor development: Recognizing our roots, charting our future. *Quest.* 1989;41:213-223.

4. Knott M, Voss DE. *Proprioceptive Neuromuscular Facilitation: Patterns and Techniques.* New York, NY: Harper and Row, Hoeber Medical Division; 1956.

5. Rood MS. Neurophysiological reactions as a basis for physical therapy. *Phys Ther Rev.* 1954;34:444-449.

6. Bobath K, Bobath B. Treatment of cerebral palsy by the inhibition of abnormal reflex action. *British Journal of Orthopedics.* 1954;11:88-89.

7. Brunnstrom S. Associated reactions of the upper extremity in adult patients with hemiplegia. *Phys Ther Rev.* 1956;36:225-236.

8. Fay T. Neuromuscular reflex therapy for spastic disorders. *Journal of the Florida Medical Association.* 1958;44:1234-1240.

9. Matthews PBC. Muscles spindles and their motor control. *Physiol Rev.* 1964;44:219-288.

10. Eldred E. Functional implications of dynamic and static components of the spindle response to stretch. *Amer J Phys Med.* 1967;46:129-140.

11. Stockmeyer SA. An interpretation of the approach of Rood to the treatment of neuromuscular dysfunction. *Amer J Phys Med.* 1967;46:900-956.

12. Knott M, Voss DE. *Proprioceptive Neuromuscular Facilitation: Patterns and Techniques.* 2nd ed. New York, NY: Harper & Row, Hoeber Medical Division; 1968.

13. Bobath K. The motor deficits in patients with cerebral palsy. *Clinics in Developmental Medicine, No 23.* London, England: William Heinemann; 1966.

14. Bobath K. A neurophysiological basis for the treatment of cerebral palsy. *Clinics in Developmental Medicine, No 75.* Philadelphia, Pa: JB Lippincott; 1980.

15. Hellebrant FE. Motor learning reconsidered: a study of change. In: Payton OD, Hirt S, Newton RA, eds. *Neurophysiologic Approaches to Therapeutic Exercise.* Philadelphia, Pa: FA Davis; 1977:33-45.

16. Delcomyn F. Neural basis of rhythmic behavior in animals. *Science.* 1980; 210:492-498.

17. Greene PH. Problems of organization of motor systems. In: Rosen R, Snell RM, eds. *Progress in Theoretical Biology, Vol 2.* New York, NY: Academic Press; 1972:303-338.

18. Kugler PN, Kelso JAS, Turvey MT. On the concept of coordinative structures as dissipative structures: I. Theoretical line. In: Stelmach GE, Requin J, eds. *Tutorials in Motor Behavior.* Amsterdam: Elsevier/North-Holland Biomedical Press; 1980:3-37.

19. Bernstein N. *The Co-ordination and Regulation of Movements.* Oxford, England: Pergamon Press; 1967.

20. Tuller B, Turvey MT, Fitch HL. The Bernstein perspective: II. The concept of muscle linkage or coordinative structure. In: Kelso JAS, ed. *Human Motor Behavior: An Introduction.* Hillsdale, NJ: Lawrence Erlbaum; 1982:253-270.

21. Geffand IM, Gurfinkel VS, Tsetlin ML, et al. Some problems in the analysis of movements. In: Geffand IM, Gurfinkel VS, Fomin SV, et al, eds. *Models of the Structural-Functional Organization of Certain Biological Systems.* Cambridge, Mass: MIT Press; 1971.

22. Schmidt RA. More on motor programs. In: Kelso JAS, ed. *Human Motor Behavior: An Introduction.* Hillsdale, NJ: Lawrence Erlbaum; 1982:189-207.

23. Keele SW. Movement control in skilled performance. *Psychological Bulletin.* 1968; 70:387-403.

24. Kelso JAS, Holt KG, Rubin P, et al. Patterns of human interlimb coordination emerge from the properties of non-linear, limit cycle oscillatory processes: theory and data. *Journal of Motor Behavior.* 1982;13:226-261.

25. Fel'dman A. Superposition of motor programs. I. Rhythmic forearm movements in man. *Neuroscience.* 1980;5:81-90.

26. Polit A, Bizzi E. Characteristics of motor programs underlying arm movements in monkey. *J Neurophys.* 1979;42:183-194.

27. Hollerbach JM. An oscillation theory of handwriting. *Biological Cybernetics.* 1981; 39:139-156.

28. Davis WJ. Organizational concepts in the central motor networks of invertebrates. In: Herman RL, et al, eds. *Advances in Behavioral Biology, Vol 18: Neural Control of Locomotion.* New York, NY: Plenum Press; 1976:265-292.

29. Kelso JAS, Tuller B. A dynamical basis for action systems. In: Gazzaniga MS, ed. *Handbook of Cognitive Neuroscience.* New York, NY: Plenum Press; 1984: 321-356.

30. Gleick J. Chaos. *Making a New Science.* New York, NY: Viking; 1987.

31. Fitch HL, Tuller B, Turvey MT. The Bernstein perspective: III. Tuning of coordinative structures with special reference to perception. In: Kelso JAS, ed. *Human Motor Behavior: An Introduction.* Hillsdale, NJ: Lawrence Erlbaum; 1982:271-281.

32. Rothstein JM, Echternach JL. Hypothesis-oriented algorithm for clinicians: A method for evaluation and treatment planning. *Phys Ther.* 1986;66:1388-1394.

33. VanSant AF. Concepts of neural organization and movement. In: Connolly BH, Montgomery PC, eds. *Therapeutic Exercise in Developmental Disabilities.* 2nd ed. Thorofare, NJ: SLACK Incorporated; 1993:1-8.

34. VanSant AF. Rising from a supine position to erect stance: description of adult movement and a developmental hypothesis. *Phys Ther.* 1988:68:185-192.

35. VanSant AF. Age differences in movement patterns used by children to rise from a supine position to erect stance. *Phys Ther.* 1988;68:1130-1138.

36. Richter RR, VanSant AF, Newton RA. Description of adult rolling movements and hypothesis of developmental sequences. *Phys Ther.* 1989;69:63-71.

37. Sarnacki S. Rising from supine on a bed: a description of adult movement and hypothesis of developmental sequences. Research Platform Presentation. Annual Conference of the American Physical Therapy Association, Anaheim, Calif, June 25, 1990.

38. Francis ED, VanSant AF. Description of the Sit-to-Stand Motion in Children and Young Adults: Hypothesis of Developmental Sequences. Research Poster Presentation. Joint Congress of the American Physical Therapy Association and the Canadian Physiotherapy Association, Las Vegas, Nev, June 16, 1988.

39. Nashner LM. Fixed patterns of rapid postural responses among leg muscles during stance. *Exp Brain Res.* 1977;30:13-24.

40. Gentile AM. Skill acquisition. In Carr JH, Shepherd RB, Gordon J et al. *Movement Science: Foundations for Physical Therapy in Rehabilitation.* Rockville, Md: Aspen Publishers, Inc; 1987:98-108.

41. Weber D, Easley-Rosenberg A. Creating an interactive environment for pediatric assessment. *Ped Phys Ther.* 2001;13:77-84.

42. Kleinman M. *The Acquisition of Motor Skill.* Princeton, NJ: The Princeton Book Co; 1983: 3-29.

43. Voss DE. Proprioceptive neuromuscular facilitation. Amer J Phys Med. 1967;46:838-898.

44. Fischer E. Factors affecting motor learning. *Amer J Phys Med.* 1967;46:511-519.

45. Hoberman M. The use of lead-up functional exercises to supplement mat work. *Phys Ther Rev.* 1951;31:1.

46. Adams JA. A closed-loop theory of motor learning. *J Mot Behav.* 1971; 3:111-149.

47. Schmidt RA. A schema theory of discrete motor skill learning. *Psychol Rev.* 1975; 82:225-260.

48. Winstein CJ. Motor learning considerations in stroke rehabilitation. In: Duncan PW, Badke MB, eds. *Stroke Rehabilitation: The Recovery of Motor Control.* Chicago, Ill: Yearbook; 1987: 109-134.

49. Winstein CJ. Knowledge of results and motor learning—implications for physical therapy. *Phys Ther.* 1991;71:140-149.

50. Winstein CJ. Designing practice for motor learning: clinical implications. In: Contemporary Management of Motor Control Problems. Proceedings of the II Step Conference. Fairfax, Va: Foundation for Physical Therapy; 1991:65-76.

51. Shea JB, Zimmy ST. Context effects in memory and learning movement information. In: Magill RA, ed. *Memory and Control of Action.* Amsterdam: North Holland; 1983:345-366.

52. Carr JH, Shepherd RB. *A Motor Relearning Programme for Stroke.* 2nd ed. Rockville, Md: Aspen;1987.

53. Carr JH, Shepherd RB. A motor learning model for rehabilitation. In: Carr JH, Shepherd RB, Gordon J, et al. *Movement Science: Foundations for Physical Therapy in Rehabilitation.* Rockville, Md: Aspen; 1987:31-91.

54. Shumway-Cook A, Woollacott MH. *Motor Control Theory and Practical Applications.* 2nd ed. Baltimore, Md: Lippincott, Williams & Wilkins; 2001.

55. McGraw MB. *The Neuromuscular Maturation of the Human Infant.* New York, NY: Hafner Publishing Co; 1945.

56. McGraw MB. *Growth: A Study of Johnny and Jimmy*. New York, NY: Appleton Century Co; 1935.

57. McGraw MB. Later development of children specially trained during infancy; Johnny and Jimmy at school age. *Child Dev*. 1939;10:1-19.

58. Thelen E. The (re)discovery of motor development: learning new things from an old field. *Dev Psych*. 1989; 25:946-949.

59. Clark JE, Whitall J. What is motor development? The lessons of history. *Quest*. 1989; 41:183-202.

60. Thomas JR, Thomas KT. What is motor development? Where does it belong? *Quest*. 1989; 41:203-212.

61. VanSant. AF. A lifespan concept of motor development. *Quest*. 1989; 41:224-234.

62. Jackson JH. Evolution and dissolution of the nervous system. In: Taylor J, ed. *Selected Writings of John Hughlings Jackson*. New York, NY: Basic Books; 1958:45-75.

63. Lerner RM. *Concepts and Theories of Human Development*. Reading, Mass: Addison-Wesley; 1976.

64. Wickstrom RL. *Fundamental Motor Patterns*. 3rd ed. Philadelphia, Pa: Lea & Febiger; 1983.

65. Bruner JS. Organization of early skilled action. *Child Dev*. 1973; 44:1-11.

66. Connolly KJ. *Mechanisms of Motor Skill Development*. New York, NY: Academic Press; 1973.

67. Kugler PN, Kelso JAS, Turvey MT. On the control and coordination of naturally developing systems. In: Kelso JAS, Clark JE, eds. *The Development of Movement Control and Coordination*. New York, NY: Wiley; 1982:5-78.

68. Thelen E. Developmental origins in motor coordination: leg movements in human infants. *Dev Psychobio*. 1985;18:1-22.

69. Thelen E, Kelso J, Fogel A. Self-organizing systems and infant motor development. *Dev Rev*. 1987;7:39-65.

70. Kamm K, Thelen E, Jensen JL. A dynamical systems approach to motor development. *Phys Ther*. 1990;70:763-775.

71. Heriza C. Implications of a dynamical systems approach to understanding infant kicking behavior. *Phys Ther*. 1991;71:222-235.

72. Espenschade A, Eckert H. *Motor Development*. Columbus, Ohio: Merrill; 1967.

73. Eckert HM. *Motor Development*. 3rd ed. Indianapolis, Ind: Benchmark Press; 1987.

74. Roberton MA. Developmental kinesiology. *Journal of Health, Physical Education and Recreation*. 1972;43:65-66.

75. Halverson LE, Roberton MA, Harper CJ. Current research in motor development. *Journal of Research and Development in Education*. 1973;6:56-70.

76. Woollacott MJ, Shumway-Cook A. *Development of Posture and Gait Across the Life Span*. Columbia, SC: University of South Carolina Press; 1989.

77. VanSant AF. Rising from a supine position to erect stance: description of adult movement and a developmental hypothesis. *Phys Ther*. 1988;68:185-192.

78. VanSant AF. Age differences in movement patterns used by children to rise from a supine position to erect stance. *Phys Ther*. 1988;68:1330-1338.

79. VanSant AF, Cromwell S, Deo A, Ford-Smith C, O'Neil J, Wrisley D. Rising to standing from supine: a study of middle adulthood. *Phys Ther*. 1988;68:830.

80. Leuhring S. *Component movement patterns of two groups of older adults in the task of rising from standing from the floor*. Unpublished master's thesis, Virginia Commonwealth University, Richmond, Va: 1989.

81. Sabourin P. *Rising from supine to standing: a study of adolescents*. Unpublished master's thesis. Virginia Commonwealth University, Richmond, Va: 1989.

82. Marsala G, VanSant AF. Movement patterns used by toddlers to rise from supine. *Phys Ther.* 1998; 78:149-159.

83. Richter RR, VanSant AF, Newton RA. Description of adult rolling movements and hypothesis of developmental sequences. *Phys Ther.* 1989; 69:63-71.

84. Lewis AM. *Age-related differences in rolling movements in children.* Unpublished master's thesis. Virginia Commonwealth University, Richmond, Va: 1987.

85. Boucher JS. *Age-related differences in adolescent movement patterns during rolling from supine to prone.* Unpublished master's thesis. Virginia Commonwealth University, Richmond, Va: 1988.

86. Francis ED. *Description of the sit-to-stand motion in children and young adults: hypothesis of developmental sequences.* Unpublished master's thesis. Virginia Commonwealth University, Richmond, Va: 1987.

87. McCoy JO, VanSant AF. Movement patterns of adolescents: rising from a bed. *Phys Ther.* 1993;73:182-193.

88. Ford-Smith, C, VanSant AF. Age differences in movement patterns used to rise from a bed: A study of middle adulthood. *Phys Ther.* 1993;73:300-309.

89. VanSant AF. A lifespan perspective of age differences in righting movements. *Motor Development: Research & Reviews.* 1997;1:46-63.

90. VanSant AF. Assessment of Neuromotor Developmental Status across the Life Span. In Proceedings of Neurology Section Measurement Forum. Alexandria, Va: Neurology Section, American Physical Therapy Association; 1990.

91. VanSant AF, Sabourin P, Leuhring S, et al. Relationships Among Age, Gender, Body Dimensions and Movement Patterns in a Righting Task. Poster Presentation. American Physical Therapy Association Annual Conference. Nashville, Tenn: American Physical Therapy Association; 1989.

92. Gesell A, Amatruda CS. *Developmental Diagnosis.* 2nd ed. New York, NY: Hoeber;1947.

93. Shirley MM. *The First Two Years. A Study of Twenty-Five Babies. Vol. 1: Posture and Locomotor Development.* Minneapolis, Minn: University of Minnesota; 1931.

94. Stockmeyer SA: An interpretation of the approach of Rood to the treatment of neuromuscular dysfunction. *Am J Phys Med.* 1967; 46:900-956.

95. Gesell A. *Infancy and Human Growth.* New York, NY: Macmillan & Co; 1928.

96. Gesell A. *The First Five Years of Life. Part 1.* New York, NY: Harper & Brothers; 1940.

97. Gesell A, Ames LB. The ontogenetic organization of prone behavior in human infancy. *J Genet Psychol.* 1940;56:247-263.

98. Ianniruberto A, Tajani E. Ultrasonographic study of fetal movements. *Seminars in Perinatology.* 1981;5:175-181.

99. Milani-Comparetti A. The neurophysiologic and clinical implications of studies on fetal motor behavior. *Sem Perinat.* 1981;5:183-189.

100. Prechtl HFR. The study of neural development as a perspective of clinical problems. In: Connolly KJ, Prechtl HFR, eds. *Maturation and Development: Biological and Psychological Perspectives. Clinics in Developmental Medicine, No 77/78.* Philadelphia, Pa: JB Lippincott; 1981:198-221.

101. Connolly KJ. Maturation and the ontogeny of motor skills. In Connolly KJ, Prechtl HFR, eds. *Maturation and Development: Biological and Psychological Perspectives. Clinics in Developmental Medicine, No 77/78.* Philadelphia, Pa: JP Lippincott; 1981:216-230.

102. Thelen E. Rhythmical stereotypes in normal human infants. *Animal Behavior.* 1979; 27:699-715.

103. Kravitz H, Boehm J. Rhythmic habit patterns in infancy a heir sequences, age of onset and frequency. *Child Development.* 1971;42:399-413.

104. Reed ES. An outline of a theory of action systems. *Journal of Motor Behavior.* 1982; 14:98-134.

105. Thelen E, Kelso JAS, Fogel A. Self-organizing systems and infant motor development *Developmental Review*. 1987;7:39-65.

106. Thelen E. Self organization in developmental processes: can systems approaches work. In: Gunner M, Thelen E, eds. *Systems and Development: The Minnesota Symposia on Child Psychology, Vol. 22.* Hillsdale, NJ: Lawrence Erlbaum; 1989:77-117.

107. Anokhin PK. Systemogenesis as a general regulator of brain development. *Prog Brain Res.* 1964;9:54-86.

108. Gibson JJ. *The Senses Considered as Perceptual Systems.* Boston, Mass: Houghton Mifflin; 1966.

109. Gibson EJ. The concept of affordances in development: the renascence of functionalism. In: Collins WA, ed. *The Concept of Development: Minnesota Symposia on Child Psychology, Vol. 15.* Hillsdale, NJ: Lawrence Erlbaum; 1982:55-81.

110. Thelen E. Developmental origins of motor coordination: leg movements in human infants. *Developmental Psychobiology.* 1985;18:1-18.

111. Clark JE, Phillips SJ, Petersen R. Developmental stability in jumping. *Developmental Psychology.* 1989; 25:1036-1045.

112. Getchel N, Roberton MA. Whole body stiffness as a function of developmental level in children's hopping. *Developmental Psychology.* 1989;25:1020-1028.

113. Goldfield EC. Transition from rocking to crawling: postural constraints on infant movement. *Developmental Psychology.* 1989;25:1013-1019.

114. Heriza C. Motor development: traditional and contemporary theories. In: Contemporary Management of Motor Control Problems. Proceedings of the II Step Conference. Fairfax, Va: Foundation for Physical Therapy; 1991:99-126.

115. Brazelton TB. *Neonatal Behavioral Assessment Scale. Clinics in Developmental Medicine, No. 50.* Philadelphia, Pa: JB Lippincott; 1973.

116. Campbell SK, Kolobe TH, Osten ET, et al. Construct validity of the Test of Infant Motor Performance. *Phys Ther.* 1995;75:585-596.

117. Haddars-Algra M. Evaluation of motor function in young infants by means of the assessment of general movements: a review. *Ped Phys Ther.* 2001;13:27-36.

Neural Systems Underlying Motor Control

Roberta A. Newton, PhD, PT

INTRODUCTION

Motor control is the process by which the central nervous system (CNS) receives, integrates, and assimilates sensory information with past experiences for planning and executing appropriate motor and postural responses. How the nervous system produces coordinated and complex motor behavior is of interest to both clinicians and researchers. The purpose of this chapter is to provide an overview of the neural systems underlying motor control. Principles and concepts presented provide part of the foundation for physical therapy examination, evaluation, and intervention. Changes in treatment approaches are, in part, reflections of advances in the understanding of the interworkings of the sensory-motor system.

What parameters of movement are controlled and how the CNS is organized to produce a variety of movements are not fully understood. Through observation and description of nervous system dysfunction and through research, models have been developed to assist our understanding. These models are based on different perspectives (eg, neurologic, biomechanical, and behavioral). Thus, no single model of motor control is universally accepted. Models also are based on the type of movement produced, such as fast, slow, skilled, and voluntary, or on the influence of affordances and constraints of the environment for movement. For example, a short leg cast affords walking but constrains selection of balance responses to an unexpected perturbation by limiting the degrees of freedom at the ankle.

Models may encompass the concept of motor programs. Some motor programs are inherent and contained in neural networks, such as the central pattern generators located in the spinal cord.[1] Other motor programs are developed and reside in a shared arrangement with various brain centers.

Which movement characteristics are contained in motor programs is controversial. Some researchers favor a model of a generalized motor program where spatio-temporal sequences of muscles are stored. The specific muscle synergies are supplied at the time of planning the movement. Others consider motor programs as representations of every motor act; thus, the spatio-temporal sequences of specific muscle synergies are stored. This potentially could produce a storage problem in the brain. Which parameters of movement or posture are stored in a motor program may be a reflection of the type of motor or postural behavior and the task constraints. Motor programs are discussed in more detail in Chapter 12.

SENSORY INFORMATION

Monitoring the internal (organism) and external environment is the primary function of sensory receptors. Sensory input denotes the location of the body in space, location of the body parts to one another, and aspects of the environment including temperature, location and contour of objects, and conditions of the support surface. Monitoring is necessary to detect a potentially harmful environment, resist the forces of gravity to maintain an upright position, or explore and manipulate the environment. The individual relies on a constellation of sensory cues from cutaneous and kinesthetic receptors located in the skin, joints, and muscles, as well as vestibular, visual, auditory, and olfactory information. Motor behavior resulting from sensory information may range from a simple spinal level reflex to a very complex motor pattern based on perception and memory of similar situations.

Sensation is defined as the process by which sensory receptors receive and route information to the spinal level for reflexive and automatic motor activity and to higher centers for processing. Perception is the integration of sensory input in conjunction with memory of similar situations. Sensation cannot be changed with repeated experience, whereas, perception is changed with repeated experience.[2]

Sensory information is used in at least three different modes during motor activity. First, sensory information reflects the location of body parts with respect to one another, and location of the body with respect to space and objects within the environment. This input is used during the planning phase so that the appropriate motor response with appropriate parameters is selected and executed. Second, sensory information can be used to revise the motor programs prior to and during the execution of a motor program (ie, concepts of feed-forward and feedback). These processes can occur at the spinal level by altering the excitability level of the internuncial and motoneuronal pools, or at higher levels, for example, in the cerebellum for comparing actual motor response to the expected motor behavior. Third, sensory input from movement may be reduced, synthesized, and stored in motor memory for future use. This use of information is termed knowledge of results (KR).

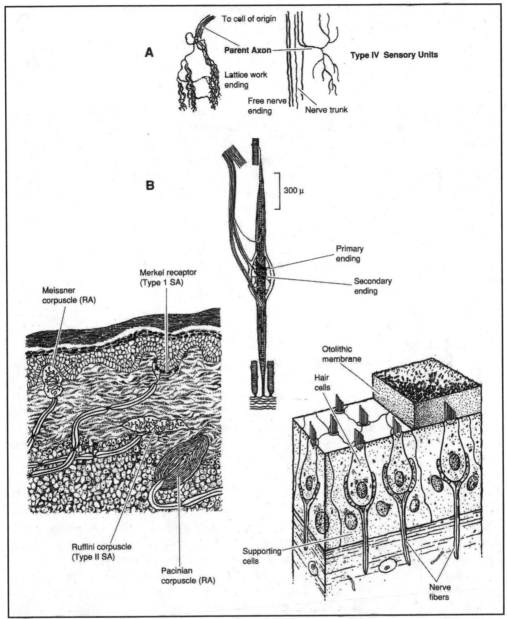

Figure 3-1. Mechano-receptors located in skin, muscle, and joint. A. Free nerve endings—type IV joint receptors. B. Encapsulated endings—cutaneous receptors, muscle spindle, vestibular receptor.

General Characteristics of Sensory Receptors

Sensory receptors are either free nerve endings or elaborate structures encased in connective tissue capsules (Figure 3-1). Although receptors tend to be modality specific, responding most efficiently to a single type of sensory stimulus, others are polymodal, responding to several types of stimuli. At the receptor level, sensory information is encoded by a pattern of action potentials. The pattern, or code, is related to the intensity and duration of the stimulus. Sequential activation of receptors indicates direction of the moving stimulus or moving body part. All receptors either partially or completely adapt to a stimulus. With continuous application of a stimulus, the response rate of the receptor will be initially high and, over time, will decrease to a lower level or will stop.

The sensory unit is the functional unit of sensation. This entity includes the receptor (or group of receptors) attached to a single afferent neuron. The sensory unit monitors a limited area, the peripheral field. The peripheral field for cutaneous receptors is a specific skin area. For joint receptors, the peripheral field is bounded by a specific joint range and is measured in degrees and direction of movement. Peripheral fields for vestibular receptors are bound by a specific direction of movement, acceleration, or velocity.

Processing Sensory Information

Although the majority of sensory afferents reach the spinal cord via the dorsal roots, approximately 20% of the unmyelinated pain afferents enter the spinal cord via the ventral root.[3] Sensory input is carried to higher centers via specific ascending pathways, as well as routed to various levels of the spinal cord through Lissauer's tract or short and long propriospinal tracts. Afferent connections at the spinal level influence the internuncial pool, automatic efferents, and motor efferents.

Cutaneous information reaches higher centers via the dorsal column-medial lemniscal system or the anterolateral system. Transmission of information by two distinct pathways is one method for the CNS to distinguish among different sensory modalities. The dorsal column-medial lemniscal system primarily transmits mechanoreception. This highly organized system produces sparse collateral branching. The result is a high degree of spatial orientation between the perceived stimulus and localization of the stimulus on the body. To increase the discriminatory function of this system, some collateral branching is inhibitory. These inhibitory endings block further spread of the signal, thereby enhancing the contrast of the transmitted signal. This process is called *lateral inhibition.*

The anterolateral system transmits a broad spectrum of modalities. Collateral branching occurs as this system ascends; therefore, the system lacks the discriminatory quality found in the dorsal column-medial lemniscal system.

In addition to the use of lateral inhibition to enhance the signal, enhancement also occurs through feedback control loops. Corticofugal inhibitory axons impinge on various levels of the neuraxis and are postulated to provide gain-control, that is, recurrent inhibition to increase or decrease the threshold level of ascending pathways.

Somatosensory Cortex

Somatic sensory area I is located in the postcentral gyrus of the cerebral cortex (Brodmann areas 3,1,2) (Figure 3-2). Somatosensory area SII also receives input from the periphery. SI and SII have dense reciprocal connections to enhance signal processing. Each side of the cortex primarily receives contralateral sensory input with the exception of the face. Functionally, the region is arranged somatotopically and in vertical columns; each column receives input from a specific sensory modality. Vertical columns in the anterior portion of the postcentral gyrus receive input primarily from proprioceptors, and those in the posterior portion receive input primarily from cutaneous receptors.

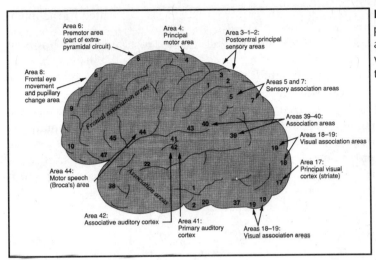

Figure 3-2. Lateral aspect of the cerebrum according to Brodmann, with functional localizations.

Widespread damage to the postcentral gyrus results in deficits in the individual's ability to gauge gradations in weight, pressure, texture of materials, and to judge shapes or forms of objects. Some ability to perceive tactile sensation may return and is believed to be due to crude perception in the thalamus.

Cutaneous Receptors

Cutaneous receptors are classified as mechanoreceptors, thermoreceptors, and nociceptors. Mechanoreceptors monitor the relative position of the stimulus on the surface of the skin, as well as assist in determining the rate of movement of body parts relative to one another or to the support surface. Mechanoreceptors provide information relative to exploring and manipulating the environment and determining the texture of the support surface. Nociceptors may be polymodal, that is, responding to two different types of noxious or potentially harmful stimuli. For example, polymodal nociceptors may respond to extremely intense temperature and intense pressure applied to the surface of the skin.

Reflexively, cutaneous input is used to provide appropriate facilitation or inhibition of the interneuronal and motoneuronal pools. Only noxious cutaneous stimuli produce reflexive stereotypic movement. Various investigators have examined the role of tactile input for manipulating the environment, particularly for precise manipulation.[4] Handling small objects between the thumb and fingertips requires refinement of muscle forces, a task that is heavily dependent on cutaneous input. A memory trace for coordinating grip and load forces is constantly updated through tactile input. The automatic adjustment through a closed loop feedback system prevents the object from slipping through the fingers. Because of this automatic feedback loop, a greater portion of the sensory processing can be used for higher level manipulatory or exploratory functions. When damage to a peripheral nerve occurs, such as in carpal tunnel syndrome involving the median nerve, there is a decrease in the amount of sensory information available for manipulation, as well as a decrease in the number of available motor units to generate appropriate forces.

Proprioceptors

Muscle, tendon, and joint receptors provide information regarding static position, movement, and sensation pertaining to muscle force. **Kinesthesia** and **proprioception** are terms describing these functions, and often are used interchangeably.

The muscle spindle is a complex receptor consisting of two major types of intrafusal muscle fibers, **afferent** and **efferent connections,** covered by connective tissue. Gamma motoneurons innervating muscle spindles adjust the sensitivity of the muscle spindle to respond to stimuli. The location of the muscle spindle in series with extrafusal muscle fibers permits the receptor to monitor muscle stretch. The muscle spindle also is sensitive to externally applied vibratory stimuli. At the spinal level, this receptor type produces autogenic facilitation of motoneurons. Antagonist muscles receive reciprocal inhibition. Spindle information to higher centers pertains to velocity and length of muscle stretch.

A proprioceptive illusion is created with muscle vibration.[5,6] Vibration activates muscle spindles, resulting in reflexive contraction of the muscle, perception of muscle stretch, and distortion of position sense. The apparent conflict can be resolved in an individual with an intact CNS, however, resolution of the conflict may not occur in the patient with CNS dysfunction.

The Golgi tendon organ monitors muscle tension for a group of muscle fibers rather than sampling muscle tension for the entire muscle. Early research suggested that the function of the Golgi tendon organ was to prevent a joint from exceeding its range. A recently hypothesized role for this receptor and the muscle spindle is to regulate muscle stiffness. That is, by monitoring the length and tension of a muscle, these receptors activate feedback loops to influence the amount of muscle tension or stiffness.[7]

Four types of receptors are considered joint receptors, three true joint receptors and one pain receptor.[8] These receptors signal specific direction and velocity of joint movement, as well as static position. Reflexively, they either facilitate or inhibit the internuncial pool. During passive joint movements, receptor input appears to be facilitory. During active movement, joint receptor input appears to facilitate antagonists and inhibit agonists to ensure joint movement in a working range and to provide control when the joint begins to move outside normal physiological range.[9]

The role of joint receptors in kinesthesia has not been fully elucidated. For example, an individual's ability to detect passive movements of the fingers and toes is diminished with nerve blockage; however, direction is detected with an increase in the velocity of passive movement. This detection could be reflective of the contribution of muscle receptors. In other studies, intracapsular anesthesia of the knee joint did not affect detection of joint position. Location of anesthesia and the differences in velocity of passive joint movement could cause the apparent discrepancies found in the outcomes of these studies. More recent studies have documented impaired proprioception in individuals with joint pathology.[10]

The role of proprioceptive feedback for the development of motor programs, particularly learning a new task, is well documented. Object manipulation is a widely used paradigm for examining this role. A patient with a sensory neuropathy may be unable to sustain a grip with the affected hand. However, he may be able to drive a car with a manual gear (providing he has done so for years) in the absence of peripheral feedback. This example demonstrates that a learned movement strategy can be executed without peripheral feedback. However, during repetitive manipulation activities performed without visual guidance, motor performance deteriorates due to undetected and uncompensated errors.[4],[11] Although peripheral feedback may not be necessary for execution of stored motor programs, feedback is necessary for the automatic adjustments that accompany movement, particularly adjustments related to load compensation, error detection, and correction. Furthermore, feedback is necessary for learning new motor programs and refining motor output during execution.

Vestibular, Visual, and Auditory Systems

The vestibular and visual systems function optimally when the head provides a stable platform; that is, the coordination between the head and trunk permit the head to maintain gaze stability.[12] Sensory end organs of the otoliths and semicircular canals respond to movement of the head (rotary, tilt, or linear translation). The three pairs of semicircular canals are arranged such that direction and velocity of movement in any plane are detected. The *otoliths* detect gravity, as well as movement including tilting. Information carried by the *vestibular nerve* is selectively transmitted to the vestibular nuclei. The *superior* and *medial nuclei* coordinate eye movement for gaze stability. The *lateral nuclei* coordinate head and eye movement and play a role in axial and limb control. The *inferior nuclei* connect with nuclei in the reticular formation, including those associated with autonomic functions. The *vestibular nuclei* are connected intimately with the cerebellum and have complex connections to other brain centers including the parieto-insular cortex and the medial superior and middle temporal areas of the cortex.[13] The integration of vestibular input with visual and somatosensory input also subserves postural and balance control, as well as the perception of verticality.[14],[15] The descending vestibulospinal pathways are implicated in the coordination of neck, trunk, and limb musculature for maintaining postural control against gravity, as well as subserving movement.

The vestibulo-ocular reflex (VOR), triggered by head movements, permits coordination of eye and head movements.[16] Activation of the VOR by the semicircular canals is termed *angular VOR* and results in the eyes moving in the opposite direction and at the same speed as head turning. Tilting or linear translation of the head, resulting in stimulation of the otoliths, can also activate the VOR. The result is the stabilization of gaze such that the visual image does not slip across the retina (oscillopsia). The cerebellum is involved intimately with regulation of oculomotor control. For example, the VOR needs to be cancelled in order for visual smooth-pursuit tracking to occur. The cerebellar cortex also is involved in voluntary gaze and eye-hand coordination.

The visual system provides sensory information pertinent to location of objects, as well as to depth perception and motion. This system also detects color, texture, and the contour of objects. Vision is useful for the individual to navigate through the environment, provide spatial orientation, recognize other individuals, judge the movement of objects, and recognize potentially harmful situations. *Focal* or *central vision* contributes to perception of object motion, verticality, object identification and location in the environment, and location of self in the environment. *Ambient* or *peripheral vision* contributes to perception of self-motion. *Microsaccades*, small oscillations of the eye, keep the visual receptors from quickly adapting when gaze is fixed on an object. *Rods* are specialized receptors that mediate vision under dimly lit conditions (scotopic vision). *Cones* are the receptors specialized for color vision (photopic vision).

Visual input from the periphery is carried over optic tract fibers to the lateral geniculate nucleus and to the superior colliculus. Visual processing occurs in the primary visual cortex (Brodmann's area 17), as well as other visual areas of the cortex (V1, V2).

Visual images are analyzed for color, linear contours, boundaries, and movement. Disorders of the visual system include primary visual deficits, as well as visual-perceptual dysfunction.[17,18]

The auditory system plays an important role in motor control by alerting, identifying, and orienting the organism to environmental sounds, particularly novel and potentially harmful ones. Receptors in the cochlea convert sound waves into action potentials that are carried by the cochlear nerve. Each receptor responds to a narrow range of frequency and intensity of sound waves. The ascending pathways from the cochlea to the cerebral cortex are complex and include the cochlear nucleus, superior olivary complex, inferior colliculus, and medial geniculate nucleus. Pathways are crossed and uncrossed to allow for bilateral integration of information. The primary auditory cortex, located on the dorsal surface of the superior temporal lobe, and several surrounding auditory cortical fields process the information. Although not completely understood, it is hypothesized that the multiple areas process different aspects of the auditory stimuli. Lesions to the auditory cortex in animals affect the ability of the animal to localize the source of the sound in the environment, as well as to discriminate among complex patterns of sound. Humans with bilateral temporal lobe damage generally demonstrate recovery of tone. The remaining deficiencies are usually related to decreased ability to detect changes in the temporal order, sequence of sounds, or in localization of sounds in space.[19]

Summary

The role of sensory receptors in regulating motor behavior is extensive at both spinal and higher center levels. Depending on the type of movement, the role varies. Rather than examining individual receptors and their roles in motor behavior, future examination should be directed toward functional classifications. For example, how all types of mechanoreceptors contribute to assessing the internal and external environment. Integration of sensory information for balance, movement, and learning is continuing to be investigated at various macroscopic and microscopic levels. Lastly, the role of sensory degradation and abnormal motor control seen in patients with chronic pain or focal hand dystonia needs to be elucidated (see Chapter 4). Continued repetitive movements (stereotypic movements) provide continued sensory information (stereotypic sensory input), which decreases the variability of movement patterns and can cause changes in the primary sensory cortex.[20-22] These changes may further compromise the patient's motor control system.

SPINAL MECHANISMS

Contributions of the spinal level to motor control occur through reflexive activity, as well as through regulation of muscle length and force.[23,24] Skeletal muscle has a dual role because it serves as a force generator due to its elastic or spring-like qualities and as a mechanical impedance due its viscous qualities. When a muscle is stretched, an increase in force occurs until a maximal physiologic length is reached. This force is stored as potential energy. The relationship between force and length is similar to properties of a spring and is depicted in length-tension diagrams. The advantage to such a mechanism is that energy can be stored, as well as used as a shock absorber (eg, when the foot hits the ground). Skeletal muscles, however, do not act singularly, but are coupled at the spinal level through various neuronal circuits to form functional synergies.

The motor unit defines the motor neuron and the muscle fibers associated with it.

The motor unit is considered the smallest functional element of motor control. Motor units vary in size according to the number of muscle fibers associated with the motor neuron. This is termed *innervation ratio*. Generally, the higher the innervation ratio, the more force produced by that motor unit. Another factor that influences the force-generation capacity is the type of muscle fiber associated with the motor unit. Motor units termed *S-type* (slow) are easy to activate and maintain a small amount of force activation for relatively long periods. They are considered fatigue resistant. The *F-type* (fast) motor units generate proportionally larger amounts of force and are divided into two subclasses—those that are unable to sustain a tetanic contraction (fast-twitch, fatigable, FF) and those that are more fatigue resistant (fast-twitch, fatigue-resistant FR).[25]

Motor units are regulated by spinal level and descending connections. At the spinal level, interneurons provide the complex integrative element for spinal level information processing. Both inhibitory and excitatory interneurons exist to either dampen or amplify the ongoing processing. Several types of interneurons have been identified and are involved in regulation of movement.[26] Renshaw neurons receive excitatory input from collaterals of motoneurons, synapse on motoneurons, and other interneurons (Ia inhibitory neurons) in the area surrounding them. The Ia inhibitory interneuron receives excitatory input from the Ia afferents of the muscle spindles and provides inhibitory connections to the antagonist motoneurons. Ia-Ib interneurons receive synaptic input from Golgi tendon organ afferents and produce inhibition of synergistic motoneurons. The functional role of the Group II excitatory interneurons is not fully understood. The last group is presynaptic inhibitory interneurons located in the dorsal gray matter. These neurons release GABA (gamma aminobutyric acid) and decrease the electrical activity of afferents with which they synapse.

The role of the spinal level connections for reflexive behavior is well known. The stretch reflex contributes to the stiffness of muscles. It also provides the "spring-like" properties. When a muscle is stretched, there is an increase in the firing of action potentials in motor units of that muscle, which increases force. Another approach to understanding spinal level control is the equilibrium point hypothesis.[27] The premise is that the resting position of the limb is the result of the spring-like properties of antagonist muscles. The stiffness of muscles is regulated by the nervous system such that the trajectory of the limb indicates successive equilibrium points. Other factors that affect muscle stiffness include the strength of the cross bridges, the contractile elements of skeletal muscle, and connective tissue in muscle, including tendons.

Although the motor unit is considered the smallest functional unit for motor control, the pattern generator may be a more encompassing model at the spinal level. Clusters of neurons at the spinal level can produce repetitive discharge to produce locomotor-like patterns. This pattern of activity has been demonstrated in animal preparations following removal of the cerebral cortex. In the presence of norepinephrine or other alpha-adrenergic agonists, the interneuronal systems continued to demonstrate rhythmic bursting. If the animal was supported and placed on a treadmill, locomotor patterns were generated.[28]

Energy costs are another consideration when examining locomotion. Changing gait speed or switching from one gait to another changes the rate of oxygen consumption. Higher energy consumption also is noted if locomotor speed is higher or lower than the usual or preferred rate.[29,30]

Altered gait patterns have been examined in individuals with peripheral and deficits. Rhythmic output persists in the absence or decrease of sensory feedback. Spinal level generators, or stepping generators, have been inferred in humans with partial spinal

Figure 3-3. The anatomical connections of the basal ganglia.

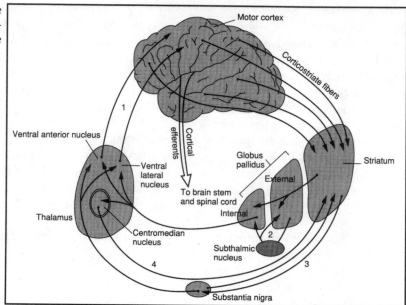

transactions.[31-34] Descending and peripheral input fine-tune the spinal generator networks. Peripheral input refines rhythmic activity, initiates compensatory changes when stepping is perturbed (eg, stumbling corrective reaction), and provides other postural and balance information to alter the rhythm of the generator. Higher center input shapes the spinal generator, producing locomotion by varying the amplitude, timing, and force parameters. Therefore, the changes seen with CNS dysfunction cannot be explained solely on the basis of muscle weakness.

BASAL GANGLIA

The basal ganglia, by virtue of their interconnections, represent an extremely complex area. Disorders such as Parkinson's disease, hemiballism, and Huntington's chorea confirm this center's role in motor control. Movement deficits include abnormalities of righting (labyrinthine and body righting reactions), equilibrium, sequencing, and velocity of movement. To consider the basal ganglia's only role to be related to motor function is too simplistic. More recently, the basal ganglia have been demonstrated to be involved in complex behaviors including cognitive and motor learning functions.

Neuroanatomical Connections

Neuroanatomical connections demonstrate the complexity of this area and the difficulty attributing functions to the basal ganglia. The three primary nuclei are the putamen, globus pallidus, and caudate nucleus. Other associated nuclei include the substantia nigra and subthalamic nucleus. The putamen and caudate nucleus are primary receiving areas, and the globus pallidus is the primary output area. The term *striatum* collectively identifies the putamen and caudate nucleus. Figure 3-3 demonstrates several circuits involving the basal ganglia, cortical, and subcortical centers.

A major circuit arises in the cerebral cortex, projects to the basal ganglia via corticostriate pathways, and returns to the cortex via the thalamus. Neurons arise from all areas of the cortex, including the primary motor, premotor, and association areas and terminate on neurons in the striatum. The terminations are somatotopically organized with functionally related neurons from different parts of the cerebrum terminating in close proximity. The arrangement of these terminations suggests an integrative role for the basal ganglia. Neurons from the striatum terminate on the globus pallidus and subthalamic nucleus. Neurons traverse to the ventroanterior and ventrolateral thalamus then back to all areas of the cerebral cortex, particularly to prefrontal and premotor areas.

This major circuit is subdivided into the *complex (association) loop* and the *motor loop*.[32,33] The complex loop is identified with frontal association areas of the cerebral cortex and uses the caudate nucleus as the major input area. The motor loop originates in the premotor and motor areas of the cerebral cortex and uses the putamen as the major input area. Both loops project to different areas of the globus pallidus, substantia nigra, and thalamic nuclei. These loops also are integrated with the internal circuit between the striatum and substantia nigra. The striatum releases GABA (an inhibitory substance) on neurons of the substantia nigra, which in turn release dopamine (an inhibitory substance at its termination in the striatum). This striatal-substantia nigra circuit is a mutual inhibitory pathway. Damage to the substantia nigra fibers produces chemical transmitter imbalance within the striatum. Thus, cholinergic pathways from the cerebral cortex are totally or partially unchecked when damage occurs to these inhibitory pathways.

Other loops run from the globus pallidus to the subthalamic nucleus and from the globus pallidus to the centromedial nucleus of the thalamus. Other efferent pathways from the basal ganglia, not necessarily forming circuits, project to the brainstem and superior colliculus.

Role in Motor Control

The role of this area in motor control has been examined through research and analysis of movement deficits associated with pathologies. Based on recordings of cellular activity in unanesthetized and unrestrained animals performing rapid movements, slow movements, and self-paced alternating movements, it can be assumed that the basal ganglia are involved with a wide variety of movements. More specifically, these nuclei control specific parameters of movement. Early studies demonstrated that basal ganglia cells were active prior to the onset of cortical activity or movement.[34] Movement-related cells were also noted to be preferentially active relative to specific movements or postures. More recently, recordings have been conducted in primates and humans performing pursuit tracking and step tracking tasks.[35] From these studies, researchers concluded that these nuclei are not involved in the initiation of a stimulus-triggered movement, but are involved with initiation of self-generated or voluntary movement.[36] Moreover, their role includes scaling parameters of movement including velocity, amplitude, and direction.

Parkinson's disease is considered the hallmark of basal ganglia dysfunction and is the first documented example of pathology related to neurotransmitter deficiency. As described in classical works by Marsden[37] and Martin,[38] individuals with Parkinson's disease have bradykinesia, tremor at rest, and cog-wheel rigidity. To examine the role of the basal ganglia using a disease model such as Parkinsonism, patients need to be observed during early onset. With progression, other cortical and subcortical areas become involved, thereby contaminating observed motor behavior attributed to the basal ganglia.

Individuals self-exposed to MPTP (1-methyl-4-phenyl-1,2,3,6 tetrahydropyridine) develop symptoms similar to Parkinson's disease.[39] This toxin selectively damages dopamine-producing neurons of the substantia nigra. The three cardinal signs of Parkinson's disease (akinesia, tremor, rigidity) demonstrated in these patients are produced solely by loss of the nigrostriatal projections.

Bradykinesia is a slowing of movement due, in part, to the inability of the patient to generate sufficient amplitude in the agonists, although the normal triphasic electromyography (EMG) pattern is intact. This finding supports the role of the basal ganglia in a scaling function, particularly in relationship to amplitude or magnitude of the initial burst of EMG activity in the agonists.

Akinesia denotes impaired initiation of movement. To date, the pathophysiologic mechanism for akinesia is not completely understood. Continued, tonic inhibition of thalamic neurons by the internal portion of the globus pallidus is a potential mechanism. Rigidity is believed to be due to loss of the nigrostriatal dopamine system since dopamine agonists reverse rigidity. The pathophysiologic basis of tremor also is not clearly understood, but may involve either cerebellar-thalamic pathways or pallidum-thalamic pathways.

Pursuit tracking paradigms have been used in patients with Parkinson's disease to delineate the basal ganglia's role in motor control, and more recently the role of the putamen in motor learning.[40] Reaction times to these tasks are increased with variability attributed to medication. This delay is believed to be due to the inability to deliver the correct initial motor command to the agonist muscle, as well as the inability to generate appropriate agonist force. These phenomena were demonstrated in standing balance responses to linear perturbation. Horak noted the activation of two movement strategies in response to linear perturbation[41] (see Chapter 11). The observed motor behavior could be the result of the inability to issue a correct initial motor command.

Generally, patients with Parkinson's disease do not achieve high velocity movements during high amplitude excursions. When tracking targets requiring initial fast movements, patients move slowly to the target using a pause-error correction mode throughout the excursion of the movement, rather than smooth pursuit movement. The faster the speed needed for target pursuit, the greater the impairment. Additionally, slowness and intermittency of movement have been documented with EMG. Alternating activity between agonists and antagonists produces intermittent bursts of activity as the patient follows or approaches the target. Patients demonstrate an increasing delay to producing faster movements and a higher error rate than normal when performing tracking tasks. Reduced predictive capabilities and reduced improvement with practice are noticed with step tracking tasks or tracking tasks containing reversals in movement. Patients are able to learn new motor tasks and learn to predict the course of a target.[42] This is indicative that the patient is able to select a sequence of motor programs necessary to carry out a movement.

In addition, patients with Parkinson's disease have been observed to be dependent on visual input for guidance of limb movements, an indication of impaired kinesthetic mechanisms.[43] Early research documented that the majority of basal ganglia cells of nonhuman primates responded preferentially to joint rotations rather than cutaneous stimulation.[44]

Patients with Parkinson's disease have difficulty performing two simultaneous movements or switching from one motor task to another. "Freezing" in the middle of a motor sequence is common. Deficits in motor performance of complex movements demonstrate the integral involvement of the basal ganglia in motor control. No single patho-physiologic mechanism can explain movement deficits in Parkinson's disease. It appears that patients perceive the motor task and select and sequence the necessary motor programs, but are unable to execute the motor programs. This is further evidenced by:

- Breakdown of simultaneous tasks into sequential tasks
- Selection of inaccurate parameters during the initial activation of the agonists
- Pause-run mode rather than a smooth running sequence of the motor program

Postural abnormalities also are evident in Parkinson's disease. The classical flexed posture is due to increased activity of axial and limb musculature. Decreased righting and equilibrium reactions produce postural instability. Since postural instability appears later in the course of the disease, it may be due to damage in other areas of the brain in concert with progressive damage to the basal ganglia. Anticipatory and compensatory postural reactions, as well as protective reactions, also are compromised.

Other motor dysfunction associated with the basal ganglia include chorea, an involuntary movement characterized by rapid, involuntary movements that flow from one body region to another in a nonstereotypic manner. Chorea is associated with metabolic imbalance seen with hyperthyroidism, use of medications including levodopa, or Huntington's disease which is an autosomal dominant condition resulting in the loss of GABA-enkephalin neurons, particularly associated with the head of the caudate nucleus. Ballism, a high amplitude movement associated with the proximal parts of the extremities, is associated with damage of the subthalmic nucleus. Dystonia is a twisting, often repetitive and sustained involuntary movement associated with a single body part (focal), body region (segmental), or the whole body (generalized).

Role in Cognition

Due to the extensive connections from the cerebral cortex to the basal ganglia, the basal ganglia are believed to participate in cognition.[45,46] The caudate nucleus is believed to be the predominant input for cognitive functions. Bilateral lesions to specific areas of the caudate nucleus produce deficits in an animal's ability to perform delayed alternation tasks. These tasks involve a delay between when the time instructions are given and when actual motor performance occurs. These deficits are noted when particular areas of the cerebral cortex are damaged, specifically those areas having projections to the caudate nucleus.

In summary, the basal ganglia play an important role in both motor processing and motor learning. Although early models based on pathology considered the basal ganglia to be primarily involved in the initiation of movement, it now appears that the basal ganglia also are involved in executing and completing movement sequences by using inhibitory input to increase or decrease other movements which may or may not be part of the primary movement. Lastly, basal ganglia models suggest a role in automatic execution of learned movement sequences. That is, those movements that do not need voluntary control or attention to take place.[47]

CEREBELLUM

The cerebellum contains half of all the neurons located in the brain, yet constitutes only 10% of brain weight. This highly organized structure is best analyzed from a three-

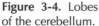

Figure 3-4. Lobes of the cerebellum.

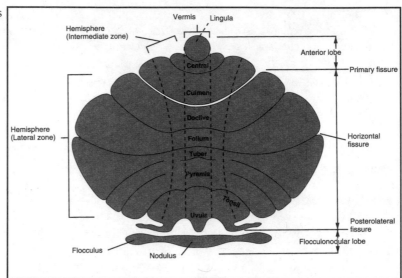

dimensional perspective. The role of the cerebellum in motor control is awesome, ranging from a comparator role to involvement in motor learning.[48]

Deep fissures serve to divide the cerebellum into the anterior, posterior, and flocculonodular lobes (Figure 3-4). The cerebellum also can be divided into three sagittal areas. The vermis is a narrow longitudinal strip located in the midline, separating the left and right cerebellar hemispheres. Each hemisphere is subdivided into an intermediate and a lateral zone. Four pairs of deep nuclei associated with this region are the fastigial, dentate, globose, and emboliform nuclei.

Input from the periphery, brainstem, and cerebral cortex terminates either in the cerebellar cortex or deep cerebellar nuclei. The raphe nuclei and locus ceruleus also send projections to the cerebellar cortex. Mossy and climbing fibers transmit all information to the cerebellar cortex. These two excitatory inputs arise from different sources. The mossy fibers originate from the brainstem nuclei and carry information from the spinal cord and cerebral cortex. Mossy fibers terminate on granule cells in the granular layer of the cerebellar cortex. Axons of the granular cells project to the outermost cortical layer, bifurcate, and become parallel fibers. By this axonal arrangement, mossy fibers influence a large number of Purkinje cells. Purkinje cells are the sole output neurons from the cerebellar cortex. The second projection system, climbing fibers, originates from the inferior olivary nucleus. These fibers impinge directly on a limited number of Purkinje cells. The mossy fiber-climbing fiber interactive arrangement on the Purkinje cell has been implicated in the cerebellum's role in learning.

The excitatory activity of the mossy and climbing fiber input on the Purkinje cell is offset by inhibitory interneurons, termed *stellate*, *basket*, and *Golgi cells*. When a group of Purkinje cells are activated, Purkinje cells bordering the active group are inhibited. The function of this lateral or surround inhibition is not clearly understood.

The major output from the cerebellar cortex is to the deep nuclei with some projections to the vestibular nuclei. By virtue of its development, the cerebellum can be considered as three distinctive regions, each with specific efferent projects and each with specific motor functions. In addition to the roles played by the cerebellum in assisting other

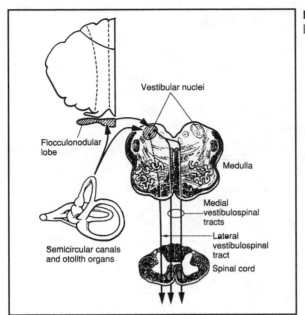

Figure 3-5. Projections of the vestibulocerebellum.

higher centers to coordinate motor behavior, the cerebellum also regulates some autonomic functions including pupillary size, respiration, and cardiovascular functions.

Neuroanatomical Connections and the Role of Cerebellar Areas in Motor Control

The vestibulocerebellum encompasses the flocculonodular lobe, which is termed the *archicerebellum* (see Figure 3-4). This area receives input from and projects to the vestibular nuclei and thus is intimately involved with regulation of balance and eye-head movement (Figure 3-5). Input to this area signals changes in head position and orientation of the head with respect to gravity. Visual information also indicates orientation of the head in space. Output from this area regulates axial muscles used to maintain balance and controls eye movement for coordination of eye-head movement.

Damage to this area is generally due to a medulloblastoma. Patients with this condition may be unable to maintain balance even in a seated position with eyes open, thereby demonstrating a lack of postural stabilization. Patients use a wide base of support during stance and gait to compensate for decreased intersegmental stability.[49]

The spinocerebellum (paleocerebellum) runs rostro-caudal to include the vermis and intermediate zones of the cerebellar hemispheres (see Figure 3-4). Sensory information is received from the periphery through the spinocerebellar tracks (hence its name) and from the visual, auditory, and vestibular systems. Input is somatotopically organized, one map lying in the rostral region and the other map in the caudal region. Auditory and visual information are directed more toward the posterior aspect of this region.

Output from the spinocerebellum terminates on different deep cerebellar nuclei, thereby forming two different projection systems (Figure 3-6). The vermis projects to the fastigial nucleus, which in turn sends bilateral projections to the lateral vestibular nuclei and the brainstem reticular formation. These latter areas form the medial descending system that regulates axial and proximal musculature. The fastigial nucleus also sends

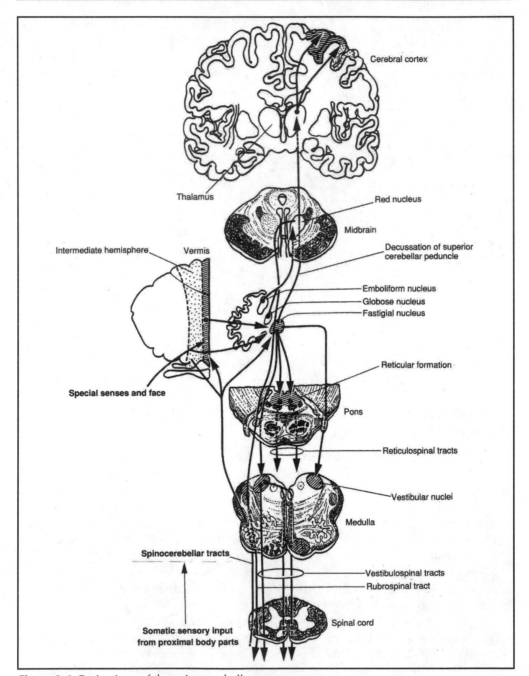

Figure 3-6. Projections of the spinocerebellum.

crossed ascending projections to the motor cortex. The intermediate part of the cerebellar hemispheres impinges on the emboliform and globose nuclei, which project to the red nucleus and the cerebral cortex. Thus, the cerebellum influences the lateral descending system, containing in part, the rubrospinal tract system which affects musculature of the distal portions of the extremities. Projections to the contralateral red nucleus then to extremity areas of the motor cortex assist in regulating the corticospinal tract.

Functions of the spinocerebellum include a regulatory role in the execution of movement and regulation of muscle forces to compensate for variations in load encountered during movement. This comparator function is dependent on information received from the cerebral cortex regarding the intended movement. This function is also dependent on feedback from the periphery regarding the actual movement. A mismatch between the actual and intended movement produces an error signal, which is corrected by revising the motor program.

Damage to the spinocerebellum results in an abnormal sequence of muscle contraction. Agonist muscle activity is prolonged, and timing of antagonist contraction for limb deceleration is delayed. When deceleration and stop commands are disrupted, movements become inaccurate and tremor occurs, particularly at the end of movement.

Damage usually entails the upper vermal and intermediate parts of the anterior lobe, such as that observed in patients with chronic alcoholism. Patients demonstrate extremely large antero-posterior sway paths in standing, but rarely exceed sway limits and fall. When tested on sudden tilt of a movable platform, a relatively normal latency of onset with increased sway amplitude of the compensatory balance response occurs.[50] Patients rely heavily on vision to maintain balance.

The cerebrocerebellum receives widespread input from the cerebral cortex, but does not receive direct input from the periphery. The major inputs arise from the premotor, motor, sensory, and posterior parietal lobes of the cerebral cortex. The lateral parts (zone) of the hemispheres define this portion of the cerebellum (see Figure 3-4). Because this is the last cerebellar area to evolve, it is also known as the *neocerebellum*. Phylogenetically, this region increased in size in relationship to increases in the size of the cerebral cortex.

Output from this area terminates on neurons in the dentate nucleus, which in turn project to the ventral lateral nucleus of the thalamus, then to premotor and motor areas of the cerebral cortex (Figure 3-7). A feedback loop is evident as fibers of the dentate nucleus project to the red nucleus, then to the inferior olivary nucleus and back to the cerebellum.

Both lesion studies and cell recordings have been used to document contributions of this area to motor control, which include a decrease in control of distal extremity musculature. Furthermore, delays in the initiation of movement, hypotonia, and motor incoordination are evident. These deficits are attributed to the loss of spatio-temporal organization necessary for movement. A delay in initiation has been hypothesized to occur either with loss of the dentate nucleus' participation in commands for initiating movement, or loss of its influence on activation of other centers.

Another possible role for the cerebrocerebellum, along with the premotor cortex, is programming of movement. Thus, this area could serve two purposes:

1. The decision to move and the initiation of movement
2. The coordination of eye-hand movements for manipulation and exploring the environment.[51]

Individuals with tumors or vascular lesions to this region demonstrate some reduction in postural stability, but no abnormal sway characteristics. These individuals may demonstrate a jerky, ataxic path that represents their center of mass when trying to follow a cursor on a computer screen. This observation further confirms the role of this area in spatio-temporal organization necessary for pursuit tasks, either whole extremity or whole body.

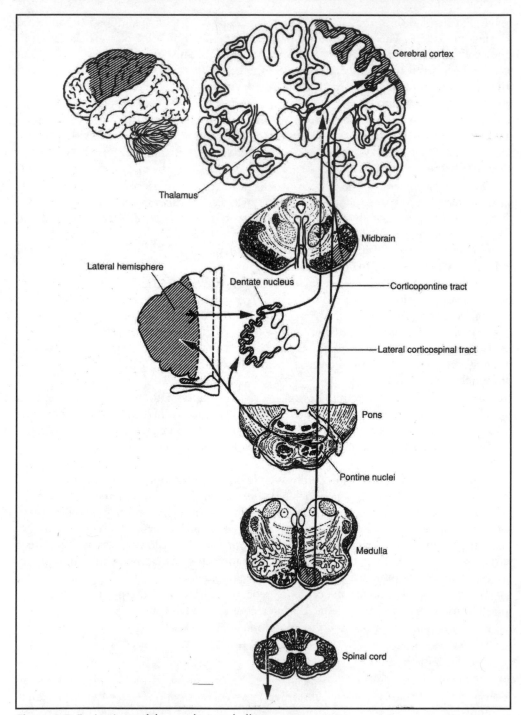

Figure 3-7. Projections of the cerebrocerebellum.

Role of the Cerebellum in Motor Learning

In the 1970s, the role of the cerebellum in motor learning was based on mathematical models exploring cerebellar circuitry.[51,52] Further evidence was obtained when researchers noted that the visual fields and the direction of the VOR could be reversed by wearing prismatic lenses. Both humans and nonhuman primates adapted to the reversal, which was considered a learning phenomena by some researchers. Cerebellar damage prevented adaptation. Based on these and other observations, it was postulated that over a period of time, climbing fiber inputs modified Purkinje's cell response to mossy fiber input. This modification (ie, adaptation) produced the learned changes observed in the VOR.

Changes in Purkinje's cell activity occur during learning of skilled motor acts. Neuronal activity was recorded during motor learning tasks in primates, such as altering the task of moving a lever by suddenly adding a new load. As the cerebellum detected mismatch between the intended and actual movement, adjustments occurred in the motor program. These adjustments were associated with neuronal activity in the cerebellum. One can question if this is a learning phenomenon or adaptation to a new situation, such as identified in the classical conditioning experiments. Learning represents a permanent change in motor behavior, whereas adaptation represents a temporary change in motor performance. In either case, learning is essential because the individual needs to respond to continuing changes in both the internal and external milieu.

Summary: Parameters of Motor Control

As stated earlier, the cerebellum's role in motor control extends beyond that just involved with movement. The cerebellum is involved with planning and executing movement, as well as serving a comparator and corrector role. Parameters of the motor program under cerebellar influence are evident in disease processes.[53] One feature is the loss of smooth coordinated movement (asynergia), which entails a decrease in accurate prediction of force, range, and direction of movement. Many complex movements are broken down into various components that produce a more irregular pattern of alternating movements. The break or stop command also is diminished, causing the extremity to overshoot the end range and rebound.

The cerebellum also regulates postural adjustments. The extent to which these postural abnormalities are evident depends on the site of damage. Parameters of balance abilities may be near normal, have near normal latency of onset with an increase in sway amplitude, or may be so impaired that the patient is unable to maintain balance even in a seated position.

The cerebellum therefore has generated many models in an attempt to explain its role in motor control, including a timer role, a comparator role between the actual movement and feedback, a coordinator role, and a motor learning role. These roles encompass the cerebellar-cortical integrative mechanisms associated with cognition and other mental operations.

CEREBRAL CORTEX

Events necessary for purposeful movement include the goal of movement, a strategy for accomplishing the movement, and execution of the motor program via coordinated activity occurring in the different descending pathways. Roles of areas other than the cerebral cortex have been described above.

Motor Cortex

The motor cortex influences alpha motoneurons through both indirect and direct neuronal connections. Since the descending neurons terminate on the same internuncial pool as afferent reflexive connections, the motor cortex participates in motor control through descending pathways, as well as by regulating spinal level reflexive or oscillatory activity. The somatotopical organization of the motor cortex is widely recognized. It now is viewed as an area containing overlapping regions representing the control of muscles in a body part rather than a specific one-to-one mapping associated with isolated muscles.

The motor cortex tends to be more involved with the production of skilled movement. This area regulates the rate of force development and maintains a steady level of force. Since this area receives and projects to the periphery, these long-loop or servo-assist loops assist with small load compensations that oppose movement excursion. When the load is large, this loop and other circuits, particularly those associated with the cerebellum, become operational.[54]

The role of the motor cortex for development of the motor program is a shared role with the premotor cortex, the supplementary motor area, the posterior parietal region, and various subcortical centers.

Supplementary Motor Area

This region lies in front of the motor cortex and has a less developed somatotopic map (see Figure 3-2). The major subcortical input is from the basal ganglia. Generally, electrical stimulation in this area produces bilateral movements. This region's role in programming complex movements in humans has been analyzed by cerebral blood flow studies.[55] When an individual compresses a spring between the thumb and index finger, an increase in blood flow occurs bilaterally in the motor and sensory cortex, but not in the supplementary motor area. When the individual performs a more complex movement sequence involving all the fingers, cerebral blood flow in the supplementary motor area significantly increases. A similar increase occurs with mental practice. These results suggest that the supplementary motor area plays a role in the sequencing of movements.

Premotor Cortex

This area is located on the lateral surface of the cerebral hemisphere anterior to the motor cortex and under the supplementary motor area (see Figure 3-2). It projects mainly to the brainstem and influences the reticulospinal system, suggesting a regulatory role of proximal and axial muscles, particularly during the early phase of limb movement toward a target.

The premotor area may be involved in response preparation, particularly related to the "go" command. Premotor cortical neurons are activated between the stimulus, "go," and the actual movement. Damage to this area produces a grasp response, the significance of which needs further delineation.

Posterior Parietal Cortex

This region lies posterior to the primary somatic sensory cortex and is interconnected with the premotor area. The posterior parietal cortex is involved intimately with processing sensory information necessary for movement. Most particularly, this area is responsible for spatial awareness. Many of the functions attributed to spatial cognition have been identified through lesions in the posterior parietal cortex. For example, some individuals experience difficulty in seeing multiple objects simultaneously. This disorder of spatial awareness is termed *simultanagnosia.* Objects appear fragmented and isolated in space and have no discernable or meaningful relationship among them.[56]

Damage in this area produces apraxia, which also is seen with damage to the frontal association areas. Neglect of one side of the body or an extremity is noted in patients with damage to this area. Unilateral neglect is believed to be a deficit in the ability to assimilate information from the contralateral side of the body into body percept. Optic apraxia is associated with impairments in visually guided arm movements necessary to reach a target (ie, failure to use visuospatial information). These individuals may have deficits in manipulating objects for exploratory purposes. Physiologic studies have confirmed that cells in the parietal cortex respond to the approach or contact of the desired target, and other cells fire in response to hand manipulation.

In summary, the motor systems of the cortex tend to function as modules. Depending on the movement, a different module will be the predominant functioning unit along with subcortical areas. This concept is termed *distributed processing*. It is evident that a motor program does not reside within a single structure but is an emergent property. That is, the motor program is a function of cortical and subcortical centers assimilating, planning, and coordinating synergies that contain appropriate velocity, direction, and amplitude parameters. The generation of the motor program also includes the selection and regulation of movements relative to specific behavioral contexts.

DESCENDING PATHWAYS

Three major descending pathways impinge on the spinal cord. They are the ventromedial system, lateral system, and the corticospinal system. The *ventromedial system* is comprised of the vestibulospinal, reticulospinal, tectospinal, and interstitiospinal tracts (see Figure 3-6). These tracts terminate on axial and limb girdle musculature. Due to the high degree of collateralization, the ventromedial system represents the fundamental descending system by which the nervous system regulates movement. This system is involved with regulation of axial musculature for maintenance of intersegmental spinal stabilization for righting, balance, and postural control. Since the ventromedial system also regulates proximal musculature, this system is involved with integration of body-extremity movements and orientation of the body and head with the direction of movement of the organism.

The *lateral system* (see Figure 3-6) arises from the contralateral rubrospinal, rubrobulbar, and ventrolateral pontine tegmentum and terminates on musculature in the distal portions of the extremities. This system is involved with independent movements of the shoulder, elbow, and hand, particularly those associated with flexion. The third descending system, the corticospinal system, comprises the corticospinal and corticobulbar pathways (see Figure 3-7). This system terminates at all levels of the spinal cord with some direct synaptic connections on alpha motoneurons. This system is involved with fine finger fractionation and regulatory control over the other two descending systems. Delineation of these two systems and their role in motor control have been obtained primarily through research on nonprimates.[57]

MODELS OF MOTOR CONTROL

Models of motor control have evolved from simple dichotomies to extremely complex interrelationships. Early technology enabled researchers to lesion various areas of the brain and examine remaining motor function. Observed motor and postural patterns were attributed to imbalances between intact and damaged structures. One such model based on ablation studies that, unfortunately, still pervades neurology is that of the extrapyramidal and pyramidal motor systems. These two systems were divided into two independent entities: the extrapyramidal system represented by the basal ganglia and the pyramidal system represented by the cerebral cortex. This division permitted early neurologists to classify nervous system diseases. Paralysis and spasticity were signs of pyramidal system damage, whereas rigidity, bradykinesia, and involuntary movements were signs of extrapyramidal system damage. This motor control model should no longer be used for the following reasons. First, by virtue of the extensive interconnections and feedback loops between cortical and subcortical systems, these centers cannot function independently. Second, the basal ganglia, cerebellum, brainstem, and red nucleus—all subcortical structures—play an important role in voluntary movement. And, third, disease or injury does not involve just one area of the brain. For example, Parkinson's disease may initially involve basal ganglia structures, but over time other subcortical and cortical areas become involved. Or, a middle cerebral infarct damages ascending and descending pathways of the cerebrum and transverse fibers of the basal ganglia. While segregating brain centers was an attempt to understand diseases or damage of the CNS, this model has outlived its usefulness and should be viewed from a historic perspective.

Hierarchy is another simplistic model attempting to replicate control of movement. In this model, a commander issues commands and the motor program is carried out by subordinate structures. This model, developed by Jackson, was based on the evolution and dissolution of the nervous system.[58] This model is not useful to study control of extremely complex movements involving feedback or motor learning, however, it is useful to explain those movements operating in an open loop fashion. That is, the motor program is initiated and runs without constant feedback. This model is useful in examining quickly executed movements.

A model that is useful for complex movements, motor learning, and for examination of the role of feedback is the systems model.[59] By virtue of its name, a single commander does not exist, but rather, depending on the particular type of movement, different systems participate. Since no single commander exists and centers participate in different functions depending on the motor act, the element of redundancy is evident. This model can support the concept of the motor program as an emergent property. That the motor program does not reside in one specific brain center is another concept of the systems model. The tripartite model for motor control is an example of a systems model. The basal ganglia, cerebellum, and cerebral cortex form the three major centers. The medial, lateral, and corticospinal descending pathways and the spinal level integrative mechanisms can be added to form a more comprehensive systems model. As is evident, the different centers serve different functions depending on the type of movement. The concept of emergent properties fits well with this model. Further delineation of these concepts are found in Chapter 2.

SUMMARY

In order to examine the complexity of neural systems underlying motor control, each element was discussed separately. To fully understand motor control, these elements need to be examined in concert with one another. The models for individual nervous system centers and for the interactive and coordinating actions of these various brain centers remain dynamic and are constantly being modified. By understanding neural systems underlying motor control, alternative therapies can be developed to evaluate and plan intervention for the patient with CNS pathology. The efficacy of these therapies then can be determined and the scientific bases for physical therapy interventions better established.

REFERENCES

1. Grillner S. Neurobiological bases of rhythmic motor acts in vertebrates. *Science*. 1985; 228:143-149.

2. Sage GH. *Introduction to Motor Behavior: A Neuropsychological Approach*. 2nd ed. Reading, Mass: Addison-Wesley Publishing Co; 1977.

3. Yaksh TL. Hammond DL. Peripheral and central substrate involved in rostrad (ascending) transmission of nociceptive information. *Pain*. 1982;13:1-85.

4. Johansson RS. Sensory control of dexterous manipulation in humans. In: Wang AM, Haggard P, Planagan J, eds. *Hand and Brain: The Neurophysiology and Psychology of Hand Movements*. New York, NY: Academic Press; 1996:381-414.

5. Matthews PBC. Where does Sherrington's "muscular" sense originate? Muscles, joints, corollary discharges. *Ann Rev Neurosci*. 1982;5:189–219.

6. Gandevia SC. Neurophysiological mechanisms underlying proprioceptive sensations. In: Struppler A. Weindl A, eds. *Clinical Aspects of Sensory Motor Integration*. Berlin, Germany: Springer-Verlag; 1987;14-24.

7. Floeter MK. Muscle, motor neurons and motor neuron pools. In: Zigmond MJ, Bloom FE, Landis SC, et al, eds. *Fundamental Neuroscience*. New York, NY: Academic Press; 1999: 863-887.

8. Newton RA. Joint receptor contributions to reflexive and kinesthetic responses. *Phys Ther*. 1982;62:22-29.

9. Schaible HG, Schmidt RF, Willis WD. New aspects of the role of articular receptors in motor control. In: Struppler A, Weindl A, eds. *Clinical Aspects of Sensory Motor Integration*. Berlin, Germany: Springer-Verlag; 1987:34-45.

10. Sharma L. Proprioceptive impairment in knee osteoarthritis. *Rheumatic Diseases Clinics of North America*. 1999;25:299-314.

11. Marsden CD, Rothwell JC, Day BL. The use of peripheral feedback in the control of movement. In: Evans ED, Wise SP, Bousfeld D, eds. *The Motor System in Neurobiology*. New York, NY: Elsevier Biomedical Press; 1985:215-222.

12. Cromwell RL, Newton RA, Carlton LG. Horizontal plane head stabilization during locomotor tasks. *J Motor Behavior*. 2001;33:49-58.

13. Brandt T, Dieterich M. The vestibular cortex. Its locations, functions, and disorders. *Ann NY Acad Sci*. 1999;871:293-312.

14. Brandt T, Dieterich M, Danek A. Vestibular cortex lesions affect the perception of verticality. *Ann Neurol.* 1994;35:403-412.

15. Shepard NT. Functional operation of the balance system in daily activities. *Otolaryngol Clin North Am.* 2000; 33:4554-4569.

16. Leigh RJ, Brandt T. A reevaluation of the vestibulo-ocular reflex: new ideas of its purpose, properties, neural substrate, and disorders. *Neurology.* 1993;43:1288-1295.

17. Mendola JD. Visual discrimination after anterior temporal lobectomy in humans. *Neurology.* 1999;52:1028-1037.

18. Bartolomeo P. Left unilateral neglect or right hyperattention? *Neurology.* 1999;53:2023-2027.

19. Clarke S, Bellmann A, Meuli R, et al. Auditory agnosia and auditory spatial deficits following left hemispheric lesions: evidence for distinct processing pathways. *Neuropsychologia.* 2000;38:797-807.

20. Byl H, Merzenich MM, Jenkins WM. A primate genesis model of focal hand dystonia and repetitive strain injury: I. Learning-induced deafferentiation of the representation of the hand in primary somatosensory cortex in adult monkeys. *Neurology.* 1996; 47:508-520.

21. Flor H, Braun C, Elbert T, et al. Extensive reorganization of primary somatosensory cortex in chronic back pain patients. *Neurosci Letters.* 1997; 224:5-8.

22. Bara-Jimenez W, Catlan H, Hallett M, et al. Abnormal somatosensory homunculus in dystonia of the hand. *Ann Neurol.* 1998;44:828-831.

23. Sharma K, Peng CY. Spinal motor circuits: merging development and function. Neuron. 2001;29:321-324.

24. Bizzi E, Tresch MC, Saltiel P, et al. New perspectives on spinal motor systems. *Nat Rev Neurosci.* 2000;1:101-108.

25. Jami L, Pierrot-Desilligny, E, Zytnicki D, eds. *Muscle Afferents and Spinal Control of movement.* New York, NY: Elsevier; 1992.

26. Fetz EE, Perlmutter SI, Prut Y. Functions of mammalian spinal interneurons during Movement. *Curr Opin Neurobiol.* 2000; 10:699-707.

27. Bizzi E, Hogan N, Mussa-Ivaldi FA, Giszter S. Does the nervous system use equilibrium-point control to guide single and multiple joint movements? *Behav and Brain Sciences.* 1992; 15:603-613.

28. Jankowska E, Edgley S. Interactions between pathways controlling posture and gait at the level of spinal interneurons in the cat. *Prog Brain Res.* 1993;97:161-71.

29. Hoyt DF, Taylor CR. Gait and the energetics of locomotion in horses. *Nature.* 1981;292:239-240.

30. Heglund NC, Willems PA, Penta M, et al. Energy-saving gait mechanics with head-supported loads. *Nature.* 1995;375:52-54.

31. Calancie B, Needham-Shropshire B, Jacobs P, et al: Involuntary stepping after chronic spinal cord injury. Evidence for a central rhythm generator for locomotion in man. *Brain.* 1994; 117:1143-1159.

32. Mello LE. Neuroanatomy of the basal ganglia. *Psychiatr Clin North Am.* 1997;20:691-704.

33. Rauch SL. Neuroimaging and neuropsychology of the striatum. Bridging basic science and clinical practice. *Psychiatr Clin North Am.* 1997;20:74174-74176.

34. De Long MR. Activity of basal ganglia neurons during movement. *Brain Res.* 1972; 40:127-135.

35. Rektor I. Parallel information processing in motor systems: Intracerebral recordings of readiness potential and CNV in human subjects. *Neural Plast.* 2000;7:65-72.

36. Cunnington R, Iansek R, Johnson KA, et al. Movement-related potentials in Parkinson's disease. Motor imagery and movement preparation. *Brain.* 1997; 120:1339-1353.

37. Marsden CD. The enigma of the basal ganglia and movement. In: Evarts ED, Wise SP, Bousfield D, eds. *The Motor System in Neurobiology.* New York, NY: Elsevier Biomedical Press; 1985, 277-282.

38. Martin JP. *The Basal Ganglia and Posture*. London, England: Pitman; 1967.

39. Ballard PA, Tetrud JW, Langston JW. Permanent human Parkinsonism due to 1-methyl-4-phenyl-1 ,2,3,6-tetrahydropyridine (MPTP): Seven cases. *Neurology*. 1985;35:949-956.

40. Soliveri P, Brown RG, Jahanshahi M, et al. Learning manual pursuit tracking skills in patients with Parkinson's disease. *Brain*. 1997;120:1325-1337.

41. Horak FB. Effects of dopamine on postural control in Parkinsonian subjects: Scaling, set, tone. *J Neurophysiol*. 1996;75:2380.

42. Bloxham CA, Mindel TA, Frith CD. Initiation and execution of predictable and unpredictable movements in Parkinson's disease. *Brain*. 1984;107:371-384.

43. Cooke JD, Brown JD, BrooksVD. Increased dependence on visual information for movement control in patients with Parkinson's disease. *Can J Neurol Sci*. 1978;5:413-415.

44. Crutcher MD, DeLong MD. Single cell studies of the primate putamen. II. Relations to direction of movement and pattern of muscular activity. *Exp Brain Res*. 1984;53:244-258.

45. Middleton FA, Strick PL. Basal ganglia output and cognition: evidence from anatomical, behavioral, and clinical studies. *Brain Cogn*. 2000;42:183-200.

46. Cotterill RM. Cooperation of the basal ganglia, cerebellum, sensory cerebrum and hippocampus: possible implications for cognition, consciousness, intelligence and creativity. *Prog Neurobiol*. 2001;64:1-33.

47. Brotchie P, Iansek R, Horne MK. Motor function of the monkey globus pallidus. 2. Cognitive aspects of movement and phasic neuronal activity. *Brain*. 1991;114:1685-1702.

48. Doya K. Complementary roles of basal ganglia and cerebellum in learning and motor control. *Curr Opin Neurobiol*. 2000;10:732-739.

49. Dichgans J, Diener HC. Different forms of postural stasis in patients with cerebellar diseases. In: Bles W, Brandt T, eds. *Disorders of Posture and Gait*. New York, NY: Elsevier Biomedical Press; 1986:207-215.

50. Diner HC, Dichgans J, Bacher B, et al. Characteristic alterations of long loop "refexes" in patients with Friedreich's disease and late atrophy of the cerebellar anterior lobe. *J Neurol Neurosurg Psychiat*. 1984;47:679-685.

51. Miall RC, Reckess GZ, Imamizu H. The cerebellum coordinates eye and hand tracking movements. *Nat Neurosci*. 2001; 4:638-644.

52. Albus JS. A theory of cerebellar function. *Math Biosci*. 1971; 10:25-61.

53. Earhart GM, Bastian AJ. Selection and coordination of human locomotor forms following cerebellar damage. *J Neurophysiol*. 2001;85:759-69.

54. Evans EV. Role of motor cortex in voluntary movement in primates. In Brookhart M, Mountcastle VB, eds. *Handbook of Physiology, Section I: The Nervous System, Vol II, Motor Control*. Bethesda, Md: American Physiological Society; 1981:1083-1120.

55. Roland PE, Larsen B, Lassen NA, et al. Supplementary motor area and other cortical areas in organization of voluntary movements in man. *J Neurophysiol*. 1980;43:118-136.

56. Coslett HB, Saffran, E. Simultanagnosia: to see but not two see. *Brain*. 991;114:1523-1545.

57. Kuypers HGHM. Anatomy of the descending pathways. In: Brookhart JM, Mountcastle VB, eds. *Handbook of Physiology, Section 1. The Nervous System, Vol II. Motor Control, Part 2*. Bethesda, Md: American Physiological Society; 1981:597-666.

58. Jackson JH. The Croonian lectures on evolution and dissolution of the nervous system. *Br Med J*. 1884;1:591-593.

59. Davis WJ. Organizational concepts in the central motor networks of invertebrates. In: Herman RM, Grillner S, Stein PSG, et al, eds. *Neural Control of Locomotion: Advances in Behavioral Biology, Vol 18*. New York, NY: Plenum Press; 1976:265-292.

CHAPTER 4

Neuroplasticity: Applications to Motor Control

Nancy N. Byl, PhD, PT, FAPTA

INTRODUCTION

Neural adaptation is the foundation of learning. The potential for neural change has been most extensively studied in the young of various species, specifically during development. However, it is now clear that changes in the structure and function of the nervous system can occur across the life span through engaging in highly attended, repetitive, and rewarded behaviors.[1-16] Goal-directed, repetitive behaviors may not only slow down the deterioration of cognitive, sensory, and motor processes associated with aging, but also may enable us to restore function following neural insults such as anoxia, traumatic brain injuries, cerebrovascular accidents (CVAs), surgery, or disease.

The challenge for physical therapists is to integrate advances in basic science with clinical practice. Frequently, clinicians are not aware of new basic neuroscience findings, and researchers lack practical insight regarding the potential application of their findings to clinical practice. As a consequence, there often is little effort by the researchers to share basic science findings with clinicians. In addition, clinicians who try to stay knowledgeable of research findings in the neurosciences may have difficulty translating theory into clinical practice. Another major barrier to effective intervention may be a lack of third-party reimbursement for adequate frequency of services. In some instances, progress is limited because the patient is not motivated to comply with the necessary

Figure 4-1. Normal hand representation. A. Hand zone in area 3b of the anterior parietal cortex. B. Outline of normal receptive fields on the hand, as correlated with the marked cortical penetration sites in C. C. Topographical representation of the hand on the somatosensory cortex, area 3b, with sample cortical penetration sites (eg, the numbers moving from distal to proximal and the letters moving from digit 5 to digit 1) correlated with the receptive fields on the hand. Area 3b hand zones representing dorsal hand surfaces are shaded black. The letter "P"

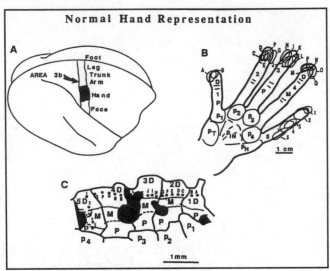

refers to the proximal segment of the digit, "M" refers to the middle segment, and "D" refers to the distal segment (reprinted with permission from the American Physical Therapy Association. Byl N. A primate model for studying focal dystonia and repetitive strain injury: Effects on the primary somatosensory cortex. *Phys Ther.* 1997;77:3:269-284).

goal-oriented repetitions that are needed to drive neural adaptation. In other cases, psychological and cognitive impairments (eg, depression, aphasia, learning disabilities) resulting from life stresses or physical impairment interfere with the potential for neural adaptation. Lastly, clinicians may be insensitive to situations where dysfunctional adaptation occurs following immobilization or compensation, or where habitual, automatic behaviors develop early following injury (eg, poorly aligned posture, abnormal gait patterns surrounding pain, or abnormal or maladaptive synergies). These motor behaviors are repeated frequently until they are learned and stereotypic, thus dominating patient movement behaviors even when voluntary control returns or when other motor behaviors are available.

NEUROPLASTICITY RESEARCH

General Issues

The hand has been the target of research in fine motor studies, as well as in studies of neuroplasticity.[1-4,7,8,17-30] Most of the tasks humans perform with their hands not only require highly articulated movements,[6,20,21,31,32] but also require coordinated, synergistic muscle recruitment and timing across multiple joints of the extremity, as well as the trunk.[33-37] The hand is highly differentiated and distinctly represented in the brain[38] (Figure 4-1). The hand allows us to express our emotions, explore our environment, manipulate objects, take care of our personal needs, feed ourselves, and perform delicate fine motor, rhythmical, and gross motor movements.

Efficient action of the hand is complemented by supplementary actions of the trunk and proximal shoulder and distal upper extremity muscles. These integrated reaching and prehension movements begin early in development.[37,39-42] For example, reaching out for an object requires preliminary alignment of the trunk to stabilize against gravity,[43,44] movement of the shoulder and elbow to orient the hand, and positioning of the wrist to maximize length tension relationships of the muscles serving the hand. It also requires contraction of the extrinsic muscles for gripping and rapid alternating digital movements. In addition, contraction of the intrinsic muscles stabilizes the hand and allows selective, individual movements of each digit. Vision also may be used to modify adaptations.[45,46] Practice has been shown to improve all aspects of preparation and performance.[44,47] Research findings on the neuroplasticity of the hand are applicable to all other topographical and functional representations of other body parts (eg, leg, trunk) and other tasks not performed with the hand (eg, walking, running).

Fine motor, flexible, differentiated, and variable movements are enabled but also can be limited as a consequence of the anatomic construction of joints (ie, bones, ligaments, fibrocartilage, fascia, retinaculi). Other factors include arthrokinematics of joint movement, the alignment and osteokinematics of bone movement, the force and direction of pull of the muscles, as well as the alignment, stretch, and direction of pull of the tendons and fascia.[36] The intricate complex of muscles of different sizes, shapes, and fiber types (ie, slow- and fast-twitch fibers) in addition to rapidly and slowly adaptive sensory fibers[48] originate both within and outside the area of the moving part. Based on a systems approach[33] or a dynamic systems model,[34,49-52] planning, preparation, sequencing, execution, and modification of movements are based on the interaction of movements controlled by the motor and sensory systems with the limbic system (eg, personal motivation, attention, sensory-motor integration) and the cognitive control systems. These neural systems interact to modify the efficiency, quality, and effectiveness of the movement. Precise, accurate, sensorimotor feedback, as well as the coordination of excitatory and inhibitory pathways from the spinal cord, brainstem, thalamus, motor cortex, supplementary cortex, primary sensory cortex, basal ganglia, and cerebellum also are critical for fine motor control.[53-56]

The parts of the body that are used most frequently for sensory processing and motor movement have a disproportionately large somatotopic representation on the sensory and the motor cortex (eg, lips, mouth, tongue, larynx, and hand)[38,53] (Figure 4-2). The density and the complexity of blood flow to the brain also are proportional in this geographical area. This extensive representation heightens the sensitivity of these parts and the ability to perform fine motor movements. It also is associated with more extensive dysfunction following an injury. For example, a disruption of blood flow to the brain usually leaves a person more impaired in the upper extremity than the lower extremity or trunk and more impaired in fine motor control than in gross motor and rhythmic movements.[53,57]

More recently, neuroscience researchers have documented that the cortex is not only mapped topographically but also is mapped by function (ie, by well-learned skilled tasks and rhythmical voluntary movements).[58] Using the technology of magnetic resonance imaging, it has been shown that blood flow increases in the specific areas of the brain that are recruited for a task. Researchers have documented increased blood flow in both a topographical area (eg, the part of the body performing the task) and in a functional area (eg, an area in the sensorimotor cortex for writing). It is clear that it is possible to perform the same functional task in different ways, referred to as motor equivalency.[59]

Using similar technology, it has been documented that about 30% of the neurons that fire when performing a task can be recruited when one imagines performing a task

Figure 4-2. Somatic sensory and motor projections from and to the body surface and muscle are arranged in the cortex in somatotopic order. Sensory information from the body surface is received by the postcentral gyrus of the parietal cortex (areas 3a and 3b, and 1 and 2). The map for area 1 is illustrated here. Areas of the body that are important for tactile discrimination, such as the tip of the tongue, the fingers, and the hand, have a disproportionately larger representation, reflecting their more extensive innervation (adapted with permission from Kandel E. *Principles of Neural Science*. New York, NY: McGraw-Hill; 2000).

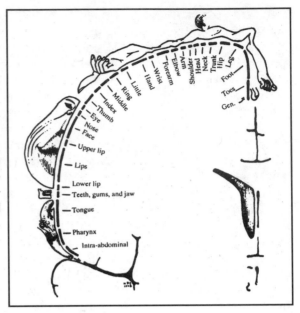

(explicit imaging).[60-69] Similarly, unconscious, implicit task performance also can be measured in terms of the latency of the cortical response.[64,65,70-75] Thus, even when there is an impairment that interferes with the ability to carry out a physical task, it is still possible to mentally image the task and generate neuronal activity.

Developmental Considerations

Over the past few years, we have expanded our understanding of human motor development through detailed analysis of various types of movements and muscular activation patterns during different stages of development. In 1967, Bernstein introduced a systems model of motor control. He also formulated the degrees of freedom problem for the complexity of fine motor control[49,50] and suggested that motor control systems could not exert control by explicit mapping of the neural commands and movement trajectories.

At birth, newborn infants have repertoires of motor behavior that are necessary for survival. Infants have feeding, respiratory, and protective reactions, and they display transient movement patterns such as stepping, postural and righting reactions, and general movements. These movement patterns emerge in the fetal stage.[76] During fetal development, the rate of sucking movements is already the same as that of a term infant during breast feeding. It is noteworthy that, from the beginning, fetal movements are patterned into recognizable forms. Many fetal movement patterns continue virtually unchanged in form and shape after birth.[76] From studies of other vertebrates, we know that innate movement behaviors are governed by central pattern generators. The most frequent movement patterns of the human fetus and newborn infant are referred to as general movements. These have been studied extensively over the last decade using video techniques.[77,78]

Examining the quality of general movements in infants at high risk for developing cerebral palsy helps predict the neurological outcome. Abnormal movement patterns have been documented to be strongly associated with lesions of the immature brain and with later development of cerebral palsy. In addition, minor disturbances of the CNS influence the quality of general movements, and even mildly abnormal general movements appear to be associated with an increased risk of minor neurological dystonia.[43] During development, the postural control system strives to achieve a stable vertical posture of the head and trunk against the force of gravity and to establish a base for adequate reaching, sitting, standing, and walking. Even a slight perturbation in equilibrium elicits direction-specific postural activity in the trunk muscles of the infant.[43,44] The infant also exhibits a large repertoire of muscle combinations, including patterns that are present in adults. With increasing age, experience-dependent selection takes place, with the most functional patterns being favored. After selecting the most functional patterns at 9 to 10 months of age, infants become able to modulate muscle activity according to external constraints. Before the infant can stand independently, the necessary muscle responses emerge at the ankle and then the knee and hip, using distal to proximal control,[47] suggesting that the postural patterns are built up through experience.

In toddlers, all direction specific leg, trunk, and ankle muscles are activated in conjunction with a high amount of coactivation. The postural adjustments become more efficient with increasing age because of shorter latencies and faster muscle contractions. Subsequently, interaction among different sensory systems (eg, the somatosensory, visual, and vestibular) develops resulting in a dynamic adaptation of the response pattern that is dependent on external conditions and visual monitoring.[79,80] The development of anticipatory postural mechanisms that stabilize the moving body is a prerequisite for improved gait.

Fetuses and newborn infants also exhibit locomotor-like behavior. The infant stepping on a slowly moving treadmill belt shares many characteristics with locomotion in spinal cats and with adult human gait (eg, adaptation to speed, to loading, and to external perturbations). The stepping activity also increases with practice. However, infant stepping movements differ markedly from adult plantigrade gait which is characterized by prominent heel strike at foot contact due to strong dorsiflexion of the foot at the end of the swing phase. Adult gait also includes out of phase movement; knee flexion during the stance phase, pelvic rotation and tilting, and a specific nonsynchronous muscle activation pattern. Infant stepping lacks these determinants and the infant displays, instead, synchronous flexion or extension in all joints, uniform muscle activity with a high degree of antagonist coactivation, and short latencies.[81,82]

Human locomotor activity is generated by spinal pattern generators. The development of bipedal plantigrade gait, however, seems to involve some supraspinal influence which shapes and fine tunes the locomotor activity.[83] This may be the reason why only a basic locomotor rhythm can be induced in human adults after traumatic spinal cord transections.

Development of Fine Motor Control: Example of Massive Neuroplasticity

Fine motor skills develop later than ambulation skills. Reaching begins to develop around 4 months of age. The development of reaching and grasping seems to involve a step wise change in neural control. Anticipation develops and becomes more efficient, as well as better coordinated with age. While reaching for movable objects by 6 months of age, infants provide evidence of their ability to extrapolate motion.[42] They need to finish a programmed movement before they can redirect their reach to a new destination.[37]

In humans, the connectivity of the corticospinal system now can be studied using transcranial magnetic stimulation. There is an increase in the density of neurons up to 10 years of age, with an increasing central conduction velocity.[84] When children start to use their hands, they use a highly variable and sequential coordination of the fingertips. They also establish an automatized coupling of grip and load forces. This synergy is not fully mature until around the age of 10 years. With age, grasp control shifts from a system involving feedback control to an anticipatory strategy with unimodal force rate trajectory targeted to an object's weight and size. By 8 to 10 years, grasping is based on internal neural representation of the object. Grip force is adapted to the friction of the digit-object interface and sensory triggered grip. Sensory triggered grip responses induced by sudden load perturbations gradually grow in amplitude and shorten in latency.[85] This takes place in parallel with developmental changes of the cutaneous-muscular reflex which initially contains a dominating spinal short latency excitatory component.[86,87]

Current evidence indicates that repetitive motor behavior during motor learning paradigms can produce changes in representational organization in the motor cortex.[88] With a pellet retrieval task in adult squirrel monkeys, there were consistent task-related changes in movement representations in the primary motor cortex in conjunction with the acquisition of a new motor skill. The monkeys then were trained to take pellets from a larger diameter well. The larger diameter well task was designed to produce repetitive use of a limited set of distal forelimb movements in the absence of motor skill acquisition. Motor activity levels were estimated by recording the total number of finger flexions performed during the training. The experiment was intended to evaluate whether simple, repetitive motor activity alone is sufficient to produce representational plasticity in cortical motor maps. The monkey retrieval behavior was highly successful and stereotypical throughout the training period, suggesting that no new motor skills were learned during the performance of the large well retrieval task. Comparisons between pretraining and posttraining maps of primary motor cortex movement representation revealed that task-related changes in the cortex were devoted to individual distal forelimb movement representations. It was concluded that repetitive motor activity alone does not produce functional reorganization. Motor skill acquisition or motor learning is a prerequisite factor in driving representational plasticity.[88] When there is a neural injury, the question is whether the nervous system responds to this injury by developing abnormal branching of inputs to motor neurons creating abnormal muscle contractions, as in children with cerebral palsy, thereby prolonging motor impairments after neural injury.[87]

Dynamic Interdependency of Fine Motor Control Skills and Sensory Processing

Fine motor control depends on an exquisite balance of motor control and sensory feedback. Sensory and motor functions are intimately interrelated for fine motor skills, and less so for automatic, rhythmic, voluntary movements or reflex motor movements. In fact, reflex motor movements are so rapid that corticosensory feedback is not possible. There is a predictive feed-forward sensory control system with contextual, cognitive, and movement phase-dependent interpretations of multisensory inputs. The sensory signals mediate, update, and support motor outputs to help regulate and grade movement, as well as minimize excessive forces. The development of skilled motor performance such as precision gripping, coordinated prehension, and individual digitated movements is complex as evidenced by the development of this skill and the observation of increased dendritic branching in the motor and somatosensory cortex.[89] Even minor disruptions in the sensory or motor cortex can interfere with individuated finger movements.[90]

Somatosensory information and feedback can modify further ongoing motor behavior. In addition, mechanical events inform the CNS about the completeness of the succinct phases of the task which trigger preprogrammed corrective action. The sensorimotor feedback loop must provide accurate information to provide the foundation for controlled movement. If there is a degradation of the somatosensory representation, the gain of the feedback mechanisms also may be degraded, creating abnormal uncontrollable patterns of movement.[91-94] Additionally, if there is damage to the primary motor cortex, animals will increase their dependency on visual monitoring of reaching, reinforcing the interrelationship of sensory processing and fine motor control.[95]

In human primates, the primary somatosensory cortex (SI) (Figure 4-3) has unique input to the motor cortex through the thalamus. Area 3b of the primary sensory cortex also projects directly to areas 1, 2, and 3a which project directly to area 4 (primary motor cortex). Interestingly, tactile perception is better when there is movement of the stimulus on the skin or movement of the skin over the stimulus. Paradoxically, from the perspective of evoked neural firing, voluntary movement may reduce the transmission of tactile inputs to SI. This is referred to as movement-related gating of sensory transmission.[35,96] This limits the amount of afferent input that must be processed at higher levels.

Selective attention also modifies firing. In the secondary somatosensory cortex (SII), neurons depend on behavioral context in the motivational state. Consequently, firing rates are modified by reward. SII is the gateway to the temporal lobe via the insular cortex and the hippocampus. However, movement itself is not essential to produce gating, since the same decline in the amplitude of somatosensory firing also is seen with isometric contractions. This modulation is nonspecific in terms of direction of movement.

The motor cortex appears to be the major source of the centrally originating gating signal. Intracortical microstimulation in area 4 can diminish the SI cortical somatosensory evoked responses (SEPs).[53] Movement itself produces a widespread nonspecific reduction in transmission of cutaneous inputs. The fusimotor system allows dynamic adjustments of muscle length and velocity. However, it is difficult to predict fusimotor discharges that may compensate for muscle shortening during movement to maintain discharge (eg, slow movements against an external load, but not rapid unloaded movements). This feedback of the muscle afferents is low at rest and increases with exploratory movements, learning a new motor task, and in conditions of increased attention or arousal. Depending on the task, sensory feedback is scaled up or down, with the gain control system acting through the effect of motor pathways. This also is applicable to feedback from joint receptors and muscle afferents.[97-99] Joint afferent discharge also is modulated by activation of muscle insertions into the joint capsule and the state of muscle contraction.[97,98]

Touch fires SI neurons and the firing covaries with texture, features, force, direction, and velocity of stimulation.[100] Some SI neurons are sensitive to cutaneous inputs in areas 3b, 1, and 2. These neurons fire with active touch, with an insensitivity to velocity.[35] SI discharge stops when there is deafferentiation. Additionally, peripheral feedback is linked to the performance of the task. For example, neurons also stop firing when the sensory information is not relevant to a texture task or to a motor task. SI neurons fire

Figure 4-3. Sites of somatosensory processing in the cortex. A. This lateral view of the cerebral hemisphere shows the locations of the primary (S-I) and secondary (S-II) somatic sensory cortices and the posterior parietal cortex. B. This cross section (at level B in part A) shows the several cytoarchitecturally distinct areas of the region: S-I (Brodmann's areas 3a, 3b, 1, 2), part of the motor cortex (area 4), and part of the posterior parietal cortex (areas 5 and 7) (reprinted with permission from Kandel E. *Principles of Neural Science.* New York, NY: McGraw-Hill; 2000).

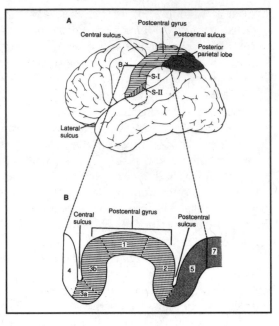

less during active exploration compared to passive exploration of textures. About 40% of SI cortical neurons show gating with responses during passive but not active touch.[35,101] Inhibitory feedback allows active output neurons to limit their activity and to create rings of less active neurons. Inhibitory interneurons also can be activated at more distant sites. Unfortunately, our sensory discrimination diminishes with aging and this also could decrease fine motor control.[102]

Sensory information is processed in the CNS in stages, sequenced in the spinal cord, brainstem, thalamus, and cortex. For example, when reading Braille, the Merkel and Meissner's corpuscles transmit the neural image of the pattern to 3b, signaling shape and sharpening the shape as a result of a pause in firing (excitatory and inhibitory).[103] When there is a spike burst, the letters stand out from the noisy background. Neurons in 3a and 3b project to areas 1 and 2 and respond to complex features like shape. Direction sensitive feature detection neurons are sensitive to direction in cortical areas 1 and 2 with stereognosis, a function of the posterior parietal cortex.[99] Areas 5 and 7 are complex somatosensory areas producing graded movements. All areas are organized functionally.[101,104]

Perception of an object (eg, weight, surface friction) appears to be centrally mediated. For example, a smooth object automatically facilitates a frictional force to overcome the load lifted against gravity that is greater than the force generated to lift the same object with a rough surface. When the surface is smooth, the person perceives the object as heavier, even if the weight is the same. Weight, surface texture, object position, and contact force at the interaction point impact object prehension and manipulation. Finally, explicit planning and control of a desired movement require a transformation of hand impedance into actual muscle and joint movement.[65,66,105-109]

Injuries of afferent pathways lead to defects in sensory/tactile discrimination, direction, sensitivity, two-point discrimination, and graphesthesia. Natural hand movements become distorted, and problems controlling force and finger movements occur. The functional role of SI can only be appreciated when studied in relation to various behavioral factors that modify access of sensory information to central processing for movement, attention, motivation, motor set, and arousal. Removal of SI (3b, 3a, 1, 2), leads to deficits in position sense, as well as an inability to discriminate texture and shape. It also is associated with motor deficits. Lesions in Brodmann's area 3b lead to deficits in discrimination of texture of objects as well as shape. Lesions in SII lead to impairments in discrimination of shape and texture, and patients cannot learn new skills. Disabling SII by injecting musimol (GABA, an inhibitory transmitter) results in a temporary loss of the ability to manipulate small objects and poor hand eye coordination, with the dysfunction simulating dystonic-type movements.[110]

The most extensive research on neuroplasticity and the effects of attended, repetitive behaviors has been focused on the somatosensory cortex (area 3b), most specifically the topography of the hand. However, the findings are equally applicable to the sensory motor interactions across task and body location. This close interaction of sensory and motor processing also has been documented in research studies where monkeys demonstrated poorer performance at grasping tasks after a focal ischemic lesion. The monkey had to visually guide the hand, demonstrating that the primary motor cortex plays a significant role in somatosensory processing during the execution of motor tasks. Motor deficits are not purely motor but partially due to a sensory deficit or a sensory motor disconnection.[95]

PRINCIPLES OF NEUROPLASTICITY

The last decade has produced seminal research in the areas of neuroscience and neuroplasticity. It has been clearly demonstrated that the nervous system is adaptable. Although accentuated during the period of development, neural plasticity has been documented across all levels of the nervous system across the life span. The scale of plasticity in progressive skill learning is massive. Enduring cortical plasticity changes appear to be accounted for by local changes in neural anatomy. Cortical plasticity processes in child development represent progressive, multiple-staged skill learning. In older individuals, cortical plasticity processing represents more efficient and effective integration of neurological processes.

In order to maximize neural adaptation, behaviors which drive changes in the nervous system require attention, repetition over time, and positive feedback.[24,26] The behaviors should be goal directed and interesting to facilitate motivation and commitment.[7,111,112] The learned behaviors must be repetitive, but not stereotypical. Ideally, the behaviors must be accurate and progressed in complexity. The behaviors also must be repeated and coordinated in time, but the behaviors or the stimuli should not be delivered simultaneously. Complexity of adaptation and learning also can be extended if behaviors are different but complementary and coincident in time.

There are important behavioral conditions that must be met in the learning phases of plasticity. With learning, the distributed cortical representations of inputs and brain actions specialize in their representations of behaviorally important inputs and actions for skill learning.[2,3,24] Behaviorally important stimuli must repeatedly excite cortical neuron populations. As a consequence, the number of neurons involved should progressively increase.

Repetitive, behaviorally important stimuli processed in skill learning also lead to progressively greater specificity in spectral (spatial) and temporal dimensions. With learning, a number of selectively responding neurons discharge with progressively stronger temporal coordination (distributed synchronism).[17,18,28-31,113] Selection of behaviorally important inputs is a product of strengthening input-coincidence-based connections (ie, synapses).[111]

Cortical field-specific differences in input sources, distributions, and time structured inputs create different representational structures.[114] Temporal dimensions of behaviorally important inputs influence representational "specialization." The integration time (ie, processing time) in the cortex is itself subject to powerful learning-based plasticity. For example, musicians can learn to alternate their digits within 60 milliseconds while the average person can only alternate his digits at the rate of 100 milliseconds. In addition, this learning can be modulated as a function of behavioral state.[115,116] For example, a person under conditions of high arousal and excitement can perform extraordinary tasks (eg, lifting a car off the leg of an injured man) that seem impossible during normal states of attention.

We are most familiar with positive neural adaptations surrounding behavioral and structural outcomes of practice, such as improved proficiency in task performance, efficient learning of new tasks, and enhanced recovery following neural insults. In studies when animals train in sensory discrimination and fine motor tasks, such as retrieving pellets out of small graded sized wells, neurons show impressive structural changes. The cortical representations are expanded, the receptive fields are smaller than normal, columnar specificity is 600 μm or less, and there is co-selection of complementary inputs. The number of excitable neurons is increased, the salience and specificity of feedback is enhanced, myelination is increased, the synapses between coincident inputs is strengthened, the integration time is shortened, or the complexity of dendritic branching is enhanced.[117,118] For example, extensive cortical representations of the digits are seen in Braille readers and musicians who use their hands precisely and extensively.[119]

We also know that we can train one sensory system (eg, somatosensory discrimination) in interval discrimination and demonstrate that learning in one sensory modality is generalized to other sensory modalities (eg, auditory discrimination).[5] This finding has powerful applications for retraining. For example, a targeted somatosensory retraining could be initiated with auditory or visual retraining.

It is known that motor imagery recruits a measurable neuronal response. Thus, repeated implicit or explicit imagery also can be associated with learning.[61-65,68-75,120] During motor imagery, this increase in cortical excitability is not associated with changes in spinal excitability.[121] There does appear to be a relationship between objects and components of potential action.[72] Also, mental rehearsal of a motor task recruits only alpha motoneurons and not fusimotor neurons,[122] potentially because there is no sensory feedback. In the presence of impairment, the repeated imagined tasks may be more or less accurate than the actual performance of the task, which may vary by the state of the neural insult. But, given the proportional neuronal recruitment of imagery versus actual task performance, greater intensity of the imagery and longer duration of imagery practice may be required to facilitate an equivalent amount of learning compared to actual task practice. However, imagery has been used regularly and effectively to improve performance at sports. Mirror imagery also has been used to manage difficult problems of phantom limb pain.[123] It is only since the development of magnetic imaging that imagery has been accepted as a legitimate intervention technique for patients with neural insults.

LIMITATIONS OF NEURAL PLASTICITY

Naturally, plasticity is constrained by anatomical structures and convergent-divergent spreads of inputs.[5,25] Plasticity also is constrained by the time constants which govern coincident input co-selection and by the time structures that allow the achievement of coherent extrinsic and intrinsic cortical inputs.[124,125] Complicated as well as simplistic inputs also can constrain cortical representational plasticity.[126] However, the most important factor that controls learning progressions is representational consolidation. For example, the trained cortex creates progressively more specific and more salient distributed representation of behaviorally important inputs through specialization. This limitation is particularly important since the power of cortical mechanisms to effectively drive changes in the nervous system wherever outputs are distributed increases with growing representational salience.

Another constraint in neural adaptation may be related to the development of mature sleeping patterns, especially within the first year of life. Sleep enables the strengthening of learning-based plastic changes. Sleep resets the learning machinery by erasing temporary nonreinforced and nonrewarded input-generated changes generated over the preceding waking periods.

Progressive myelination is another potentially powerful basis for sequenced learning. Myelination controls the conduction time and therefore the temporal dispersions of input sources to and within cortical areas. Competition between neural structures for isolated and shared functions, hard wired programs, neurochemical processes, myelin, and cellular mechanisms limit infinite expansions of new dendritic branching and synaptic linkages.[127-129]

Top down modulation controls attentional windows and learned predictions. Expectations and behavioral goals are constructed by learning. The modulatory control systems that enable learning also are plastic. The modulatory control systems change with maturation. They can constrain progressive learning because they are signaled by complex information feedback from the cortex itself. Thus, these limitations of neurophysiology also limit neural adaptation.

Competition exists among neuronal pools and time constants, defined integration time, and reflex inhibition limit adaptation.[27,130] When inputs occur regularly within the inhibitory or integration period, they may no longer be registered as temporally distinct. Digit representational borders also can be broken down by amputation, syndactyly, surgical fusion, simultaneous touching of multiple digits, or stereotypical, repetitive inputs including multifinger Braille reading.[15,22,91,92,131-133] The stimulated skin surfaces form a unified rather than a distinct representation in the cerebral cortex.[131]

Negative learning can occur when an individual performs repetitive tasks in abnormal or atypical ways. This may be a result of compensation that occurs as a result of failure of normal development or compensation that occurs following injury, chronic pain, surgical reconstruction, neural insults such as a CVA, or neural degenerative conditions such as multiple sclerosis or Parkinson's disease. Although most of these impairments are thought to be static, often the magnitude of disability increases with age, as well as with time. For example, it is not uncommon to observe the patient who achieves good return of voluntary movements post-CVA, but who persists in using the lower extremity in an immature synergistic pattern during ambulation. Despite the most careful, precise surgical correction, a release of the hamstrings to enable more knee extension may not result in the patient obtaining full function despite anatomic and biomechanical normality. In other cases, surgery to deafferent a hypertonic limb for purposes of improving gait may be associated with an inability to walk postsurgery. Change in structure can create more disability if delicate balances are altered. Further, there is increasing evidence that extensive repetition of abnormal patterns of movement creates a cortical representation that is learned and becomes the dominant pattern. In order to change the behavior, one must unlearn the abnormal and restore the normal topographical and functional representation in the cortex, basal ganglia, cerebellum, and thalamus. Central changes may not be corrected with peripheral modifications.

Despite the infinite number of degrees of freedom and permutations of movement variability, much of what we do in life is repetitive. We learn new skills and perfect old ones with practice. Learning is the culmination of neural adaptation. We perform some activities so regularly that they become nearly automatic and are stable, reproducible, and secure (eg, postural righting in standing, swallowing, talking, running, writing, typing). Once automatic, very little new learning takes place and tasks can be accomplished with minimal effort and minimal learning. However, this condition presents a risk for negative learning.

Spatial and temporal separateness of noncoincident inputs is essential to the maintenance of the normal sensory organization of the hand, and good distinct digital borders are absolutely essential for fine motor control of the digits. There are instances in automatic, well-learned tasks when highly attended repetitive behaviors clearly exceed the capacity of neural processing. If attended repetitive behaviors become stereotypical and near simultaneous in time, the nervous system is unable to distinctly record information from individual digits or generate precise outputs.

Thus, repetitive, stereotypical, related, competitive, or coincident inputs occurring nearly simultaneously in time can degrade the topographical representation of the involved body part. This has been measured with electrophysiological techniques,[91,92] as well as magnetoencephalography.[134,135] Abnormal representation of the somatosensory representation of the body part can interfere with normal sensorimotor feedback and disrupt fine motor control[91,92,115] (Figures 4-4a and 4-4b).

Another limitation in neural adaptation relates to the timing of the injury and the retraining. Initially, following an acute injury, every effort needs to be directed at decreasing the extent of the damage. For the most part this means using pharmacologic agents to limit the damage, immobilization to rest the part, and appropriate chemotherapeutic agents to facilitate healing and repair. There appears to be a delicate balance in this early phase of injury when aggressive physical training may exacerbate brain damage. In other words, like any other injury, there must be a balance of immobilization and mobilization. Thus, the timing for beginning physical retraining postacute injury must be individually determined for each patient.[136]

The functional limitations and disability that may result from impairment(s) also will vary depending on the personality and the motivation of the individual. In addition, we know that there does not need to be any pathology (ie, an injury or a lesion) to create neural learning or neural dysfunction.[91,92,115,116] In other words, compensatory behaviors can follow temporary impairments, where excessive, intensive, repetitive overuse of an extremity can lead to an imbalance of postural righting, as well as to peripheral and central changes in the nervous system.

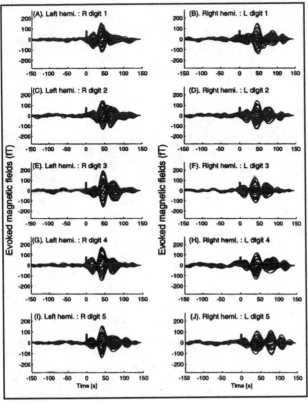

Figure 4-4a. Somatosensory evoked magnetic responses measured by magnetoencephalography for digits 1 thought 5 in a normal female flutist. These images represent normal patterns of somatosenosry evoked responses following a tap on the finger (the tap stimulus indicated by the rectangle at 00 msec). The peak amplitude responses (60-67 fT on the left side and 83-92 fT on the right) occurred between 40 and 44 msec and were the second oscillation after stimulus. The neuronal pool was consistent in its response, and the activity quieted quickly after stimulation. On average, three half-cycle oscillations occurred over 150 msec, the defined data collection period. The evoked neuronal response was similar on both sides for latency and density, but the amplitudes of the firing were greatest on the dominant (right) side (reprinted with permission from Byl N, McKenzie A, Nagarajan S. Differences in somatosensory hand organization in a healthy flutist and a flutist with focal hand dystonia: a case report. *J Hand Ther.* 2000;12(4):302-309).

IMPLICATIONS OF NEUROPLASTICITY FOR CLINICAL PRACTICE

The good news is that the CNS is massively adaptable. If we can drive both spontaneous and purposeful changes in structure and function with attended, repetitive, rewarded behaviors, then we should be able to reverse negative musculoskeletal and neurological behaviors through focused, selective, goal-directed repetitive behaviors (see Table 4-1 at the end of the chapter). Although the most extensive research on neuroplasticity and the effects of attended, repetitive behaviors has been focused on the somatosensory cortex (area 3b), most specifically the topography of the hand, the findings are equally applicable to the rest of the body.

The bad news is that only part of neural adaptation is automatic. Maximum neural adaptation only occurs in individuals who are committed to learning. Only attended, planned, behaviors repeated and progressed in difficulty over time will capture the potential of the nervous system for change. Automatic, stereotypical behaviors are not associated with measurable learning. As therapists, we will not be able to provide our patients with the individualized, supervised repetitive practice that is needed to drive the changes in structure and function of the nervous system. Instead we must mentor, guide, motivate, and teach our patients about the potential of their nervous system to adapt. Every patient needs to know that, despite the magnitude of the impairment challenging

Figure 4-4b. The degradation of the evoked somatosensory response on the right and the left hands of a flutist with focal hand dystonia. Two fingers were considered involved, the left ring and little fingers (digits 4 and 5) of the left hand. Some background neuronal activity was evident even during the resting state, making it difficult to see the stimulus onset marker at 00 msec. Bilaterally, the peak amplitude of the first response occurred early (approximately 26 to 32 msec on the involved side and 35 to 36 msec on the uninvolved side). The amplitudes of the responses were reduced for the affected digits and increased for the unaffected digits of the involved hand. The evoked magnetic responses were variable, even in the uninvolved digits. On average, four half-cycle oscillations occurred between 0 and 150 msec. The pattern of firing was the least well-organized for the involved digits (4 and 5) on the left side (reprinted with permission from

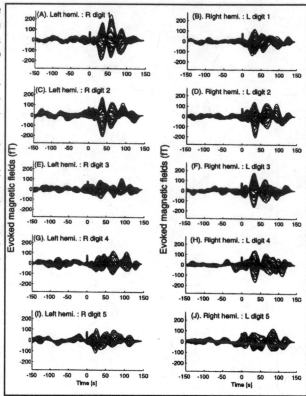

Byl N, McKenzie A, Nagarajan S. Differences in somatosensory hand organization in a healthy flutist and a flutist with focal hand dystonia: a case report. *J Hand Ther.* 2000;12(4):302-309).

him or her, motivated individuals can make impressive changes in their nervous system with selective, goal-directed, and challenging repetitive behaviors.

Our challenge as physical therapists is to design innovative programs that include timely, creative applications of basic neuroscience research to practice. In some cases, continued research in neuroscience should help us define the underlying neurophysiological pathways that are dysfunctional and to understand mechanisms of the neurotransmitters, the hormones, and the growth factors that are essential to learning. We also need a better understanding of the role of emotions and the limbic system in modifying structure and function. Increased knowledge also will help physicians prescribe the most appropriate drugs to facilitate the behavioral adaptation program as well as to prevent unnecessary damage as a result of direct injury, hypoxia, swelling, and scarring. However, medications cannot replace the essential element of goal-directed, challenging, repetitive, and normal (even though potentially incomplete) behaviors for learning.

The ideal practitioner will be committed to reading the basic science literature which has potential for clinical applications, collaborating in research with basic scientists when possible, or, at a minimum, bringing challenging clinical research questions to the basic scientist. Clinicians also should try to build cohorts of patients to follow over time to enable a more complete understanding of functional outcomes, as well as changes with maturation and aging. In addition, the ideal practitioner must review the evidence that supports a specific therapeutic approach to the management of a clinical problem and make a commitment to share this research evidence with third party payers to facilitate legitimate financial support for medical care reimbursement.

Despite the possible economic limitations in health care, the patient/practitioner relationship must be stronger than ever. The patient and the family must be engaged in the process of decision-making regarding care. The clinician must be aware of new clinical approaches and set up methodological designs in clinical practice that contribute to evidence in support of intervention. Examples are: random assignment of patients with a specific impairment to two different treatment approaches, sequential clinical trials noting which of two treatment approaches achieved measurable outcomes earlier, single case designs repeated over multiple subjects, and cross over designs where all subjects receive both treatments. These interventions may not necessarily have to be considered formal research, as, in some instances, they could be incorporated into the quality assurance program for the practice site. In other instances, the patient would need to be informed regarding the data analysis plan and consent would need to be obtained for participation and to have relevant data included in an analysis of effectiveness. This type of evidenced-based practice requires a commitment to the profession beyond the expected commitment to high quality care that is ethical and sensitive to the needs of the individual. It also will be a challenge to achieve these goals in a managed health care environment where visits may be limited and reimbursement for care may be capitated.

The ideal practitioner will make sure that every patient and family understands the principles of neuroplasticity, whether the patient has a musculoskeletal, cardiopulmonary, and/or a neuromuscular problem that interferes with control of voluntary movement. The ideal practitioner also will make sure that every patient understands the benefits of mental practice and the role of integration of visual, motor, and mirror imagery in terms of initiating recruitment and firing of the neuronal networks that can begin to facilitate improved structure and function even when normal motor control may not be possible. The opportunities for physical therapists to contribute to neurological rehabilitation in the 21st century are exciting and infinite.

TABLE 4-1
Restoring the Somatosensory Hand Representation and Fine Motor Control: Example of Applying the Principles of Neuroplasticity

A. Problem

Degradation of the somatosensory representation of the hand associated with loss of fine motor control or involuntary movements during performance of a target task (eg, a musician, a data entry clerk, a computer scientist, a secretary).

B. Purpose

Restore the differentiation of the somatosensory representation of the hand and fine motor control.

C. Specific Neurosensory Retraining Activities

Active stimulation: Active exploration of objects

1. Nontarget Sensory Tasks
   - Read Braille (workbooks and regular books) and play card games using Braille cards, using one finger at a time
   - Scan embossed letters through a windowed opening (4 to 8 mm) (eyes closed)
   - Palpate plastic discs created with matched pairs of indented symbols of letters, figures/shapes
   - Play games with eyes closed (Scrabble and dominos)
   - Put shapes into matched holes with eyes closed
   - Place small party objects in a plastic bag and try to match objects with eyes closed
   - Identify alphabet soup letters by exploration with target fingers
   - Place small objects in large boxes of rice and beans; with eyes closed, bury hand in rice and find matching objects

2. Target Sensory Tasks (without any tension in the hand)
   - Feel the musical instrument; do not use it or play it
   - Identify everything about the surface of the instrument, eyes closed (eg, strings, fret, white keys, black keys)
   - Place raised letters on the keys of the computer keyboard; palpate to determine if matched to underlying key
   - Explore target surface with each finger individually while keeping all other fingers relaxed

3. Nontarget Sensory Motor Tasks
   - Introduce a distinctive stimulus (eg, sharp, dull, soft, design); subject must bend the metacarpal joint following the stimulus
   - Palpate different alphabet magnet letters (eyes closed) and spell words by placing letters on the refrigerator
   - Look at a picture on the wall, then close the eyes and feel selected objects in a box that match the picture; with the unaffected side, feel the picture on the wall and

with the affected digits place the objects appropriately on the picture where you remember they should go (eg, pin the tail on the donkey)

- Smoothly and efficiently remove small objects from wells of different sizes, progressing the task from easy to hard and from slow to fast
- Smoothly and efficiently, lightly hold a pen or pencil (just barely preventing it from dropping) and write using the proximal muscles of the shoulder and elbow; increase the difficulty and speed of what is being written
- Working with puzzles with raised surfaces, put puzzles together with eyes closed
- Eyes closed, feel pegs, lightly hold them, and efficiently place pegs into holes; progress difficulty by getting pegs of different sizes and increasing speed
- Forearms supinated, resting on the legs, hands relaxed, bend elbow and shoulder and take each finger to feel different parts of the body. Start slowly and then increase speed. Be accurate and only lightly feel area

4. Target Sensory Motor Tasks
- Close eyes and balance posture with gravity while holding and lightly exploring the feel of the musical instrument
- Letting the hand be like a dead weight, use large, slow, free-flowing circular movements of the shoulder to bring the hand to contact the playing surface of the instrument (eg, dropping the finger on the key of the piano, the string of the guitar, or the fret of the violin). Progressively decrease the range of proximal movement and increase the speed
- With the hand as a dead weight, drop one finger at a time on the playing surface, creating a strong sound on the piano or from the string of the guitar
- With the weight of the hand relaxed on the playing surface, one finger at a time, initiate the pressure down on the key using the muscles inside the hand; then release the pressure down, but do not lift up
- Begin sequencing movements of the digits on the instrument without tension, moving from muscles at the shoulder or elbow to muscles inside the hand
- Begin to learn new music or type unfamiliar passages on the instrument
- Put hand in shaving cream and begin making large circular movements, making the movements smaller and smaller and ultimately making the movements faster
- Put Velcro on a pen and hold the pen between digits 2 and 3 (D2 and D3) and move the pen between the fingers
- With the pen between D2 and D3, practice placing the pen in the writing position
- Holding the pen very lightly, practice making large circular movements from proximal shoulder and elbow muscles and progress to making letters and writing sentences, slowly increasing the speed

Passive stimulation: Stimuli delivered to the skin

1. Place raised surfaces of different configurations on finger pads; patient has to identify (eg, alphabet soup letters)
2. Have a friend or family member write different numbers, letters, shapes, and symbols on the involved fingers of the patient's affected hand (eyes closed) (Figure 4-5)

Figure 4-5. Making a symbol on the patient's affected hand (patient's eyes are closed).

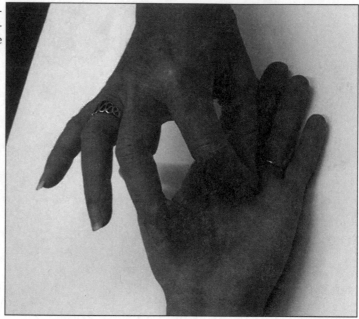

a. In the simple case, the patient must name the letter or word drawn

b. For complex designs, the patient must draw what he or she felt (angles, intersections, curves must be accurate)

c. When the patient interprets the stimulus incorrectly, the friend will provide the stimulus again. If missed a second time, the friend will have the patient look at the design delivered, then have the patient close his or her eyes and deliver the stimulus again. This repetition and feedback are designed to increase the potential for learning

D. Selective Sensorimotor Training: Fine Motor Control

Let the weight of the hand drop across the surface with the wrist in a stable position and all other fingers relaxed with gravity

Do simple tasks that are embedded in the target specific task

Do functional tasks (activities of daily living) centering and stabilizing the movement at the proximal shoulder paired with the elbow muscles and the muscles inside the hand

Combine the movement at the shoulder with the desired outcome of the digit on the instrument

1. Position the trunk and the shoulder on the instrument with the trunk and upper limb balanced and comfortable with gravity

2. Drop a digit onto the playing surface from the elbow with the wrist and finger stable with gravity; let this natural weight create the ideal sound from the instrument (eg, key of piano, key of keyboard, string of guitar, opening of flute)

   • First drop the index finger, eyes closed

   • Second drop the middle finger, eyes closed

- Progress to dropping the ring and 5th finger
- Then drop combinations of the fingers

3. On the guitar, reverse the movement by bending the elbow, keeping the wrist stable, and bringing the weight of the hand and one digit in a stable position, up past the string

4. Contact the target surface, slowly match the tension in the key or the string. Initially, be careful not to exceed the natural force and quality of the key or string. When you develop a clear recognition of the match of force needed between the finger and the key or string, then learn to add the additional force necessary to activate the string or the key

With forearms supinated (palms and forearms up), move one finger at a time from the base joint, using only the muscles inside the hand rather than the muscles from the forearm which serve the fingers

1. Bend each finger individually and then bend all fingers together at the base (MP) joint, Increase the speed and shorten the range

2. Alternate fingers by bending at the base joint

3. Straighten the interphalangeal (IP) joints and keep the MP joints flexed

4. Pair finger movements together (eg, index and 4th; index and 5th)

Place forearms in pronation (palm down) with no surface contact and with forearm muscles quiet

1. Lift each individual finger by straightening the small joints of the fingers (IP joints) without extending the large MP joint

2. Lift digits in sequence by extending IP joints

Place forearms palm down, with surface contact

1. Lift each individual finger by straightening the IP joints without extending the MP joints

2. Lift digits in sequence by extending IP joints

3. Lift pairs of digits by extending IP joints

Begin to do more complex fine motor tasks such as manipulating coins in the hand, manipulating the pen such as twirling with the fingers, playing a trill, weaving, beading, perhaps even juggling, but feel the center of control as your shoulder with the base joints of the fingers feeling as if they are connected to that shoulder point (Figure 4-6)

On the target instrument, eyes closed, let the fingers fall by dropping the elbow into extension and then lift the fingers by flexing the elbow. Keep the fingers and wrist in a stable, functional position. Increase the speed by shortening the range of movement at the elbow. From the base joint perform flexion and extension movements of the digits including alternating movements simulating a trill

1. Balance posture with gravity

2. Keep forearm muscles quiet

3. Center of movement, posterior shoulder extended to elbow with individual finger movement as needed occurring at the base joint (not the distal finger joints)

Figure 4-6. Determining the outcome of the roll of dice with eyes closed.

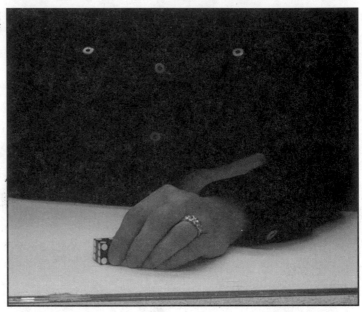

E. Biofeedback

Learning must be reinforced through reward (eg, auditory, tacile, or visual biofeedback)

Auditory and visual biofeedback should be integrated into the training program

Emphasis will be placed on retraining the most involved fingers

1. Patients in retraining should be given a biofeedback unit to take home for a month
2. Biofeedback can be used to help individuals learn to:
   - Inhibit the co-contraction of agonists and antagonists (particularly the extrinsic finger extensors and flexors)
   - Use the intrinsic muscles of the hand to initiate flexion at the MP joint without recruiting additional finger flexors
   - Abduct the fingers and extend the IP joints using the intrinsic muscles while keeping the extensor digitorum quiet
   - Release digit downward pressure without lifting and extending the fingers with the extensor digitorum
   - Alternate and sequence adjacent digits by using the interossei and the lumbricals (on as well as off the instrument)
   - Complete common personal care and household activities, writing, keyboarding, and the target specific task using the intrinsic muscles inside the hand and minimizing the use of the extrinsic muscles
3. A two-channel biofeedback is beneficial for retraining. Place one electrode on the flexor surface of the forearm and the second on the extensor surface. Show the patient how to use tape to increase sensory feedback and consequently serve as a biofeedback mechanism. If the finger is excessively curling, place the tape on the

extensor surface; when the tape is stretched, it gives the individual feedback that excessive flexion is occurring

F. Mental Imagery, Visualization Techniques, Mental Rehearsal, and Mental Practice

Mental imagery, visualization, mental rehearsal, and mental practice can reinforce learning

Audio and audiovisual training tapes should be made for the patient to use to develop skills of imagery

As soon as possible, the patient should be encouraged to image without the assistance of the tapes since self-imagery provides the most viable image. These tapes will initially focus on: a) healing, b) relaxation, c) balancing the posture with gravity, d) normalizing all hand functions in activities of daily living, e) normalizing sensory processing (eg, ability to discriminate all textures, letters, figures normally), f) eliminating abnormal movements, g) freely moving the upper limb using proximal shoulder and elbow joints, and h) normalizing the target task (eg, writing, computer, keyboard, instrument). Some of the tasks the patient will be asked to image include: a) lifting a glass, b) using utensils, c) brushing teeth, d) cooking, e) cleaning house, f) picking up and manipulating small objects, g) washing dishes, h) writing, i) using a keyboard, j) picking up, retrieving, and manipulating small objects, and k) playing a musical instrument

The mental imagery must be reinforced with mental practice

1. The patient is asked to reflect back to the time when the hand was working normally
2. The patient constantly reminds him- or herself how easy it was to do the task, how warm the hand felt, how each individual digit felt absolutely controlled, how easy it was to control each digit separately, and how coordinated the hand felt
3. The patient is asked to review the pleasure of performance in his or her job or on the target instrument including the satisfaction of the tone, accuracy, speed, and tension-free movements as well as the confidence of knowing the hand position, the quality of the sensation, and the control of fine motor movement

G. Mirror Imagery

Mirror imagery also can be used to change the strategy for writing, keyboard techniques, handling objects, and instrument play

Use mirrors as a type of "virtual reality" to restore the somatosensory function of the involved part

The affected hand is placed out of view (eg, behind the mirror). The subject concentrates on the mirror image (eg, the right hand looks like the left hand in the mirror). The subject tries to replicate the mirror image with his affected side. The mirror will be placed on a table surface, the keyboard, or the target instrument

REFERENCES

1. Merzenich MM, Wright B, Jenkins WM, et al. Cortical plasticity underlying perceptual, motor and cognitive skill development: implications for neurorehabilitation. *Cold Springs Harbor Symposium in Quantitative Biology.* 1996;61:1-8.

2. Merzenich MM, DeCharms RC. Neural representations, experience and change. In: Llinas R, Churchland P, eds. *The Mind-Brain Continuum.* Boston, Mass: MIT Press; 1996: 61-81.

3. Merzenich MM, Jenkins WM. Cortical representation of learned behaviors. In: Andersen P, Hvalby O, Paulsen O, et al, eds. *Memory Concepts.* Amsterdam: Elsevier; 1993.

4. Merzenich MM, Jenkins WM. Reorganization of cortical representation of the hand following alterations of skin inputs induced by nerve injury, skin island transfer and experience. *J Hand Ther.* 1993;6:89-94.

5. Nagarajan SS, Blake DT, Wright BA, et al. Practice-related improvements in somatosensory integral discrimination are temporarily specific but generalize across skin location, hemisphere and modality. *J Neuroscience.* 1999;18:1559-1663.

6. Nudo RJ, Jenkins WM, Merzenich MM, et al. Neurophysiological correlates of hand preference in primary cortex of adult squirrel monkeys. *J Neuroscience.* 1992;12:2918-2947.

7. Nudo RJ, Millikin GW, Jenkins WM, et al. Use dependent alterations of movement representations in primary motor cortex of adult squirrel monkeys. *J Neuroscience.* 1996; 16:785-807.

8. Nudo RJ, Plautz EJ, Millikin GW. Adaptive plasticity in primate motor cortex as a consequence of behavioral experience and neuronal injury. *Seminars in Neuroscience.* 1996;9:13-23.

9. Nudo R, Wise BS, Fluentes F, et al. Neural substrates for the effects of rehabilitative training on motor recovery after ischemic infarct. *Science.* 1996;272:1791-1795.

10. Nudo RJ, Millikin GW. Reorganization of movement representations in primary motor cortex following focal ischemic infarcts in adult squirrel monkeys. *J Neuroscience.* 1996; 75:2140-2149.

11. Spengler F, Roberts TPL, Poeppel D, et al. Learning transfer and neuronal plasticity in humans trained in tactile discrimination. *Neurosci Letters.* 1997;232:151-154.

12. Taub E. Somatosensory deafferentiation research with monkeys: implications for rehabilitation medicine. In: Ince LP, ed. *Behavioral Psychology in Rehabilitation Medicine: Clinical Applications.* New York, NY: Williams and Wilkins; 1980:371-401.

13. Taub E, Crago JE, Uswatte G. Constraint-induced movement therapy: a new approach to treatment in physical medicine. *Rehabil Psychol.* 1988;43:152-170.

14. Taub E, Miller NE, Novak TA, et al. Techniques to improve motor deficit after stroke. *Arch Phys Med Rehabil.* 1993;74:347-354.

15. Taub E, Flor H, Knecht S, et al. Correlation between phantom limb pain and cortical reorganization. *J NIH Research.* 1995;7:49-51.

16. Wolf SL, Lecraw DE, Barton L, et al. Forced use of hemiplegic upper extremities to reverse the effect of learned nonuse among chronic stroke and head-injured patients. *Exp Neuro.* 1989;104:125-132.

17. Jenkins W, Allard T, Nudo R. Cortical representational plasticity. In: Raskic P, Singer W, eds. *Neurobiology of the Neocortex.* New York, NY: John Wiley; 1988:41-67.

18. Jenkins W, Merzenich M, Ochs M, et al. Functional reorganization of primary somatosensory cortex in adult owl monkeys after behaviorally controlled tactile stimulation. *J Neurophysiol.* 1990;63:82-104.

19. Kaas JH, Merzenich MM, Killackey HP. The reorganization of somatosensory cortex following peripheral nerve damage in adult and developing mammals. *Ann Rev Neuroscience.*

1983; 6:325-356.

20. Merzenich MM, Kaas JH, Wall J, et al. Progression of change following median nerve section in the cortical representation of the hand in areas 3b and 2 in adult owl and squirrel monkeys. *Neuroscience*. 1983;10:639-665.

21. Merzenich MM, Kaas JH, Wall J, et al. Topographic reorganization of somatosensory cortical areas 3b and 1 in adult monkeys following restricted deafferentiation. *Neuroscience*. 1983;8:33-55.

22. Merzenich MM, Nelson RJ, Stryker MP, et al. Somatosensory cortical map changes following digit amputation in adult monkeys. *J Comp Neurol*. 1984;224:591-605.

23. Merzenich MM. Development and maintenance of cortical somatosensory representations: functional "maps" and neuroanatomic repertoires. In: Barnard KE, Brazelton TM, eds. *Touch: The Foundation of Experience*. Madison, Wis: Intl Univ Press; 1991:47-71.

24. Merzenich MM, Allard T, Jenkins WM. Neural ontogeny of higher brain function: implications of some recent neurophysiologic findings. In: Franzen O, Westman P, eds. *Information Processing in the Somatosensory System*. London: McMillan Press; 1991:293-311.

25. Merzenich MM, Sameshina K. Cortical plasticity and memory. *Current Opin Neurobiol*. 1993;3:187-196.

26. Merzenich MM, Jenkins WM. Cortical plasticity, learning and learning dysfunction. In: Jules B, Kovacs I, eds. *Maturational Windows and Adult Cortical Plasticity*. New York, NY: Addison-Wesley; 1995:247-272.

27. Merzenich MM, Schreiner C, Jenkins WM. Neural mechanisms underlying temporal integration, segmentation, and input sequence representation: some implications for the origin of learning disability. *Ann NY Acad Sci*. 1995;682:1-22.

28 Recanzone G, Jenkins W, Hradek G, et al. Progressive improvement in discriminative abilities in adult owl monkeys performing a tactile frequency discrimination task. *J Neurophysiol*. 1992;67:1015-1030.

29. Recanzone GH, Merzenich MM, Jenkins WM, et al. Topographic reorganization of the hand representation in cortical area 2b of owl monkeys trained in a frequency-discrimination task. *J Neurophysiol*. 1992; 67:1031-1056.

30. Recanzone GH, Merzenich MM, Jenkins WM. Frequency discrimination training engaging in a restricted skin surface results in an emergence of a cutaneous response zone in cortical area 3a. *J Neurophysiol*. 1992;67:1047-1070.

31. Yang TT, Gallen C, Schwartz B, et al. Sensory maps in the human brain. *Nature*. 1994; 368:592-593.

32. Iwamura Y, Tanaka M, Sakamoto M. Diversity in receptive field properties of vertical neuronal arrays in the crown of the post central gyrus of the conscious monkey. *Exp Brain Res*. 1985;58:400-411.

33. Bernstein N. *The Coordination and Regulation of Movements*. Oxford, UK: Pergamon Press; 1967.

34. Sporns O, Edelman GM. Solving Bernstein's problem: a proposal for the development of coordinated movement by selection. *Child Dev*. 1993;64:960-981.

35. Jiang W, Chapman CE, Lamarre Y. Modulation of cutaneous responsiveness of neurons in the primary somatosensory cortex during conditioned arm movements in the monkey. *Exp Brain Res*. 1991;84:324-354.

36. Leijinse JA. Anatomical factors predisposing to focal dystonia in musicians' hand: principles, theoretical examples, clinical significance. *J Biomechanics*. 1996;30:659-669.

37. Savelsberg G, von Hofsten C, Jonsson B. The coupling of head, reach and grasp movements in nine month old infant prehension. *Scand J Psyc*. 1997;38:325-333.

38. Penfield W, Rasmussen T. *The Cerebral Cortex of Man: A Clinical Study of Localization of Function*. New York, NY: MacMillan; 1950.

39. Konczak J, Dichgans J. The development toward stereotypic arm kinematics during reaching in the first 3 years of life. *Exp Brain Res.* 1997;117:346-354.

40. Konczak J, Borutta M, Dichgans J. The development of goal directed reaching in infants. II. Learning to produce task-adequate patterns of joint torque. *Exp Brain Res.* 1997; 113:465-474.

41. Kuhtz-Buschbeck JP, Stolze H, Johak K, et al. Development of prehension movements in children: a kinematic study. *Exp Brain Res.* 1998;122:424-432.

42. von Hofsten G, Vishton P, Spelke ES, et al. Predictive action in infancy: tracking and reaching for moving objects. *Cognition.* 1998;67:255-333.

43. Hadders-Algra M, Brogren E, Forssberg H. Training affects the development of postural adjustments in sitting infants. *J Physiol.* 1996;493:289-298.

44. Hadders-Algra M, Brogen E, Forssberg H. Ontogeny of postural adjustments during sitting in infancy: variation, selection and modulation. *J Physiol.* 1996;493:273-288.

45. Forssberg H, Nashner LM. Ontogenetic development of postural control in man: adaptation to altered support and visual conditions during stance. *Neuroscience.* 1982;2:545-552.

46. Wannier TMJ, Maier MA, Hopp-Rayond MC. Contrasting properties of monkey somatosensory and motor cortex neurons activated during the control force in precision grip. *J Neurophysiol.* 1991;65:572-587.

47. Sveistrup H, Woolacott MH. Practice modifies the developing automatic postural response. *Exp Brain Res.* 1997;114:33-43.

48. Mriganka W, Wall JT, Kaas JH. Modular distribution of neurons with slowly adapting and rapidly adapting responses in area 3b of somatosensory cortex in monkeys. *J Neurophysiol.* 1985;52:724-727.

49. Thelen E, Kelso JAS, Fogel A. Self-organizing systems and infant motor development. *Dev Rev.* 1987;7:39-65.

50. Ulrich BD. Dynamic systems theory and skill development in infants and children. In: Connolly KJ, Forssberg H, eds. *Neurophysiology and Neuropsychology of Motor Development.* London: MacKeith Press;1977:319-345.

51. Schoner G, Kelso JAS. Dynamic pattern generation in behavioral and neural systems. *Science.* 1988;239:1513-1520.

52. Changeux JP. Variation and selection in neural function. *Trends Neurosci.* 1997;20:291-299.

53. Kandel ER, Schwartz JH, Jessel TM. *Principles of Neural Science.* 4th ed. New York, NY: Elsevier Science; 1999.

54. Mushiake H, Inase M, Tnaji J. Selective coding of motor sequence in the supplementary motor area of the monkey cerebral cortex. *Exp Brain Res.* 1990;82:208-210.

55. Preston JB, Whitlock DG. Intracellular potentials recorded from motoneurons following precentral gyrus stimulation in primate. *J Neurophysiol.* 1961;24:91-100.

56. Roland PE, Larson B, Lassen NA, et al. Supplementary motor area and other cortical areas in organization of voluntary movement in man. *J Neurophysiol.* 1980;43:118-136.

57. Ghez C, Vicario O. Discharge of the red nucleus neurons during voluntary muscle contraction activity patterns and correlation with isometric forces. *J Physiol (Paris).* 1978;74: 283-285.

58. Rijntjes M, Dettmers C, Buchel C, et al. A blueprint for movement: functional and anatomical representations in the human motor system. *J Neurosci.* 1999; 19:8043-8048.

59. Hebb DO. *The Organization of Behavior.* New York, NY: John Wiley; 1949.

60. Abbrazese G, Trompeto C, Schieppati M. The excitability of the human motor cortex increases during execution and mental imagination of sequential but not repetitive finger movements. *Exp Brain Res.* 1996;111:476-482.

61. Decety J. Do imagined and executed actions share the same neural substrate? *Brain Res Cogn Brain Res.* 1996;3:87-93.

62. Decety J, Perani D, Peannerod M, et al. The neurophysiological basis of motor imagery. *Behav Brain Res.* 1996;77:45-52.

63. Decety J, Jeannerod M. Mentally simulated movements in virual reality. Does Fitts law hold in motor imagery? *Behav Brain Res.* 1996;72:127-134.

64. Jeannerod M. To act or not to act. Perspectives on representation of actions. *O J Exp Psychol.* 1999;52:1-29.

65. Jeannerod M. Mental imagery in the motor context. *Neuropsychologia.* 1995;33:1419-1432.

66. Jeannerod M. Object oriented action. In: Bennett KMB, Castillo U, eds. *Insights Into The Reach to Grasp Movement.* Amsterdam: Elsevier-North Holland; 1994.

67. Jeannerod M, Frak V. Mental imaging of motor activity in humans. *Curr Opin Neurobiol.* 1999;9:735-739.

68. Jeannerod M, Decety J. Mental motor imagery: a window into the representational stages of action. *Curr Opin Neurobiol.* 1995;5:727-731.

69. Porro CA, Francescato MP, Cettolo V, et al. Primary motor and sensory cortex activation during motor performance and motor imagery: a functional magnetic resonance imaging study. *J Neurosci.* 1999;16:7688-7698.

70. Parsons LM, Fox PT. The neural basis of impicit movements used in recognizing hand shape. *Cogn Neuropsych.* 1998;15:583-615.

71. Parsons LM, Fox PT, Downs JH, et al. Use of implicit motor imagery for visual shape discrimination as revealed by PET. *Nature.* 1995;375:54-58.

72. Tucker M, Ellis R. On the relations between seen objects and components of potential actions. *J Exp Psychol (Hum Perc Perf).* 1998;24:830-846.

73. Schwartz DL Black T. Inferences through imaged actions. Knowing by simulated doing. *J Exp Psychol (Hum Perc Perf).* 1999;25:116-136.

74. Sirigu A, Cohen L, Duhamel JR. Congruent unilateral impairments for real and imagined hand movements. *Neuroreport.* 1995;6:997-1001.

75. Sirigu A, Duhamel JR, Cohen L, et al. The mental representation of hand movements after parietal cortex damage. *Science.* 1996;273:1156-1154.

76. Prechtl HFR. The importance of fetal movements. In: Connolly KJ, Forssberg H, eds. *Neurophysiology and Neuropsychology of Motor Development.* London: MacKeith Press; 1997: 42-53.

77. Hadders-Algra M, Groothius AMC. Quality of general movements in infancy is related to the development of neurological dysfunction attention deficit hyperactivity disorder and aggressive behavior. *Dev Med Child Neurol.* 1999;41:381-391.

78. Hadders-Algra M, Klip-Van den Nieuwendijk A, Martijn A, et al. Assessment of general movements: towards a better understanding of a sensitive method to evaluate brain function in young infants. *Dev Med Child Neurol.* 1997;39:88-98.

79. Hadders-Algra M, Brogren E, Forssberg H. Postural adjustments during sitting at preschool age: presence of a transient toddling phase. *Dev Med Child Neurol.* 1998;40:436-447.

80. Sundermier L, Woollacott MH. The influence of vision on the automatic postural muscle responses of newly standing and newly walking infants. *Exp Brain Res.* 1998;120: 537-

540.

81. Ledebt A, Bril B, Breniere Y. The build-up of anticipatory behavior. An analysis of the development of gait initiation in children. *Exp Brain Res.* 1998;120:9-17.

82. Forssberg H. Neural control of human motor development. *Curr Opin Neurobiol.* 1999;9:676-682.

83. Yang JF, Stephens MJ, Vishram R. Infant stepping: a method to study the sensory control of human walking. **J Physiol.** 1998;507:927-937.

84. Muller K, Kass-Iliyya F, Reitz M. Ontogeny of ipsilateral corticospinal projections: a developmental study with transcranial magnetic stimulation. *Ann Neurol.* 1997;42:705-711.

85. Eliasson AC, Forssberg H, Ikuta K, et al. Development of human precision grip. V: Anticipatory and triggered grip actions during sudden loading. *Exp Brain Res.* 1996; 106:425-433.

86. Gibbs J, Harrison LM, Stephens JA, et al. Cutaneomuscular reflex responses recorded from the lower limb in children and adolescents with cerebral palsy. *Dev Med Child Neurol.* 1999; 41:456-484.

87. Gibbs J, Harrison LM, Stephens JA, et al. Does abnormal branching of inputs to motorneurones explain abnormal muscle contraction in cerebral palsy? *Dev Med Child Neurol.* 1999;41:465-472.

88. Plautz EL, Milliken GW, Nudo RJ. Effects of repetitive motor training on movement representations in adult squirrel monkeys: Role of use versus learning. *Neurobiol of Learning and Memory.* 2000;74:27-55.

89. Withers GS, Greenough WT. Reach training selectively alters dendritic branching of subpopulations of layer II-III pyramidals in rat motor-somatosensory forelimb cortex. *Neuropsychologica.* 1989;27:61-69.

90. Schieber MH, Poliakov AV. Partial inactivation of the primary motor cortex hand area: effects on individuated finger movements. *J Neurosci.* 1998;18:9038-9045.

91. Byl N, Merzenich M, Jenkins W. A primate genesis model of focal dystonia and repetitive strain injury: I. Learning-induced de-differentiation of the representation of the hand in the primary somatosensory cortex in adult monkeys. *Ann Neurol.* 1996;47:508-520.

92. Byl N, Merzenich M, Cheung S, et al. A primate model for studying focal dystonia and repetitive strain injury: effects on the primary somatosensory cortex. *Phys Ther.* 1999;79: 727-739.

93. Wilson F, Wagner C, Homberg V, et al. Interaction of biomechanical and training factors in musicians with occupational cramps/focal dystonia. *Neur.* 1991 4:(3 supp 1) 292-296.

94. Wilson F, Wagner C, Homberg V. Biomechanical abnormalities in musicians with occupational cramp/focal dystonia. *J Hand Ther.* 1993;6:298-307.

95. Nudo RJ, Friel KM, Delia S. Role of sensory deficits in motor impairments after injury to the primary motor cortex. *Neuropharmacology.* 2000;39:733-742.

96. Knecht S, Kunesch E, Buchner H, et al. Facilitation of somatosensory evoked potentials by exploratory finger movements. *Exp Brain Res.* 1993;95:330-338.

97. Burke D, Hagbarth KE, Lofstedt L. Muscle spindle activity in man during shortening and lengthening contractions. *J Physiol (London).* 1978;277:131-142.

98. Burke D, Gandevia SC, Macefield G. Responses to passive movement of receptors in joint, skin and muscle of the human hand. *J Physiol (London).* 1988;402:347-361.

99. Hyvarinen J, Poranen A. Movement-sensitive and direction and orientation-selective cutaneous receptive fields in the hand area of the post-central gyrus in monkeys. *J Neurophysiol.* 1978;283:523-537.

100. Costanzo RM, Gardner EP. A quantitative analysis of responses of direction-sensitive neu-

rons in somatosensory cortex of awake monkeys. *J Neurophysiol*. 1980;43:1319-1341.

101. Vega-Bermudez F, Johnson KO, Hsiao SS. Human tactile pattern recognition: active versus passive touch, velocity effects, and patterns of confusion. *J Neurophysiol*. 1996;65:531-546.

102. Shimokata H, Kuzuya F. Two point discrimination test of the skin as an index of sensory aging. *Gerontology*. 1995;42:267-272.

103. LaMotte RH, Lu C, Srinivasan MA, et al. Cutaneous neural codes for shape. *Can J Physiol Pharmcol*. 1994;72:498-505.

104. Mountcastle V, Talbor ULT, Sakata H, et al. Cortical neuronal mechanisms in flutter vibration studied in unanesthetized monkeys: neural periodicity and frequency. *J Neurophysiol*. 1969;32:452-481.

105. Jeannerod M. The timing of natural prehension movements. *J Mot Behav*. 1984;26:235-254.

106. Johansson R. Sensory input and control of grip. *Novartis Foundation Symposium*. 1988;218:45-59.

107. Johnson KO, Hsiao SS. Evaluation of the relative roles of slowly and rapidly adapting afferent fibers in roughness perception. *Can J Physiol Pharmcol*. 1994;72:488-497.

108. Warren S, Hamalainen HA, Gardner EP. Objective classification of motion and direction-sensitive neurons in primary somatosensory cortex of awake monkeys. *J Neurophysiol*. 1986; 56:598-622.

109. Wei JW. Signalling of kinesthetic information by peripheral sensory receptors. *Ann Rev Neurosci*. 1982;5:171-187.

110. Hikosaka O, Tnaka M, Sakama M, et al. Deficits in manipulative behaviors induced by local injections of muscimol in the first somatosensory cortex of the conscious monkey. *Pain Res*. 1985;328:375-380.

111. Xerri C, Coq JO, Merzenich MM, et al. Experience-induced plasticity of cutaneous maps in the primary somatosensory cortex of adult monkeys and rats. *J Physiol (Paris)*. 1996;90:277-287.

112. Xerri C, Merzenich MM, Jenkins W, et al. Representational plasticity in cortical area 3b paralleling tactual-motor skill acquisition in adult monkeys. *Cerebral Cortex*. 1999:9:264-276.

113. Jenkins W, Merzenich M. Reorganization of neocortical representations after brain injury: a neurophysiological model of the bases of recovery from stroke. *Prog Brain Res*. 1987;71:249-266.

114. Allard T, Clark SA, Jenkins WM, et al. Reorganization of somatosensory area 3b representations in adult owl monkeys after digit syndactyly. *J Neurophysiol*. 1991;104:1048-1058.

115. Wang X, Merzenich MM, Sameshima K, et al. Remodeling of hand representation in adult cortex determined by timing of tactile stimulation. *Nature*. 1995; 378:71-75.

116. Wang X, Merzenich MM, Sameshima K, et al. Afferent input integration and segregation in learning are input timing dependent. *Neurosci Abstr*. 1994;20:1427.

117. Kleim JA, Lussnig E, Schwarz ER, et al. Synaptogenesis and Fos expression in the motor cortex of the adult rat after motor skill learning. *J Neurosci*. 1996;16:4529-4535.

118. Rema V, Armstrong-Jones M, Ebner FF. Experience-dependent plasticity of adult rat S2 cortex requires local NMDA receptor activation. *J Neurosci*. 1998;18:10196-10206.

119. Elbert T, Panter C. Wienbruch C, et al. Increased cortical representation of the fingers of the left hand in string players. *Science*. 1995;270:305-307.

120. Schnitzler A, Salenius S, Salmelin R, et al. Involvement of primary motor cortex in motor imagery: a neuromagnetic study. *Neuroimage*. 1997;6:201-208.

121. Yahagi S, Shimura Y, Kasai T. An increase in cortical excitability with no change in spinal excitability during motor imagery. *Percept Mot Skills*. 1996;83:288-290.

122. Gandevia SC, Wilson LR, Inglis JT, et al. Mental rehearsal of motor tasks recruits alpha motoneurons, but fails to recruit human fusimotor neurons selectively. *J Physiol*. 1997;505: 259-266.

123. Ramachandran VS, Rogers-Ramachandran D. Synaesthesia in phantom limbs induced with mirrors. *Proc Soc London B*. 1996;263;377-386.

124. Buonomano TV, Merzenich MM. Temporal information transformed into a spatial code by network with realistic properties. *Science*. 1995;267:1028-1030.

125. Buonomano TV, Hickmott PW, Merzenich MM. Context-sensitive synaptic plasticity and temporal-to-spatial transformations in hippocampal slices. **Proc Natl Acad Sci USA.** 1997; 94:10403-10408.

126. Ahissar E, Vaadia E, Ahissar M, et al. Dependence of cortical plasticity on correlated activity of single neurons and on behavioral context. *Science*. 1992;257:1412-1415.

127. Greenough WT, Change FF. In Peters A, Jones EG, eds. *Cerebral Cortex Vol 7*. New York, NY: Plennum; 1988:335-392.

128. Engbert F, Bonhoeffer T. Dendritic spine changes associated with hippocampal long term synaptic plasticity. *Nature*. 1999;399:66-70.

129. Keller A, Arissan K, Asanuma H. Synaptic proliferation in the motor cortex of adult cats after long-term thalamic stimulation. *J Neurophysiol*. 1992;168:295-308.

130. Byl N, Merzenich MM. Principles of neuroplasticity: implications for neurorehabilitation and learning. In: Gonzales EG, Myers JS, Edelstein JE, at al, eds. *Downey and Darling's Physiological Basis of Rehabilitation Medicine*. Boston, Mass: Butterworth & Heinemann;2001:609-628.

131. Sur M, Merzenich MM, Kaas JH. Magnification, receptive-field area and "hypercolumn" size in area 3b somatosensory cortex in owl monkey. *J Comp Neurol*. 1980;44:295-311.

132. Pascual-Leone A, Wassermann Em, Sadato N, et al. The role of reading activity on the modulation of motor cortical outputs to the reading hand in Braille readers. *Ann Neurol*. 1995;38:910-915.

133. Flor H, Braun C, Elbert T, et al. Extensive reorganization of primary somatosensory cortex in chronic back pain patients. *Neuroscience Letters*. 1997;224:5-8.

134. Rowley HA, Roberts TPL. Functional localization by magnetoencephalography *Neuroimaging Clinics of North America*. 1995;5:695-710.

135. Roberts TPL, Poeppel D, Rowley HA. Magnetoencephalography and magnetic source imaging. *Neuropsych Neuropsychol Behav Neur*. 1998;11:49-64.

136. Risedal A, Zeng J, Johansson BB. Early training may exacerbate brain damage after focal brain ischemia in the rat. *J Cerebral Blood Flow Metab*. 1999;19:997-1003.

Musculoskeletal Considerations in Production and Control of Movement

Mary M. Rodgers, PhD, PT

INTRODUCTION

The intent of this chapter is to provide a basic scientific foundation for an understanding of movement, which includes consideration of the laws of mechanics as they relate to the description and production of movement, the musculoskeletal structures that produce movement, and specific interactions between the human body and the environment that require movement control. Any study of the production and control of movement requires a consideration of the interaction of many different systems whose final outcome is biomechanically measurable. This chapter is organized in three sections. In the first section, biomechanical terms and concepts used in the dynamic analysis of motion are introduced. Specific musculoskeletal components and their mechanical characteristics are described in the second section. The final section brings together biomechanical concepts and musculoskeletal structures as they interact in different movements such as walking.

BASIC BIOMECHANICAL TERMS AND PRINCIPLES

Static analysis simplifies the process of analyzing movement. With large accelerations or masses, however, static analysis would be inaccurate. To more accurately analyze movement of the human body, an understanding of the principles of dynamics is necessary. Dynamics is the study of motion (eg, the relationships between factors causing motion and the motion itself). In statics, bodies are in static equilibrium or in dynamic equilibrium with no great acceleration. In dynamics, bodies are in motion but not in equilibrium.

Dynamics is further subdivided into the areas of kinematics and kinetics. Kinematics is the study of characteristics of motion, or motion descriptors. Kinematics is used to relate displacement, velocity, acceleration, and time without reference to the cause of motion. For example, in the analysis of gait, the pattern of the center of mass of the body, the range of motion of the different segments, and the speed and direction of their motion are all examples of kinematics.

Kinetics is the study of the relationship existing among forces acting on a body, the mass of the body, and the motion of the body. Kinetics is used to predict the motion caused by given forces or to determine the forces required to produce a given motion. Examples of forces which affect the motion or a body are gravity, friction, water and air resistance, muscle contraction, and elastic components. Applying Newton's laws of motion to the characteristics of motion enables the determination of the force characteristics involved in the motion.

The study of dynamics is invaluable in the field of medicine as evidenced by the role biomechanical investigations have played in the analysis of gait patterns, development of prosthetics and orthotics, analysis of muscle function in different activities, analysis of the effect of water and air resistance on the moving body, prediction/evaluation of effects of surgical intervention (eg, tendon transfer), and the analysis of mechanism of injury (eg, sport injuries).

The analysis of temporal factors is basic to dynamic assessment of human movement. Examples of factors which relate to time include cadence, duration of a movement phase, and the temporal pattern. Cadence is measured by count (strikes per minute) and can be used to determine slow versus fast walking or running. The duration of a movement is important in muscle activity. For example, in a ballistic motion, a larger amount of muscle tension would be required than in a slower motion. Tension requirements may exceed the material strength of the musculotendinous components, causing rupture. In electromyographic studies of the lower extremity muscles during walking, the knowledge that certain muscles are active or inactive is useless unless the time of activity also is known and can be related to the pattern of gait. Changes in position always are connected with changes in time, so that knowledge of timing is essential in kinematic and kinetic analyses of motion.

KINEMATICS

Dynamic assessment requires an understanding of linear and angular kinematic parameters. A discussion of these parameters follows.

Position and Displacement

Motion involves a continuous change in position, which in the case of a moving body is called *displacement*. A change in position may be translatory or linear so that every point of the body is displaced along parallel lines. In translation, a point is moved from

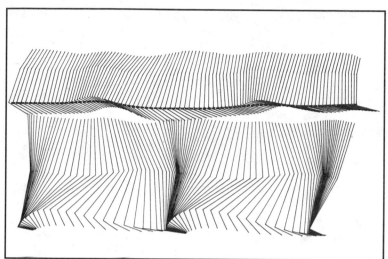

Figure 5-1. Translation and rotation movements during walking. The stick figure is reconstructed from three-dimensional motion analysis. It shows the combination of angular movement of the limbs about the joints and translation of the center of mass (darker dashed line) which occurs during walking.

one position to another and can be determined as in static analysis. The straight line distance between the two points is the magnitude of the displacement, and the direction must be indicated. Displacement is, therefore, a vector quantity while distance is a scalar quantity (magnitude without direction).

Change in position also may be rotational or axial, causing angular motion. In the body, movement around an axis may occur in a rotational pattern. Motion may be a combination of linear and rotational movement (Figure 5-1). For example, movements in gait represent a combination of translation (in the general movement of the body) and rotation (as the extremities rotate around many joints to achieve the end result of walking). Human motion can be described as a translatory motion which has major contributions from linear, angular, and curvilinear movements. The motion that a body has in translation along a straight course or rotation about a particular axis constitutes one degree of freedom. The joints of the body often have many degrees of freedom in that they permit motion in more than one plane.

Kinematic analysis has a wide range of applications in physical therapy. Angular displacement is probably the most common kinematic measurement taken for human motion. Because of the structure of the human body as a linked system of rigid segments moving about joint axes, an understanding of the kinematics of the body often is accomplished by analysis of rotational motion. Measurement of joint angles, documentation of deformities, assessment of fracture, planning of osteotomies, and examination of joint stability are just a few of the medical applications of kinematic analysis.

Velocity

Displacement per unit time gives the rate of displacement or velocity. The average velocity of a body over a time interval is defined as the quotient of the displacement (s) and the time interval (t). Speed or velocity provides an account of both the spatial and temporal elements of motion. However, velocity is a vector quantity (includes direction of movement), whereas speed is scalar only (shows magnitude of the velocity vector without regard for change in direction). Average velocity can be used when the velocity is relatively constant. Additionally, average velocity calculated over a short period of time will approach the value for instantaneous velocity (ie, velocity at a specific instant of time or at a certain point on its path).

Linear velocity is the time rate of change of position and displacement. The units are expressed as meters per second (m/s). Graphically, velocity refers to the slope of the position time graph. A change in the slope of the position line depicts a change in the relationship (or velocity). Angular velocity is the time rate of change of angular positions and is expressed in radians per second (rad/s) or degrees per second.

Acceleration

When an object moves from one location to another, its velocity may not be constant over the entire distance. The magnitude of the velocity may increase or decrease relative to its straight line of displacement, or the direction of velocity may change. These changes in velocity are referred to as acceleration and deceleration (negative acceleration). Since change in velocity takes place over a certain time interval, acceleration is considered the rate of change in velocity.

Linear acceleration is expressed in meters per second squared (m/s^2). If the final velocity is greater than the initial velocity, the object is accelerating or has positive acceleration. If the final velocity is less than the initial velocity, the object is decelerating or has negative acceleration. Instantaneous acceleration would be approximated by using small time intervals in the analysis. Angular acceleration (alpha) is the time rate of change of angular velocity. The units for angular acceleration are radians per second squared (rad/s^2) or degrees per second squared.

As an example, suppose a patient is moving her arm through a range of 105 to 135 degrees of shoulder abduction. The angular displacement would be 30 degrees or .52 radians. If the starting position were stationary and the movement occurred in 2 seconds, the average angular velocity of shoulder abduction would be .26 rad/s (15 deg/s). If the patient continues to abduct the arm, and at 2.5 seconds the arm is traveling at a velocity of 1.57 rad/s (90 deg/s), the average angular acceleration would be .63 rad/s (36 deg/s).

Relative Motion

In many applications of dynamics, the description of a frame of reference is necessary in order to relate motion at different locations. For example, motion of the ankle joint occurs in several different planes. Motion at the knee joint occurs primarily in one plane. The three-dimensional motion of the ankle during locomotion cannot be compared to that of the knee unless the kinematics and kinetics are described in the same planes for each joint. Similarly, the coordinate systems must be defined when analysis involves more than one technique.

If two bodies are moving along the same straight line, the position coordinates can be measured from the same origin. The difference in their positions defines the relative position coordinate of point A to point B and is denoted as $s_{A/B}$. The relative linear velocity between the points is the rate of change of relative displacements ($v_{A/B}$). Similarly, the relative linear acceleration between the points is the rate of change of relative velocities ($a_{A/B}$). Relative motion also may be angular, in which case the same relationships are expressed using angular terms.

The applications for relative motion analyses are many. The effects of reconstructive surgery on joint motions can be documented using motion analysis prior to and following surgery. Additionally, basic research involving the effects of total joint kinematics on ligaments uses motion analysis.

Three-Dimensional Motion

Planar motion is movement in which all points of a rigid body move parallel to a fixed point. This motion has three degrees of freedom, including sliding anteriorly or posteriorly, sliding laterally, and rotating about an axis perpendicular to the translatory axes. The movements of vertebrae in trunk flexion illustrate planar motion as they rotate forward and translate simultaneously.

Plane motion is described by the position of its instantaneous axis of rotation and the motion's rotational magnitude about this axis. In cervical flexion, for example, as a vertebra moves in a plane, there is a point at every instant of motion somewhere within or without the body that does not move. If a line is drawn from that point so that it perpendicularly meets the line of motion, the point of intersection is called the ***instantaneous axis of rotation*** (or ***screw axis***) for that motion at that point in time. Most joint movement is primarily rotatory motion, but the axis of motion may change its location and/or its orientation during a complete range of motion.

The term ***three-dimensional motion*** implies that an object may move in any direction by combining multidirectional translation and multi-axial rotation. In the human body, most movements are three-dimensional in that they move in more than one plane. The normal range of motion of joints denotes the extremes of rotation and translation of the joint. An articulation may have several degrees of freedom and a limited range of motion. Degrees of freedom refer to the ability to move in planes (number of axes), while the range of motion is dependent on soft tissue restraints, the number of joint axes, the joint architecture, and the size and position of adjacent tissue that may affect motion of a part. For example, the knee joint has one degree of freedom and a large range of motion, while the L5 vertebrae has six degrees of freedom and a limited range of motion. A range of motion can be expressed for each degree of freedom in a joint.

KINETICS

So far, only the movement itself without regard for the forces that cause the movement has been discussed. The study of these forces and the resultant energetics is called ***kinetics***. The forces that cause motion can be internal or external. Internal forces may result from muscle activity, ligaments, or from friction in the muscles and joints. External forces may come from the ground or from external loads, or from active bodies or passive sources (eg, wind resistance). Since most of these forces are not directly measurable, they can be calculated using readily available kinematic and anthropometric data. Three forces (gravity, ground reaction forces, and muscle/ligament forces) constitute all of the forces acting on the total body system.

The force exerted on an object as a result of gravitational pull is referred to as ***gravitational force***. This force may be considered as a single force representing the sum of all the individual weights within the object. For internal force calculations, gravitational forces act downward through the centers of mass of each segment and are equal to the magnitude of the mass times acceleration due to gravity.

The forces that act on the body as a result of interaction with the ground are called ground reaction forces (GRF). Newton's third law implies that GRF are equal and opposite to those that the body is applying to the ground. GRF are external forces which can be measured using a force transducer (force platform). GRF are distributed over an area of the body (ie, under the foot). For calculation purposes, GRF may be considered to act at a point so that the forces are represented as vectors. Under the foot, the point at which GRF act is referred to as the *center of pressure.*

Muscle and ligament forces can be calculated in terms of *net muscle moments* in order to represent the net effect of muscle activity at a joint. In the case of co-contraction at a joint, the analysis yields the net effect of both agonists and antagonists. The analysis includes any frictional effects at the joint or within the muscle. Increased friction reduces the net muscle moment so that the moments created by the muscle contractile elements are higher than the tendon moments. At the extreme end of range of movement, the passive structures such as ligaments become important in limiting movement. The moments generated by these passive structures then add or subtract from those produced by the muscle.

The previously described forces act on the total body. In analysis of internal forces, body segments must be examined one at a time. Joint reaction forces are the equal and opposite forces that exist between adjacent bones at a joint caused by the weight and inertial forces of the two segments. Bone-on-bone forces are seen across the articulating surfaces and include the effect of muscle activity. In actively contracting muscles, the articulating surfaces are pulled together, creating compressive forces. In this situation, the bone-on-bone force equals the compressive force due to muscle, plus the joint reaction forces.[1]

APPROACHES TO ANALYSIS OF MOVEMENT

The kinematics of a motion can be used to examine the forces that actually cause the movement to occur. Force and motion may be studied using one of three approaches that are based on Newton's laws of motion. The law of inertia states that if a resultant force acting on a body is 0, the body will remain at rest (if originally at rest) or will move with constant speed in a straight line (if originally in motion). The law of acceleration states that if the resultant force acting on a body is not 0, the body will have an acceleration proportional to the magnitude and in the direction of this resultant force. A third law of motion, the law of action/reaction, states that forces of action and reaction between bodies in contact have the same magnitude, same line of action, and opposite sense. These three laws form the basis for kinetic analysis using the acceleration, impulse-momentum, and work-energy approaches.

Acceleration Approach

Statics is defined as having acceleration equal to 0, so that the resultant force acting on the body is also 0. In dynamics, the resultant force is not equal to 0, therefore the body will accelerate. Since mass does not change, the force is proportional to the acceleration. Mass is the quantity determining the inertia of the body, therefore a large mass will have a large inertia. Units involved in the acceleration approach include Newtons for force, kilograms for mass, and meters/per second[2] for acceleration.

The acceleration approach can be used to convert weight (a force) to mass. For example, the mass of a man who weighs 667.5 N (150 pounds) would be equal to the force divided by gravity (9.8 m/s^2) or 68 kg. In another example of the acceleration approach to problem-solving, the resultant force required for a runner weighing 620 N (139 pounds.) to reach an acceleration of 28 m/s^2 would be:

$$F = (620 \text{ N} / 9.8 \text{ m/s}^2) \times 28 \text{ m/s}^2 = 1771 \text{ N}$$

Acceleration also is involved with angular motion. A force acting through a distance from the axis of rotation causes motion since the moment is not balanced as it is in statics. The law of acceleration, therefore, has several angular analogies or correlates. In angular motion, the mass is represented by the moment of inertia, which relates resistance of a mass to its distance from an axis. In angular terms, the linear formula F=ma becomes moment or torque equals moment of inertia multiplied by angular acceleration.

If the body is divided into many particles, each has a mass (m) and a perpendicular distance (r) from the axis. The sum of all the particles (mr^2) is the moment of inertia for the entire body. In linear terms, the center of mass represents the place at which the mass of the body is concentrated. In angular motion, this location is designated using the radius of gyration (k). An increase in either mass or distance from the axis will increase resistance of the body to angular acceleration (distance more so than mass since it is a squared term). For example, the k for a below knee prosthesis will influence how easily it swings (or the amount of resistance to movement) even more so than its mass. The placement of a leg cast also will influence resistance to motion more so than the mass of the cast.

If no external torque acts on a closed system, the total angular momentum remains unchanged even when the moment of inertia is changed. This principle often is expressed in athletics. A gymnast, high diver, or free-fall parachutist can regulate speed as the body rotates about its center of gravity by changing postures. If the extremities are tucked, the radius of gyration is shorter than when the extremities are abducted, so that the moment of inertia will be small and the body will spin rapidly about a transverse axis in the coronal plane. This is how the spinning figure skater can increase rotational speed by bringing the arms toward the center of the body. Conversely, the speed of rotation can be decreased by extending the extremities to increase the radius of gyration and increase the moment of inertia.

The following is an example of the acceleration approach to solve a human motion problem. A patient is able to hold the forearm in static equilibrium (Figure 5-2) using a muscle force of 108 N. How does the muscle force requirement change if the arm is accelerating at 80 rad/s^2 into elbow flexion? Almost three times as much muscle force is required when the forearm is accelerating compared to a static position. The potential for muscle tears and strains in ballistic types of movements is evident from this example.

Impulse-Momentum Approach

This approach is useful when the force involved in a dynamic problem acts over a period of time and is essential when a collision is involved. Impulses are forces developed during impact (eg, the product of force and time). The value of momentum will increase with an increase in force, the application of force over a longer period of time, or a combination of both. The direction of the velocity vector will be that of the resultant force, so that velocity will be increased or decreased depending on the direction of

Figure 5-2. Person holding a forearm weight. In the static position, the arm and weight are balanced using a muscle force of 108 N. If the arm is accelerating at 80 rad/s^2, the force required of the muscle must increase almost three times.

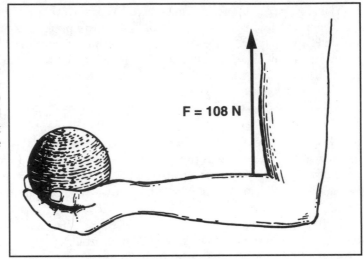

F = 108 N

the force. Whether the impact is delivered or received, its force will depend on the relative velocities of the colliding bodies. Thus, a greater impact force occurs when a hip impacts than when an elbow impacts because the trunk has a greater mass. When impact is made by elbow or knee extension (as in throwing or kicking), a greater velocity must be developed.

Applying force for a longer period of time increases the change in momentum. The impulse involved to stop a moving object corresponds directly to the change in momentum of the object so that the force and time of the impulse are inversely related. A longer time taken to stop a moving object will require less force by allowing an increased time for the momentum to change, as when the hand is allowed to go backward when catching a ball or when a person rolls to decrease the force of a fall. Conversely, an increased force will reduce the duration necessary to stop the object. Postural adjustments just prior to receiving an impact (such as using one's center of gravity, going with the direction of force, and prolonging the duration of impact) can decrease the force of impact. For example, a toppling force can be minimized by receiving impact as close as possible to the center of gravity. Impact force can be decreased by moving in the same direction as the force (eg, rolling with the punch).

Moment of inertia multiplied by the change in velocity represents the angular momentum of the rotating body. The torque applied to a rotating body is directly proportional to the product of its moment of inertia and angular velocity and inversely proportional to its duration. The angular impulse is defined as the torque times the duration of torque application, which equals the angular momentum. The change in angular momentum of a rotating body depends on the magnitude and direction of the torque and the duration of the torque applied.

A common example of angular impulse occurs during the gait cycle. Electromyographers have studied the coordinated action of the lower extremity muscles. These muscles exert a force over a period of time. The force in this case produces a torque which changes the angular momentum of the extremity. The impulse-momentum approach also may be applied to rotator cuff lesions which occur during throwing. The velocity involved in the angular momentum of the arm and ball is directed backward, then suddenly the direction of the angular velocity is changed by the internal rotator muscles as the throwing phase starts. The rapid change in angular momentum may produce immediate muscle or joint damage or a fracture of the humerus. Angular momentum also plays an important role in exercise. A quick, forceful muscular contraction at the beginning of the movement may produce sufficient impulse to allow the body part and exercise weight to move through the range of motion without further muscle contraction. This minimizes the strengthening effects of the exercise. Momentum of a body part often is used in stretching exercises. If the momentum caused by a large mass or velocity is too great, the tissues may not be capable of supplying sufficient force to stop the movement. The force needed may be greater than the rupture strength of the tissues, and they may tear. Prolonged stretching at low velocity will decrease the chances of injury.

Work-Energy Approach

When the forces acting on the system are known as a function of the position of the body, the work-energy approach is the more convenient method to solve for motion. Work is defined as a force overcoming a resistance and moving an object through a distance. Its value is determined by multiplying the force by the displacement of the object. If force is not in the same direction as the displacement, the component of force in the direction of the displacement must be used to determine the work done. The displacement must be along the same line and in the opposite direction to the resisting force of the object. For example, movement perpendicular to the force of gravity will produce no work against gravity. A component of applied force must be parallel to elastic resistance as in a spring or with friction for work to be done.

The unit of measure for work is the Newton-meter (Nm) or Joule. These units should not be confused with torque or moment which have similar units and are also defined as a force times distance. The resultant force producing work is concerned with a displacement and lies along the same line as the distance the object is moved. Conversely, the resultant force producing torque is perpendicular to a lever arm distance. A force producing torque also can produce work, but the correct distance must be used. By converting angular to linear motion, the work done during angular motion can be calculated (torque times angular displacement).

Work usually is considered a force that lifts an object against gravity, although this is not the only way to perform work. If a resultant force moves a resistance through a distance parallel to the line of action of the force, work is accomplished. For example, a spring, friction, and a balloon all resist force so that work is performed when movement occurs. Work is also performed when acceleration occurs. In Newton's second law, force causes acceleration of an object and the accelerated motion is parallel to the force. Negative work refers to the situation in which a force acts parallel to the movement but in the opposite direction. When a weight is lowered from a height with the force controlling the descent, negative work is said to occur. A spring, which is released gradually, or a moving object, which is decelerated are two additional examples of negative work.

Energy is the ability or capacity to do work. Although other forms of energy exist (eg, heat, light, nuclear, electrical), our focus is on mechanical energy. ***Potential energy (PE)*** is energy by position, due to gravity. Potential energy equals the work done to elevate an object. For example, a 20 kg barbell lifted 1 meter above the floor has a potential energy equal to the force needed to overcome gravity (F) times the height (h) above the floor (PE = F x h = mgh). Therefore, the barbell at this position has 20 kg (9.81 m/s^2) (1 m) or 196.2 J of potential energy. The units to measure energy are the same as those used to measure work, and the work done equals the potential energy of the object. When work is done to overcome gravity, the PE of the object is increased.

Kinetic energy (KE) of the body is defined as the energy of motion. The work done on an object equals the change in its kinetic energy. Any moving body must possess energy because a force must be exerted to stop it, and it cannot be stopped in zero distance. To start an object moving, force must be exerted over a distance.

The law of conservation of energy states that energy cannot be created or destroyed but may be transformed from one form to another. This law deals with the transmission, absorption, and dissipation of energy. The sum of potential energy and kinetic energy equals the total energy of the system. The principle of conservation of energy is that as potential energy decreases, the kinetic energy increases. Conversion of PE to KE in falls relates to mechanisms of injury. The KE at the instant of impact may be determined from the PE of the body before the fall, and the height of the body's center of mass at impact. For example, a 70 kg man who falls on his hip has a center of mass located at 70 cm above the floor. His PE while standing is (70 kg x 70 cm) equal to 4900 kgcm. Normally the KE at impact is dissipated by bones, ligaments, muscles, and other soft tissues so that the energy absorption is within tolerable limits. According to Frankel and Burstein, if the hip carries most of the impact, a fracture is likely to occur since the femoral neck cannot absorb over 60 kgcm.[2]

The speed of loading a body tissue is related to its energy absorption. Frankel reported that with the slow loading of a bone, a greater load will be needed to fracture it.[3] However, with a rapidly applied load, the bone will break with a high energy explosion, while slow loading produces low energy fractures. Noyes determined that the speed of loading affected the type of tissue damaged.[4] A fast loading produced more ligament failures, whereas a slow rate resulted in more avulsion fractures.

The quantity of work required for a certain task or movement does not address the amount of time needed for the task or movement to take place. For example, the same amount of work is done if a 10 kg weight is lifted 1 meter, whether the lifting is performed in 1 second or 1 minute. However, the power is different between the two situations. Power is the rate of doing work or the rate at which energy is expended. If the torque and angular velocity are known, the rotational power or development of rotational kinetic energy about an axis can be determined.

MUSCULOSKELETAL COMPONENTS

Because human movement is such a complex phenomenon, a number of simplifying assumptions are necessary for any analysis. For example, the dynamics section of this chapter describes methods of analysis in which the segments being moved are assumed to be rigid and the muscle forces are assumed to be in one direction. These assumptions ignore the complexity of both the bone and muscle structures, but allow the use of basic concepts in the study of human movement. Enoka described a "simple joint system" which is responsible for the production of human movement.[5] The system is composed of five parts: rigid link, synovial joint, muscle, neuron, and sensory receptors. The motor commands and sensory information must interact with the musculoskeletal components in order to produce and control movement. Description of these five components of the simple joint system follows.

Bone

The rigid link component of the simple joint system includes bone, tendon, and ligament. Bone has unique mechanical properties that allow it to provide rigid kinematic links and attachment sites for muscles, thereby facilitating muscle action and body movement. Strength and stiffness are the significant mechanical properties of bone. Bone strength, or the amount of force necessary to break bone, varies according to the angle and direction of force application. For example, Cowin found that a human femur has over twice as much tensile strength along the length of the bone as opposed to tensile strength perpendicular to the bone.[6] Because function has a direct effect on the mechanical characteristics of bone, it is strongest in the direction of most frequent stress. According to Alexander, bones are generally two to five times stronger than the forces they commonly encounter in everyday activities.[7]

The method of load application affects bone strength. For example, mature bone is strongest in compression. Additionally, bone increases in strength and stores more energy with increased speed of loading. The loading applied to bone through muscle activity alters the in vivo stress patterns in bone. Living bone is continually undergoing processes of growth, reinforcement, and reabsorption which together are referred to by Lanyon and Rubin as remodeling.[8] When the frequency of loading prevents the remodeling necessary to prevent failure, bone fatigues. Bone is laid down when needed and reabsorbed where not needed (Wolff's law) and remodels in response to mechanical demands. Examples are seen in the bone loss that occurs with space (no gravity) travel and with spinal cord injury (disuse osteoporosis). Conversely, bone hypertrophy often is seen in athletes who are routinely applying high loads to specific bones.

Tendon and Ligament

The tendons and ligaments surrounding the skeletal system are passive elements in the simple joint system in that they do not produce movement, but rather transmit movement. Tendons attach muscle to bone, and ligaments tie bone to bone. The structural organization of these two connecting links varies with the different function performed by each. Tendon and ligament are composed of three types of fibers: collagen, elastic, and reticulin fibers. The behavior of tendon and ligament is related to the structural orientation of these fibers, the properties of the collagen and elastic fibers, and the proportion between the collagen and elastic fibers. The function of tendon is to transmit force from muscle to bone or cartilage, therefore, its strength is needed in tension. The almost completely parallel alignment of the fibers provide tendons with high tension load tolerance (higher than that of ligament). The larger the cross-sectional area of the tendon, the more force it can withstand. Conversely, tendon can be deformed by small compressive and shear forces. Ligaments have a principle purpose of stabilizing joints, and ligament fibers are less consistently parallel than tendon fibers. Since joints may encounter forces that are tensile, compressive, or shear, the arrangement of fibers within a given ligament reflect the primary forces it must resist. They may be aligned in parallel, oblique, or spiral arrangements to accommodate forces in different directions.

The transition between bone and either tendon or ligament is gradual, creating a series of junctions instead of a marked change in structure. The bone-ligament and bone-tendon junctions are most susceptible to injury. However, all parts of the connecting links (ligament, tendon, and bony junctions) are affected by activity. Several investigators have shown that increased use results in increased strength of all parts of the connecting links and enhances the healing process.[9,10]

Synovial Joint

In the calculations made using rigid body link segments, the segments are assumed to be joined by frictionless pinned joints. Since the synovial joint most closely approximates these assumptions, it will be described as the joint component of the simple joint system. The surfaces of the bones that form the joint are lined with articular cartilage which functions to absorb impacts, to prevent direct wear to the bones, and to modify the shape of the bone to ensure better contact between the bones. The cartilage increases its thickness by increasing fluid absorption when a person goes from resting to active states. This increased thickness provides more protection during activity. The articulating surfaces are enclosed in a joint capsule that is covered internally with synovial membrane. The structure of the joint is quite variable and determines the quality of movement between two adjacent body segments. A joint will have one to three axes, referred to as degrees of freedom.

Muscle

Muscles are able to respond to a stimulus, propagate a wave of excitation, modify length, grow, and regenerate to a limited extent. Of the different types of human muscle, skeletal muscle most closely approximates the role needed in the simple joint system analysis (eg, to provide a force that interacts with those exerted by the environment on the system). Skeletal muscles act across joints to produce rotation of body segments (rigid links) about their joint.

The two most important elements of muscle function are the relationship between the sarcolemma and the sarcoplasmic reticulum and the components of the sarcomere. Sarcolemma is the cell membrane that surrounds each set of myofilaments that comprises a muscle fiber. The sarcolemma provides active and passive selective membrane transport in its function as an excitable membrane. Sarcoplasm is the fluid enclosed inside of the sarcolemma which contains fuel sources, organelles, enzymes, and contractile components (ie, myofilaments bundled into myofibrils). The sarcoplasm also contains a hollow membranous system that is linked to the surface sarcolemma and assists the muscle in conducting commands from the nervous system.

The sarcomere is the basic contractile unit of the muscle that is arranged in series, end to end, to form a myofibril. An interdigitating set of thick and thin contractile proteins, or myofilaments, comprises the sarcomere. The thin filament has two strands of actin molecules upon which are superimposed two-strand (tropomyosin) and globular (troponin) proteins. During a muscle contraction, the tropomyosin and troponin impose their influence on the activity of actin. The thick filament is comprised of the protein myosin, which can be decomposed into light meromyosin (LMM) and heavy meromyosin (HMM) fragments. The myosin molecules contain two regions of greater flexibility, so that the HMM fragment can extend from the thick filament to within close proximity of the thin filament. Because of this interaction with actin, the HMM extension has been called the crossbridge.

Neuron and Sensory Receptors

Discussion of the musculoskeletal components of the simple joint system have so far described the rigid link elements, the joint about which they rotate, and muscles that can exert a force on the rigid links. Basic information about the way muscles are activated is discussed in detail in Chapters 3 and 4, therefore, only brief mention will be made here. The nervous system is comprised of neurons which have the common functions of receiving information, determining if a signal should be transmitted, and transmitting the electrical signal. In the simple joint system, the neural elements of greatest interest are the motoneurons because they innervate the skeletal muscles. The motor end plate (neuromuscular junction) is where the electrical energy of the nerve action potential is transferred to chemical energy in the form of a neurotransmitter. On the muscle side of the junction, the neurotransmitter (chemical energy) is converted back to electrical energy with the final product being a muscle action potential. The final component of the simple joint system is the sensory receptor. The function of sensory receptors is to provide feedback to the system about its state and the environment via conversion of energy from one form to another (transduction).

APPLICATIONS TO PRODUCTION AND CONTROL OF MOVEMENT

Control of Muscle Force

Excitation Factors

Control of muscle force is dependent on the excitation of the force-generating units and the characteristics of these force-generating units (muscle mechanics and muscle architecture). Excitation factors important to regulation of muscle force include the number of motor units activated (motor-unit recruitment) and the rate at which each of the active motor units generates action potentials (rate coding). Movement is accomplished through the orderly recruitment of motor units so that as muscle force increases, additional motor units are activated. Once a motor unit is activated, it remains active until the force declines. The force reaches a plateau when no additional motor units are recruited and is reduced by the sequential deactivation of motor units. This derecruitment occurs in the reverse order of recruitment. For some muscles (eg, adductor pollicis), all motor units are probably recruited at 30% of maximum force level. According to Kukulka and Clamann,[11] other muscles (eg, biceps brachii) probably continue to recruit motor units up to 85% of maximum force level. The increase in muscle force beyond the motor-unit recruitment level is due to rate coding.

Although several hypotheses have been advanced to account for orderly recruitment, there is no agreement on a single mechanism.[12] The size principle proposed by Henneman suggests that the orderly recruitment of motor units is due to variations in motoneuron size, so that the motor unit with the smallest motoneuron is recruited first and the motor unit with the largest motoneuron is recruited last.[13] Recruitment order also may be influenced by morphological and electrical characteristics of the motoneuron. Since recruitment order is predetermined, the brain does not have to specify which motor units are to be activated, and motor units cannot be selectively activated.

Generally, the small motoneurons appear to innervate the slow-contracting, low-force, and fatigue-resistant motor units (Type S), whereas the largest motoneurons innervate the fast-contracting, high force, fatigable motor units (Type FF). According to Stuart and Enoka, the considerable overlap which occurs between the motor unit types makes selective activation of only one type of motor-unit or muscle fiber type (slow-twitch vs fast-twitch) highly unlikely.[12]

The force exerted by a muscle results from variable combinations of the number of active motor units and the rate at which these motor units discharge action potentials (rate coding). The relationship between muscle force and action potential rate (frequency) is nonlinear, with the greatest increase in force occurring at the lower action-potential rates (3 to 10 Hz). This relationship shifts depending on the length of the muscle, with the frequency affecting the greatest force changes being 3 to 7 Hz for long muscle lengths and 10 to 20 Hz for short muscle lengths. Gydikov and Kosarov[14] proposed two types of motor units (tonic and phasic) which differ in their muscle force/action-potential relationships. For tonic motor units, discharge rate increases as muscle force increases, but remains constant at high forces. Conversely, the discharge rate of phasic motor units increases over the entire range of muscle forces (linear relationship). In addition, the tonic motor units generate smaller action potentials, are recruited at lower muscle forces, and are less fatigable. The phasic motor units appear to be important for dynamic conditions and contribute more to muscle force than do the tonic units. Increases in muscle force result from increases in the concurrent processes of recruitment and rate coding. Harrison suggested that the relative contribution of recruitment and rate coding depends on the distribution of motor-unit mechanical properties.[15]

Another aspect of rate coding that affects force production is the relationship in time between an action potential and other action potentials generated by the same and other motor units (temporal patterning). Burke, Rundomin, and Zajac described the "catch" property of muscle as the discharge of two action potentials (a doublet) from one motor unit within a short time interval (ie, 10 ms) which produces a substantial increase in the force exerted by the motor unit.[16] According to Gydikov and associates, the occurrence of these doublets represents a rate coding effect which probably varies from muscle to muscle and may depend upon the task (concentric vs eccentric).[17] Milner-Brown et al[18] proposed that an increase in motor-unit synchronization (where the motor units of a muscle discharge action potentials at similar instants in time) also will result in greater muscle force.

Muscle Mechanics

The characteristics of the force-generating units in the muscle influence the force that a muscle exerts and are referred to as muscle mechanics. External mechanical variables such as length, velocity, power, and force are interdependent with the internal contractile state (ie, rate of action potential occurrence). According to the sliding-filament theory, the development of force depends on attach-detach cycles of the crossbridges extending from thick filaments to the thin filaments. The greater the number of these cycles, the greater the force generated. Since force exertion occurs only during the attachment phase, the thick and thin filaments must be close enough for the attachment to occur. In this way, the length of the muscle influences force generation since tension varies as the amount of overlap between thick and thin filaments within a sarcomere varies.

Force generation is not only dependent on the active process of crossbridge cycling via changing muscle length. The connective tissue structures within muscle (ie, sarcolemma, endomysium, perimysium, epimysium, tendon) exert a passive force when stretched. This passive force combines with the active contribution of crossbridge activity to produce the total muscle force. At shorter muscle lengths, all of the force generated is due to crossbridge activity, whereas at longer lengths most of the total muscle force is due to the passive elements. The greatest overlap of thick and thin filaments occurs at a muscle length that is about midway between the minimal and maximal lengths (typically the resting length of the muscle).

Human movement is caused primarily by rotary forces (torque), so that the relationship between muscle length and muscle torque is of primary importance. Three factors influence this relationship: fiber arrangements, number of joints, and moment arm. Most body movements are controlled by groups of muscles as opposed to a single muscle, and these muscles may have different arrangements of their fibers (eg, fusiform, pinnate, bipinnate). This means that at any specific joint position, the fibers in the muscles crossing the joint may be at different positions on their force-length curves. Since a number of muscles cross more than one joint (eg, rectus femoris, semitendinosus, gastrocnemius), their length and force-generating abilities are influenced by more than one joint. Torque is the product of force and moment arm (perpendicular distance from the line of action of the muscle force vector to the joint axis). Since this moment arm distance changes with joint position, variations in muscle torque represent the interaction of moment-arm and muscle length effects.

The relationship between the net muscle torque and the torque due to a load will determine whether the lengths of active muscles shorten (concentric), lengthen (eccentric), or remain unchanged (isometric). Torque-angle relationships have been found to remain the same regardless of whether the measurements were isometric, concentric, or eccentric muscle actions. The general effect of these muscle action types is to shift the relationship up and down the vertical axis such that the greatest torques are exerted eccentrically and the least concentrically.

Concentric and eccentric muscle torques are generated with changing muscle lengths, therefore their torques are dependent on the magnitude and direction of the rate of change in length (velocity of muscle action). Although the rate of crossbridge attachment-detachment increases as the shortening speed increases, the average force exerted by each crossbridge decreases, and there may be fewer crossbridges formed as the muscle shortens more quickly. Since the energy used by the muscle increases (due to increased crossbridge detachment) with shortening speed while the torque exerted decreases, the muscle becomes less efficient (work output/energy input) with increases in the discrepancy between the muscle and load torques. The maximum torque under the three muscle action conditions varies as eccentric is greater than isometric, which is greater than concentric.

Several theories have been advanced to explain why a muscle can exert greater torque eccentrically than concentrically, although none have been proven. The mechanism responsible for crossbridge detachment may differ, thus altering the duration of the attachment phase and the force exerted by the crossbridge. A second possibility proposed by Hoyle may involve an enhancement of the contractile machinery activity by either increasing the quantity of calcium released or by stretching the less completely activated sarcomeres within each myofibril.[19] Training studies have shown that the eccentric activation of muscle is closely associated with muscle soreness that occurs 42 to 48 hours after exercise.[20,21] Two theories commonly cited to account for the soreness are the muscle spasm and structural damage theories. The muscle spasm theory espoused by de Vries suggests that exercise induced ischemia allows the transfer of a substance (called P) across the muscle cell membrane and into the tissue extracellular fluid, activating pain nerve endings that elicit reflex activity in the form of a muscle spasm.[22] The structural damage theory suggests that damage to connective tissue and/or muscle fibers occurs which activates sensory neurons due to the accumulation of metabolites.[23-25]

Positive work by a muscle occurs when a muscle shortens and the force it exerts causes an object to move. Negative work occurs when a muscle lengthens while exerting a force on the object that is moved. As discussed previously, work is defined as the product of force and distance. Therefore, an isometric muscle action where the object is not moved involves no mechanical work. This does not address the metabolic work required for any muscle action including isometric. Since the rate of doing work is referred to as power, the rate of positive work or work done by the muscle is indicated as power production. Power absorption describes the rate of doing work on the muscle. Power production is limited by the rate at which energy is supplied for the muscle contraction (ie, ATP production) and the rate at which the myofilaments can convert chemical energy into mechanical work.[26] Power is determined as the product of the force and velocity of the muscle contraction. Maximum power occurs when the force being exerted is about one-third of the maximum isometric force. Any effect on either force or velocity will alter power. Muscle temperature mainly affects contraction speed and influences the peak power production.

Muscle architecture (how sarcomeres are arranged within the muscle) affects the force exerted by the muscle on the rigid link. The three major architectural influences are the average number of sarcomeres per muscle fiber (in-series effect), the number of fibers in parallel (in-parallel effect), and the angle at which the fibers are oriented relative to the line of pull of the muscle (ie, the degree of pinnation). The greater the number of sarcomeres in series, the greater will be the change of length of the myofibril and the rate of change in length to a given stimulus. Muscle fiber force is proportional to the number of myofibrils in parallel (cross sectional area of muscle). The advantage of pinnation (angles of muscle fiber from the line of pull of the muscle) is that a greater number of fibers, and thus sarcomeres, in parallel can be packed into a given volume of muscle.

Muscles can have fibers arranged with a common angle of pinnation (unipinnate), with two sets of fibers at different pinnation angles (bipinnate), or with many sets of fibers at a variety of angles (multipinnate). Muscle fibers aligned with a zero angle of pinnation are usually described as having fusiform or parallel arrangement. Since a muscle fiber consists of myofibrils arranged in parallel, and a myofibril represents a series arrangement of sarcomeres, the muscle fibers actually comprise an in-series and an in-parallel collection of force-generating units. A long, small diameter muscle fiber represents a dominant in-series effect and, conversely, a short, large diameter fiber mainly exhibits in-parallel characteristics. Muscles are designed to capitalize on these characteristics, as evidenced by the antigravity muscles that are generally twice as strong as their antagonists and demonstrate correspondingly larger physiological cross sectional areas.

In addition to these whole muscle effects of sarcomere arrangement, at least two other design factors influence the torque a muscle can exert. These are the points of attachment of the muscle relative to the joint and the proportion of whole muscle length that contains contractile protein. The angle of pull and thus the proportion of muscle force that contributes to rotation depends on the distances from each end of the muscle to the joint and the joint angle. The major effects of varying these parameters on the torque have been summarized by van Mameren and Drukker.[27] The torque-angle relationship has a sharper peak when the distances to each end of the muscle from the joint are equal. When either side of the muscle is a much greater distance than the other from the joint, the maximum torque values are attainable over a greater range of joint angles. Peak torque is reached closer to full extension when the muscle distances are equal and occurs closer to midrange position when the distances are markedly different. The maximum torque exerted by the muscle is greater when the distances are different and when the proportion of whole muscle length containing contractile protein is greater. Muscles that have different lengths do not gain much torque by increasing the whole muscle contractile length.

Patterns of Muscle Activation

Muscle Organization

Muscle activity patterns represent a combined effect of the type of movement desired and the functional and structural restraints of our bodies. Structural restraints refer to the organization of muscles around the joint, which varies throughout the body. The structure of the joint largely determines the quality of motion that can occur between two segments. The number of movements that a joint permits defines the degrees of freedom of the joint. Movable joints have a minimum of one (eg, elbow) and a maximum of three (eg, hip and shoulder) degrees of freedom. A minimum of one pair of muscles must cross a joint to control each degree of freedom, although usually several muscles contribute to the same action. The main difference between these groups of muscles is their points of attachment and thus their mechanical action.

The attachment points may vary in three ways: by moment arm, by action, and by postural position. In the first variation, the changes in moment arm distances are maximized for one muscle over one part of the range of motion and for another muscle over another part of the range. For example, the further a muscle attachment is from a joint, the greater the velocity of muscle shortening for a particular angular velocity of the extremity, but the greater the variation in the moment arm. In the second variation, muscles can contribute to different actions, as in the biceps brachii assisting with elbow flexion and forearm supination because of its attachment on the radial tuberosity. In the third variation, suggested by Lexell and associates, one muscle in the group may be more ideally located to assist with the maintenance of posture so that muscles involved with maintaining upright posture tend to be closer to the long bone of the segment.[28] In addition, muscles may span more than one joint. Some investigators have asserted that two joint muscles simplify the control of movement for the central nervous system (CNS).[29,30]

Net Muscle Activity

The mechanical effect of muscular activity can be quantified as resultant muscle force and resultant muscle torque. Two limitations to this approach are the method used to determine resultant muscle torque and nonmuscular contributions. Resultant muscle torque is calculated as the residual moment from the Newtonian equations of motion. Free-body and mass acceleration diagrams are composed for dynamic analysis and the moments of force are identified (Figure 5-3). Values for all of the terms are known except for the resultant muscle torque, and so the expression is rearranged to solve for the unknown. This unknown is referred to as the residual moment because it represents

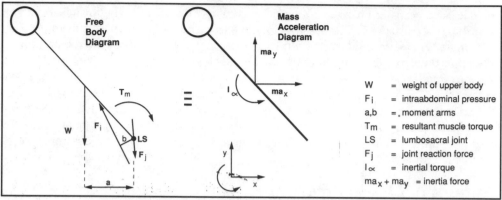

Figure 5-3. Free body diagram (FBD) and mass acceleration diagram (MAD) showing the trunk of a person standing up from a squat.

any difference in the kinematic effect and the moments of force. Two limitations associated with this procedure are that other structures (eg, ligaments, joint capsule) in addition to muscle can contribute to the residual torque, and that residual torque does not represent the absolute quantity of muscle activity.

Despite these limitations, the mechanics of movement still can be used to deduce the net muscle activity. By comparing the directions of the resultant muscle torque vector and the segment rotation in dynamic analysis, the net muscle activity can be determined as concentric or eccentric. If the directions of the resultant muscle torque vector and the segment rotation are the same, then the muscle group is experiencing a concentric muscle action. Conversely, if the directions of the resultant muscle torque vector and the segment rotation are opposite, then the muscle group is experiencing an eccentric muscle action. In addition, the orientation of the body relative to the direction of gravity will affect the pattern of muscle activation (eg, upright standing versus supine). These analyses apply only to quasistatic conditions where the accelerations of the system and its parts are very small. In fast movements, different types of contact forces (joint reaction, ground reaction, fluid resistance, elastic, inertial and muscle forces) become large and substantially alter the pattern of muscle activity necessary to control the movement. For these fast movements, a complete dynamic analysis is required.

Measurement of electromyographic (EMG) activity provides a picture of the total neural drive to a muscle and can provide information about force relationships that are difficult to measure using other means. Three examples (moment arm effects, three burst pattern, and co-contraction) provide an overview of the ways in which EMG can assist in the understanding of the neural signals sent by segmental centers. Although the relationship between muscle force and EMG is complex, EMG is related to force in a predictable manner under isometric conditions. Using the isometric condition, the EMG angle relationship is inversely related to the changes in moment arm. As a second example, a three burst pattern of EMG has been shown for both biphasic and unidirectional movements. The three burst pattern for unidirectional movements appears to be related to the stopping of a movement at a targeted position, but the control strategy adopted by the central nervous system has not yet been determined. The three burst pattern is drastically affected by the features of movement (eg, instructions given to the subject) and by the mechanical conditions (eg, orientation of the subject, inclusion of more than one muscle in a movement). Lastly, co-contraction also has been observed using EMG and is a variable characteristic of the three burst pattern. Since co-contraction has the mechanical effect of making a joint stiffer, it would seem to be a useful feature for learning novel tasks or performing high accuracy movements. According to Husan, under certain conditions co-contraction decreases the cost of performing a movement.[31] Other investigators have found that the neural strategy involved in performing co-contraction is different from that of more normal activities (eg, supporting a load).[32]

Posture Requirements and Responses

The execution of any movement must be accompanied by maintenance of postural stability and equilibrium. This postural stability may be static (maintenance of upright standing posture) or dynamic (maintenance of balance during movement). See Chapter 11 for a review of balance mechanisms.

Gait

Transfer Function of Muscles

The pattern of muscle activity during gait has been used as a way to observe muscle group interaction during walking. Inman et al[33] reported that EMG produced a waveform which reflected the muscle force waveform. Winter suggested that electromechanical delays between the neural command and the muscle response are recognized by the CNS, as evidenced by both early activation and early deactivation of muscles.[34] These patterns are evident in the tibialis anterior (TA) and soleus (S) muscles during walking (Figure 5-4). TA reaches peak activity just before heel contact (HC) so dorsiflexor tension reaches its peak just after HC (so that ground reaction forces which will attempt to plantarflex the foot are resisted). Similarly, at the end of stance, TA reaches its peak activity exactly at toe-off (TO), but dorsiflexor tension does not increase to a reasonable level until about 5% after TO, when it dorsiflexes the foot for toe clearance. At the end of stance, about 200 ms before TO, the S activity reaches its peak and suddenly drops off to near-zero 100 ms before TO. This sudden derecruitment of the plantarflexors reflects the need to decrease the plantarflexor force from its peak at about 100 ms before TO to near-zero at TO. If this plantarflexor activation had continued until TO, there would be a large plantarflexor moment into early swing which would prevent the rapid dorsiflexion of the foot necessary for safe toe clearance.

Inertia of Extremity Segments

Moments of inertia for individual segments are required for the generation of appropriate acceleration profiles. This information is especially important during the swing phase of gait when the thigh and leg/foot segments are initially accelerated and then decelerated prior to HC. The moments of force cannot be too high or too low if correct trajectories are to be achieved. For example, the foot segment must achieve a low but safe toe clearance, and the heel must decelerate to near-zero velocity prior to HC. The trajectory patterns during swing are extremely consistent as evidenced by the intra-subject repeat assessment done days apart or minutes apart by Winter.[35] This consistency suggests that the CNS accounted for the segment inertia and generated the appropriate moment of force. Ralston and Lukin added weight to the leg and reported increased kinetic energy changes of the leg and foot.[36]

Figure 5-4. Electromyographic patterns of the soleus and tibialis anterior during walking (adapted from Winter DA. *CNS Strategies in Human Gait*, with permission of Gordon and Breach Science Publishers, S.A., © 1989).

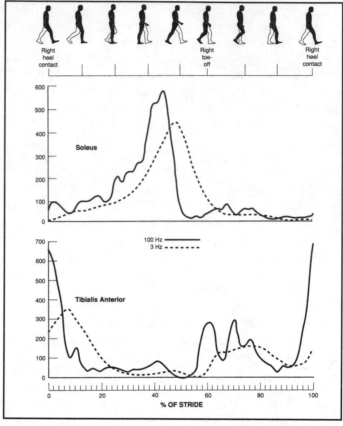

Gravitation Forces

Another factor evident from the consistent swing phase trajectories is the contribution of gravitational forces to the acceleration and deceleration of the swinging leg. During the swing phase of gait, the thigh and leg/foot form a double pendulum system which is influenced by gravitational moments. During early swing, gravity assists the forward acceleration of the leg and foot, and at the end of the swing it assists in its decelerating prior to HC. The knee's gravitational moment increases from TO to a maximum during early swing (at maximum knee flexion). Here, gravity assists in decelerating the backward rotating leg and then is the major contributor to its forward acceleration. During late swing, the leg is decelerated until HC, with the gravitational component being somewhat less, but still important. The active contribution of the knee extensors is only about 20% to the leg's acceleration with gravity adding about 50% and the knee acceleration couple about 30%. However, during the deceleration in late swing, the knee flexors are responsible for about 80% of the joint moment of force. The CNS must recognize these nonmuscular contributions since the gravitational component remains constant when walking is slow, but total inertial moment decreases.

Interextremity Coupling

A third contributor to the leg's acceleration during walking is interextremity coupling. During the swing phase, the angular acceleration of the thigh by the hip flexors/extensors causes a linear acceleration at the knee. This acceleration results in a reaction force at the knee, so that a couple is created to assist in the leg's acceleration and deceleration. This acceleration component usually is more important than the active muscle moment, so that the hip extensors must become active to create a reaction force at the knee that assists in the acceleration of the distal segments. This coupling strategy is used by persons with above-knee amputations to swing their prosthetic leg.

During the stance phase of gait, control of the knee joint is essential for safe and efficient weight bearing. The ankle and hip joints assist in the control of the knee joint, creating a total extremity synergy referred to by Winter as the support moment.[37] This support moment is calculated to recognize interextremity coupling such that above or below normal extensor moments at the hip and ankle have a direct control of the knee joint. For example, hyperactivity of the plantarflexors during mid-stance will slow down or stop the forward rotation of the leg over the foot, and thereby reduce knee flexion (or even cause the knee to hyperextend). Similarly, hyperactivity of the hip extensors early in stance will cause a backward rotation of the thigh and the knee flexion again is reduced. Such interextremity coupling gives greater flexibility to the CNS to accomplish the same knee control in more than one way.

Eccentric-Concentric Muscle Action

As previously mentioned, muscle force decreases as the velocity of shortening (concentric muscle action) increases, and increases as the velocity of lengthening (eccentric muscle action) increases. In order to generate the correct muscle force, the CNS activation must be altered depending on the lengthening or shortening velocity. The same level of activation may result in markedly different levels of force. This velocity effect is less important during slow walking than during faster walking.

Overall Control of Gait

In addition to these control factors, a total control strategy must be incorporated that supports the body during stance (prevents collapse of the lower extremity), maintains upright posture and balance of the trunk in both anterior-posterior and medial-lateral directions, and controls the foot trajectory to achieve safe ground clearance and gentle heel or toe landing. The first two tasks are regulatory, occur during the stance phase of gait, and involve high forces. The third task is cyclical, occurs primarily during the swing phase of gait, and involves low forces.

SUMMARY

The musculoskeletal system exhibits characteristics that influence the production and control of any movement. Kinematics and kinetics are basic to an understanding of the role that these musculoskeletal characteristics play in movement production and control. Three approaches can be used to solve kinetic problems with the approach of choice dependent on the information available (ie, acceleration approach, impulse-momentum approach, and work-energy approach). The role that the musculoskeletal components play also is influenced by their individual structures and by the way that the individual structures work together during different types of movement. The control of muscle force and the patterns of muscle activation create numerous strategies available to the CNS for execution of movement. Walking is an example of one activity that demonstrates the interaction of musculoskeletal components in movement production and control.

REFERENCES

1. Winter DA. *Biomechanics and Motor Control of Human Movement.* 2nd ed. New York, NY: John Wiley & Sons, Inc; 1990.

2. Frankel VH, Burstein AH. *Orthopaedic Biomechanics—The Application of Engineering to the Musculoskeletal System.* Philadelphia, Pa: Lea & Febiger; 1970.

3. Frankel VH. Biomechanics of the locomotor system. In: CD Ray, ed. *Medical Engineering,.* Chicago, Ill: Year Book Medical Publisher; 1974:505-516.

4. Noyes FR, Torvik PJ, Hyde WB, et al. Biomechanics of ligament failure. *J Bone Joint Surg.* 1974;56A:1406-1418.

5. Enoka RM. *Neuromechanical Basis of Kinesiology.* Champaign, Ill: Human Kinetics Books; 1988.

6. Cowin SC. The mechanical and stress adaptive properties of bone. *Ann Biomed Eng.* 1983; 11:263-295.

7. Alexander AM. Optimal strengths for bones liable to fatigue and accidental fracture. *J Theor Biol.* 1984;109:621-636.

8. Lanyon LE, Rubin CT. Static vs dynamic loads as an influence on bone remodelling. *J Biomech.* 1984;17:897-905.

9. Woo SL-Y, Ritter MA, Amiel D, et al. The biomechanical and biochemical properties of swine tendons—long term effects of exercise on the digital extensors. *Connect Tissue Res.* 1980;7:177-183.

10. Vailas AC, Tipton CM, Mashes RD, et al. Physical activity and its influence on the repair process of medial collateral ligaments. *Connect Tissue Res.* 1981;9:25-31.

11. Kukulka CG, Clamann HP. Comparison of the recruitment and discharge properties of motor units in human brachial biceps and adductor pollicis during isometric contractions. *Brain Res.* 1981;219:45-55.

12. Stuart DG, Enoka RM. Motoneurons motor units and the size principle. In WD Willis, ed. *The Clinical Neurosciences: Sec. 5 Neurology.* New York, NY: Churchill Livingston; 1983: 471–517.

13. Henneman E. Relation between size of neurons and their susceptibility to discharge. *Science.* 1957;126:1345-1347.

14. Gydikov A, Kosarov D. Physiological characteristics of the tonic and phasic motor units in human muscles. In: Gydikov AA, Tankov NT, Kosarov DS, eds. *Motor Control.* New York, NY: Plenum; 1973:75–94.

15. Harrison PJ. The relationship between the distribution of the motor unit mechanical properties and the forces due to recruitment and to rate coding for the generation of muscle force. *Brain Res.* 1983;264:311-315.

16. Burke RE, Rundomin P, Zajac FE. The effect of activation history on tension production by individual muscle units. *Brain Res.* 1976;109:515-529.

17. Gydikov AA, Kossev AR, Kosarov DS, et al. Investigations of single motor units firing during movements against elastic resistance. In: Jonsson B, ed. *Biomechanics X-A.* Champaign, Ill: Human Kinetics; 1987:227–232.

18. Milner-Brown HS, Stein RB, Lee RG. Synchronization of human motor units: possible roles of exercise and supraspinal reflexes. *Electroencephalogr Clin Neurophysio.* 1975; l38:245-254.

19. Hoyle G. *Muscles and Their Neural Control.* New York, NY: Wiley; 1983.

20. Armstrong RB, Ogilvie RW, Schwane JA. Eccentric exercise-induced injury to rat skeletal muscle. *J Appl Physiol.* 1983;54:80-93.

21. Komi PV, Buskirk ER. Effect of eccentric and concentric muscle conditioning on tension and electrical activity of human muscle. *Ergonomics.* 1972;15:417-434.

22. de Vries HA. Quantitative electromyographic investigation of the spasm theory of muscle pain. *Am J Phys Med Rehabil.* 1966;45:119-134.

23. Abmham DWM. Factors in delayed muscle soreness. *Med Sci Sports Exerc.* 1977;9:11-20.

24. Kuipers H, Drukker J, Frederik PM, et al. Muscle degeneration after exercise in rats. *Int J Sports Med.* 1983;4:45-59.

25. Armstrong RB. Mechanisms of exercise-induced delayed onset muscular soreness: a brief review. *Med Sci Sports Exerc.* 1984;16:529-538.

26. Weis-Fogh T, Alexander RM. The sustained power output from striated muscle. In: Pedley TJ, ed. *Scale Effects in Animal Locomotion.* London, England: Academic Press; 1977: 511–525.

27. van Mameren H, Drukker J. Attachment and composition of skeletal muscle in relation to their function. *J Biomech.* 1979;12:859-867.

28. Lexell J, Henriksson-Larsen K, Sjostrom M. Distribution of different fibre types in human skeletal muscle: 2. A study of cross-sections of whole muscles vastus lateralis. *Acta Physiol Scand.* 1983;117:115-122.

29. Fujiwara M, Basmajian JV. Electromyographic study of two-joint muscles *Am J Phys Med Rehabil.* 1975;54:234-242.

30. Mussa-Naldi FA, Hogan N, Bizzi E. Neural, mechanical and geometric factors subserving arm posture in humans. *J Neurosci.* 1985;5:2732-2743.

31. Husan Z. Optimized movement trajectories and joint stiffness in unperturbed, inertially loaded movements. *Biol Cybern.* 1986;53:373-382.

32. Gydikov A, Kossev A, Radicheva N, et al. Interaction between reflexes and voluntary motor activity in man revealed by discharges of separate motor units. *Exp Neurol.* 1981; 73:331-344.

33. Inman VT, Ralston Ad, Saunders JB, et al. Relation of human electromyogram to muscular tension. *Electroencephalogr Clin Neurophysio.* 1952;l4:187-194.

34. Winter DA. CNS strategies in human gait: implications for FES control. *Automedica.* 1989;11:163-174.

35. Winter DA. *The Biomechanics and Motor Control of Human Gait.* Waterloo, Canada: University of Waterloo Press; 1987.

36. Ralston HJ, Lukin L. Energy levels of human body segments during level walking. *Ergonomics.* 1969;12:39-46.

37. Winter DA. Overall principle of lower extremity support during stance phase of gait. *J Biomech.* 1980;13:923-927.

SUGGESTED READINGS

Beer FP, Johnston ER. *Vector Mechanics for Engineers Static and Dynamics.* 3rd ed. Baltimore, Md: Williams & Wilkins; 1986.

Cavanagh PR, Lafortune MA. Ground reaction forces in distance running. *J Biomech.* 1979; 13:397-406.

Cochran G. *A Primer of Orthopaedic Biomechanics.* New York, NY: Churchill Livingston; 1982.

Dhanjoo NG. *Osteoarthromechanics.* Washington, District of Columbia; Hemisphere Pub Co; 1982.

Frankel VH, Nordin M, eds. **Basic Biomechanics of the Skeletal System.** Philadelphia, Pa: Lea & Febiger; 1980.

Friederich JA, Brand RA. Muscle fiber architecture in the human lower extremity. *J Biomech*. 1990; 23(1):91-95.

Frost HM. *An Introduction to Biomechanics*. Springfield, Ill: Charles C. Thomas, Pub; 1980.

Fung YC. *Biomechanics: Mechanical Properties of Living Tissues*. New York, NY: Springer-Verlag; 1981.

Goldick HD. *Mechanics, Heat, and the Human Body: An Introduction to Physics*. Upper Saddle River, NJ: Prentice-Hall Inc; 2001.

Hay JG. *The Biomechanics of Sports Techniques*. 2nd ed. Englewood Cliffs, NJ: Prentice-Hall Inc; 1966.

Levangie PK, Norkin CC. *Joint Structure and Function*. 3rd ed. Philadelphia, Pa: FA Davis; 2001.

LeVeau BF. *Williams and Lissner: Biomechanics of Human Motion*. 3rd ed. Philadelphia, Pa: WB Saunders Co;1992.

Miller DI, Nelson RC. *Biomechanics of Sports*. Philadelphia, Pa; Lea & Febiger: 1976.

Radin EL, Simon SR, Rose RM, et al. *Practical Biomechanics for the Orthopedic Surgeon*. New York, NY: John Wiley & Sons; 1979.

Rodgers MM, Cavanagh PR. Glossary of biomechanical terms, concepts, and units. *Phys Ther.* 1984;64:1886-1902.

Schafer RC. *Clinical Biomechanics: Musculoskeletal Actions and Reactions*. 2nd ed. Baltimore, Md: Williams & Wilkins; 1987.

Shames IH. *Engineering Mechanics*. 2nd ed. Englewood Cliffs, NJ: Prentice-Hall Inc; 1966.

Soderberg GL. *Kinesiology: Application to Pathological Motion*. Baltimore, Md: Williams & Wilkins; 1986.

Wiktorin C, Nordin M. *Introduction to Problem Solving in Biomechanics*. Philadelphia, Pa: Lea & Febiger; 1986.

Case Studies

Patricia C. Montgomery, PhD, PT
Barbara H. Connolly, EdD, PT, FAPTA

INTRODUCTION

Students, new graduates, or clinicians inexperienced in the management of patients with pathology involving the nervous system may have difficulty integrating theory with practice. A problem-solving approach can be helpful in developing skills in the practical application of examination, evaluation, and intervention strategies. To facilitate a problem-solving approach, we have selected five case studies that represent common clinical problems encountered by the practitioner. Contributing authors were asked to identify functional limitations, impairments, treatment goals, and functional outcomes to address the problems observed in each of these patients. A brief composite clinical picture of each patient is presented in this chapter and should be reviewed before proceeding to the subsequent chapters. The conceptual framework of the *Guide to Physical Therapist Practice* is reviewed and applied to three of the patients in the case studies in Chapter 7. Additional information about all five patients gathered from the examination and specific tests and measures is provided throughout the text. In the final chapter, a summary of each patient's status, current intervention strategies, and discharge plan is provided.

CASE STUDY # 1
Jane Smith

CURRENT STATUS

Mrs. Smith is a 74-year-old woman who is 6 months post onset of her cardiovascular accident (CVA) and comes into a rehabilitation facility two times per month as an outpatient to receive physical therapy.

HISTORY

Mrs. Smith has a medical history of hypertension, peripheral vascular disease, and bilateral endarterectomies. She is retired, but has remained active with her hobbies including gardening, sewing, and bowling. She is married with two grown children and four grandchildren. She lives with her husband in a split-level home. She has to go upstairs to the bedroom and downstairs to the laundry area. There are three steps to enter the home and to reach the mailbox she has to go down a small incline in the driveway.

Six months ago, Mrs. Smith woke up in the morning with a right hemiparesis and marked aphasia. Her husband brought her into the emergency room of the local hospital where she received medical treatment.

Four days following onset of her CVA, Mrs. Smith was evaluated by physical, occupational, and speech therapists. The initial physical therapy examination noted that she was oriented and cooperative, but with severe expressive aphasia. She could say "yes" and "no," but her responses were unreliable. Her right upper extremity was flaccid; she had adductor and extensor stiffness in the right lower extremity. She needed maximal assistance to roll, for all transfers, and activities of daily living (ADLs) and could not stand and bear weight on the right leg. Her sitting balance was fair, and she had poor sensation on the right side of her body. Her occupational and speech therapy examinations indicated that her limb apraxia interfered with performance on language and ADL tasks. She had severe verbal apraxia with moderate to marked aphasia. Verbal production was limited to isolated episodes of automatic speech.

Two weeks following onset, Mrs. Smith was transferred to the rehabilitation unit in another facility. The physical therapy examination at that time indicated Grade 2 strength in the right hip and knee musculature with the muscles around the ankle and foot at Grade 1. Rolling to the right could be accomplished with minimal assistance and to the left with moderate assistance of one other adult. Mrs. Smith needed assistance in pivot transfers, coming from sit to stand, balancing in standing, and with maneuvering her wheelchair. She required frequent verbal cues because of severe neglect of the right side. A hinged ankle foot orthosis (AFO) was ordered for her right lower extremity. She also was demonstrating perseveration in dressing and difficulty with sequencing tasks. Reading comprehension was good, but she was able only to use gestures and automatic speech to communicate.

Mrs. Smith was in the rehabilitation unit for 3 months. She then returned home and was seen as an outpatient three times per week by a physical therapist, occupational therapist, and speech therapist for 2 months, then one time per week for 1 month by each therapist. She is now being seen twice monthly by physical and occupational therapists and weekly by a speech therapist.

SYSTEMS REVIEW

Arousal, Attention, and Cognition

Mrs. Smith continues to demonstrate severe verbal apraxia, with moderate aphasia. She is 85% accurate with "yes" and "no" to complex questions and 50% accurate to two-step verbal commands. She can sing familiar tunes, but cannot use sentences. She communicates via facial expressions and gestures. She demonstrates some impulsivity during treatment, is often frustrated, and occasionally will throw things. Deficits in response selection (making decisions) and response programming during motor tasks are evident. Mrs. Smith has poor balance, especially during transfers and in standing. She has a decreased awareness of her balance problems and poor appreciation of safety factors.

Sensory Integrity/Perception

Generally poor sensory appreciation of the right limbs is present to tactile and somatosensory input. She reports that her right side feels numb and tends to neglect the hemiplegic limbs and the right side of space. She has a right visual field deficit. Auditory perception appears intact.

Flexibility/Range of Motion

Passive range of motion (ROM) is within normal limits in all joints with the exception of limited ankle dorsiflexion on the right, associated with tightness in the gastrocnemius.

Muscle Performance/Strength

Weakness or difficulty recruiting the appropriate muscle group(s) is present in the right lower and upper extremities, as well as in the trunk. Mrs. Smith does not always move through the range of motion available to her.

Motor Function

Mrs. Smith has difficulty combining limb synergies within and between the upper and lower extremities. She cannot vary her speed, tending to move slowly. She has poor reciprocal limb movement (eg, flexion/extension of elbow). A flexion synergy often is observed in the right upper extremity, especially when she is physically or emotionally stressed. She has voluntary hand grasp with poor release. She is independent in feeding skills using her left upper extremity.

Balance

Balance when attempting transfers and in standing is poor. She does not regain her balance quickly and would fall if not supported by her hemi-walker or another adult.

Posture

Mrs. Smith has an asymmetrical body alignment (leaning to the left) both in sitting and in standing. She is able to only partially bear weight on the right hip during sitting and the right leg during standing.

Gait/Locomotion

Mrs. Smith is ambulating in the parallel bars and approximately 30 feet with a hemi-walker. She has active hip flexion, but poor right foot placement. Mrs. Smith lacks knee flexion during gait, circumducting the right leg. She tends to lead with the left side with the right side of her pelvis retracted. Step length on the right is decreased. Mrs. Smith continues to wear a hinged AFO on the right foot.

CASE STUDY # 2
Daniel Johnson

CURRENT STATUS

Mr. Johnson is 59 years old and has a diagnosis of Parkinson's disease. He recently had an increase in the severity of his symptoms and was referred to physical therapy for evaluation, treatment, and a home program.

HISTORY

Mr. Johnson was referred by his family practice physician to a neurologist approximately 4 years ago, at age 55. Up until that time, he had been healthy with no major surgeries or disease processes noted. His initial symptoms included left upper extremity tremor and facial masking with complaints of general fatigue. He received a diagnosis of mild Parkinson's disease at that time.

One year later, he was referred to physical therapy because of shoulder pain, apparently related to the rigidity associated with the Parkinson's disease. He was complaining of myoclonic jerking of his body, usually at night. He had a bilateral upper extremity tremor, exacerbated when he was stressed. He also was noting difficulty when rising from a low chair and had begun shuffling his feet when tired. He had a mildly stooped posture with moderate tremoring of the left hand. Grade 1 rigidity in the upper extremities was noted (slight or detectable only when activated by mirror or other movements). Performance on a finger tapping test was normal. He had decreased voice volume. At 56 years of age, Mr. Johnson continued to work as an elementary school teacher and was active in physical activities, such as swimming and walking.

Mr. Johnson was followed periodically by physical therapy and provided with a home program. Approximately 3 years after onset, Mr. Johnson noted severe problems with constipation due to decreased motility. His physician placed him on a regimen of enemas and suppositories, which relieved this problem. He also noted increased problems with hesitancy in his speech and reported bouts of frequent depression. He had a Grade 2 rigidity of the upper extremities (mild to moderate) and Grade 1 rigidity of the lower extremities. Finger tapping was mildly impaired. He reported upper back and neck pain when walking. At this point in time, Mr. Johnson began a medical leave from his teaching position.

Mr. Johnson is taking Sinemet (Merck & Co, Whitehouse Station, NJ) and bromocriptine. He reports bouts of dyskinesia about 30 minutes after taking his medication. This consists of involuntary writhing around the neck and shoulders and is thought to be a side effect of Sinemet.

Mr. Johnson lives at home with his wife. He has three children: two teenagers at home and the oldest child in college. They live in a three-bedroom rambler without stairs. However, they live in a northern state and must frequently deal with snow and ice during the winter months. He is concerned that he is having more difficulty with the recreational activities that he enjoys (ie, swimming and walking).

SYSTEMS REVIEW

Arousal, Attention, and Cognition

Mr. Johnson is displaying problems with short-term memory. Because he is noting mild memory impairment, he is not taking anticholinergic drugs, as they often exaggerate memory deficits. Mr. Johnson is showing more signs of depression, is less interested in social activities, and reports frequent insomnia.

Sensory Integrity/Perception

Responses to tests of basic sensory integrity (eg, two-point discrimination, pressure, heat, and cold) are intact.

Flexibility/Range of Motion

Although Mr. Johnson does not always use full range available during functional movement, range of motion of the extremities is within normal limits. He has decreased flexibility of the trunk and pelvis.

Muscle Performance/Strength

General strength and endurance are less than anticipated, probably due to less overall physical activity.

Motor Function

Mr. Johnson demonstrates the classic motor symptoms of Parkinson's disease including akinesia (difficulty initiating movement), bradykinesia (slow movement), and dyskinesia (poor synergistic organization of movement). He has increased bilateral tremoring, which is constant rather than intermittent. He is having more difficulty with transitional movements, such as in and out of chairs and in and out of a bed. He turns "en block," and trunk rotation is particularly difficult.

Balance

Increasing problems with balance are noted. He has slow reactions to loss of balance, particularly in standing.

Posture

Mr. Johnson's body alignment is forward, increasing his tendency to fall forward.

Gait/Locomotion

Although Mr. Johnson is still ambulating independently, he has a shuffling gait and lacks a reciprocal arm swing. He has difficulty with starting, stopping, and turning during ambulation.

CASE STUDY #3
Shirley Teal

CURRENT STATUS

Ms. Teal is a 21-year-old woman who is 4 months post motor vehicle accident (MVA). She has been in an extended care facility since 2 months post MVA. She receives physical and occupational therapy at the facility but becomes very combative in therapy and strikes out or curses at the therapist(s) frequently. It is anticipated that she will be discharged from the facility within the next 2 months. She will be living with her parents and her young child in a second-floor apartment.

HISTORY

At the time of admission to the hospital following the MVA, Ms. Teal was decerebrate, had intracranial bleeding in the right occipital horn, and was diagnosed with a traumatic brain injury (TBI). She was comatose and received a tracheotomy and a gastrostomy immediately after admission to the hospital. At 2 months post trauma, she was transferred to an extended care facility. At that time, she was able to open her eyes to verbal and tactile stimuli, but was unable to visually track an object. She was able to move her upper and lower extremities spontaneously, but not on command. The initial physical therapy examination noted that she had mild to moderate resistance to passive movement in both upper extremities (right greater than left) and severe stiffness in her lower extremities. She was limited in passive range of motion in right elbow extension (-30 degrees), right knee extension (-15 degrees), and right hip extension (-15 degrees). Other ranges of motion were passively within normal limits. She exhibited bilateral ankle clonus (right greater than left) when minimal stretch was applied. She exhibited poor head and trunk control when supported sitting was attempted.

At the time of the accident, she was a single parent with a 2-year-old child. She lived alone with her child and supported herself by working in a beauty salon. She has a high school education plus some training as a beautician.

SYSTEMS REVIEW

Arousal, Attention, and Cognition

Ms. Teal continues to demonstrate problems with cognition. She has difficulty with maintenance of concentration and demonstrates an inability to switch attention between tasks or objects within the environment. She is able to follow simple instructions but occasionally forgets what is asked of her.

Sensory Integrity/Perception

Ms. Teal is aware of sensory input to all extremities. However, she is unable to discriminate common objects that are placed in her hands. She has an excessive dependence on vision for her balance control in sitting and standing. Auditory perception appears intact. She has benign paroxysmal positional nystagmus (BPPN) and vertigo.

Flexibility/Range of Motion

She has decreased range of motion in the right lower extremity, including a 40-degree plantarflexion contracture and -10 degrees of full hip and knee extension. She has full range of motion actively in the left extremities.

Muscle Performance/Strength

Ms. Teal continues to demonstrate increased stiffness bilaterally (right greater than left) in both upper and lower extremities. Her strength is decreased in the right lower extremity, and she has an inability to sustain right knee extension during stance.

Motor Function

Ms. Teal has good head control in all positions. She is able to sit independently, although she lists to the left. She is able to come to sitting by rolling to the side and with minimal assistance from the therapist. She requires supervision and occasional minimal assist with rolling. She is able to perform standing pivot transfers with only minimal assistance from the therapist.

She is able to move her left wrist, fingers, elbow, and shoulder free of synergist patterns, but with decreased strength and coordination. She is unable to reach with her right arm directly to an object that is held out to her and she has foot placement problems with the right leg in sitting or in standing.

Balance

She tends to lose her balance easily if she moves quickly and demonstrates positional dizziness due to BPPN and vertigo.

Posture

In sitting, Ms. Teal has difficulty in maintaining weight equally on both buttocks. She tends to list to the left side while placing weight primarily on her left buttock. She is able to stand in parallel bars, but has to be reminded to place weight on her right lower extremity.

Gait/Locomotion

Ms. Teal is able to perform pivot transfers and stands in the parallel bars for 5 minutes with minimal assistance. She does not initiate ambulation on her own. She is independent in a wheelchair by using the left arm for pushing and her left leg for pulling.

CASE STUDY # 4
Shawna Wells

CURRENT STATUS

Shawna is a 4-year-old child with a diagnosis of cerebral palsy, spastic quadriparesis, and mild mental retardation. She is in a preschool program where she receives direct and indirect (consultative) physical therapy services.

HISTORY

Shawna was born at full-term to a 27-year-old mother who had experienced a normal twin pregnancy. Problems were noted at birth due to a breech position of one infant. Shawna had APGAR scores (Appearance, Pulse, Grimace, Activity, and Respiration) of three and five at 1 and 5 minutes. Her twin sibling had APGAR scores of eight and 10 at 1 and 5 minutes. Shawna has a history of failure to thrive during her first year of life.

Shawna was enrolled in an early intervention program (EIP) at 4 months of age. She has been receiving physical therapy, occupational therapy, and speech therapy each on a weekly basis through the EIP since that time. For the past 3 months, Shawna has been mainstreamed into a full-day preschool program and is continuing to receive therapies on a weekly basis.

Shawna has a history of respiratory problems. She has no difficulty with feeding but has problems with speech (breathiness) and with respiratory patterns (lacks full inspiration and expiration). She had a heel cord release on the right leg approximately 1 year ago.

Shawna lives at home with her mother, father, and typically developing 4-year-old twin brother. The family lives on a farm, and the parents rely on agriculture as their source of income.

SYSTEMS REVIEW

Arousal, Attention, Cognition

Shawna has difficulty with selective attention and perseveration of responses. Her response programming ability appears to be within normal limits. Shawna has poor short-term and long-term memory for motor learning. Her IQ on standardized tests is estimated to be about 70. She occasionally has temper tantrums during her physical and occupational therapy sessions but most of the time she is cooperative. When she is agitated, she thrusts herself into extension but can be easily calmed. She performs well if food reinforcers are offered.

Sensory Integrity/Perception

Shawna demonstrates good sensory identification ability to auditory stimuli. She is able to visually locate and point to common objects without difficulty. She has minimal difficulty in discriminating somatosensory stimuli but has avoidance reactions with some sensory inputs. Shawna does not like being handled initially in therapy but becomes less resistant as the therapy session progresses. She has had difficulties with tactile hypersensitivity since birth. Additionally, she demonstrates autonomic distress with movement. She is hesitant to play on movable toys and becomes agitated when she is moved in space.

Flexibility/Range of Motion

Resistance to passive range of motion in ankle dorsiflexion and knee extension is noted indicating tightness in the gastrocnemius/soleus and hamstrings bilaterally. She also has decreased trunk and upper extremity flexibility. She is able to reach for objects with either hand but is unable to actively flex at the shoulder beyond 115 degrees. Shoulder abduction is limited to approximately 90 degrees when she reaches out to the side. Passive range of motion is slightly better (an additional 10 to 15 degrees of motion).

Muscle Performance/Strength

Overall strength and endurance for motor activities are diminished as compared to her typically developing twin.

Motor Function

Shawna has good head control in all positions. She is able to sit on the floor independently, although with increased flexion in the trunk when her legs are extended. She is able to come to sitting independently either by rotating to the side or by assuming a "W" sitting position. She does not need her arms for support in tailor sitting unless she attempts to reach with one arm for a toy. Shawna is able to roll using trunk rotation. Shawna is able to creep on her hands and knees using a homologous pattern (eg, "bunny hopping"). She is able to use a poorly coordinated reciprocal pattern for short distances but only does so with verbal encouragement.

Balance

Shawna demonstrates adequate righting responses of her head and trunk when she is tilted slowly in space. She has ineffective protective responses in the extremities when moved forward, sideways, and backwards. She is unable to maintain her posture in any position when she is moved quickly. In standing with her walker, she is unable to maintain her balance on any surface that is not flat and firm. She uses a stepping pattern in response to external perturbation. She appears to have a decreased cone of perceived stability and relies heavily on visual inputs.

Posture

When sitting on the floor with her legs extended, Shawna demonstrates a posterior pelvic tilt with a forward head and trunk. When sitting on a bench, in a chair, or in her wheelchair, her trunk posture is more erect. She tends to hold her upper extremities flexed and close to her body. She has a generally crouched posture with ankle, knee, hip, and trunk flexion when she stands.

Gait/Locomotion

Shawna ambulates with a posterior control walker and with minimal assistance from the therapist. She demonstrates poor disassociation of the lower extremities during ambulation with particular difficulty in reciprocation. She is unable to sustain full knee extension on the stance leg during gait. Shawna wears a hinged AFO on the right and has minimal heel strike bilaterally. Shawna prefers to crawl on hands and knees as her primary means of locomotion.

CASE STUDY # 5
Robert Anderson

CURRENT STATUS

Mr. Anderson is a 38-year-old male with a diagnosis of an incomplete T9-10 spinal cord injury and residual radial nerve damage associated with an upper extremity fracture. He receives outpatient physical therapy services at a local hospital twice each week.

HISTORY

Mr. Anderson was involved in a single vehicle motorcycle accident 6 months ago when he lost control of his motorcycle on a slippery road. He sustained an incomplete T9-10 spinal cord injury. He was wearing a helmet and, although he sustained a concussion, he did not have a serious head injury. Mr. Anderson also had fractures of the right femur and left radius (now healed) with residual damage to the left radial nerve. He was an inpatient at a rehabilitation facility for the first 4 months following his injury and has been discharged to home. Mr. Anderson is a banker and has returned to work part-time. He is married with two young children (5 and 8 years of age) and lives with his family in an older two-story home with bedrooms and baths on the upper level. His wife works outside of the home as a teacher. He has a large extended family living in the area. He was in generally good health prior to the accident, and his recreational activities included running and motorcycle racing.

Systems Review

Arousal, Attention, and Cognition

Mr. Anderson is a very cooperative and motivated patient who is anxious to return to work full-time and to achieve full independence. He has no cognitive deficits.

Sensory Integrity/Perception

Loss of sensation is noted with the spinal cord injury and the residual radial nerve injury. Intermittent problems with sacral skin breakdown have occurred.

Flexibility/Range of Motion

Normal passive range of motion is present at all joints. Mr. Anderson notes occasional muscle spasms in his lower extremities.

Muscle Performance/Strength

Initially, Mr. Anderson had a flaccid paralysis of the lower extremities, but has had increasing stiffness (tone). His right upper extremity strength is normal, but he has some weakness in the left arm due to the radial nerve damage.

Motor Function

Mr. Anderson is independent in self-care (eg, dressing, bowel and bladder care). He has some difficulty with transfers, including sit to stand with knee ankle foot orthoses (KAFOs) and to the bed, floor, bath, car, and his wheelchair.

Balance

Mr. Anderson is able to sit without upper extremity support indefinitely and sustain minor balance disturbances in all directions. He cannot stand independently, but must use a walker or forearm crutches and lower leg bracing (ie, KAFO).

Posture

No difficulties or abnormal postures are noted.

Gait/Locomotion

For household ambulation, Mr. Anderson occasionally walks with a swing-through gait using his braces and forearm crutches. He does not have the endurance to use this method for community ambulation. He uses an ultralight manual wheelchair during his daily routine. He is currently driving a car that has been modified with hand controls.

Summary

The preceding descriptions of the five case studies can be used as a guide for information provided in subsequent chapters. The final chapter will provide an integrated approach to evaluation and intervention for each of the five patients used in the case studies.

CHAPTER 7

Applying the *Guide to Physical Therapist Practice*

Joanell A. Bohmert, PT, MS
Marilyn Woods, PT

The purpose of this chapter is to apply the *Guide to Physical Therapist Practice, Second Edition* (the *Guide*), to clinical practice.[1] The *Guide* is the primary resource document that describes the practice of the physical therapist. The *Guide* provides the concepts and framework with which physical therapists organize practice.

DEVELOPMENT OF THE *GUIDE*

The *Guide* was developed by the American Physical Therapy Association (APTA) based on the needs of membership to justify physical therapist practice to state legislators. This process began in 1992 with a board-appointed task force and culminated in the publication of a *Guide to Physical Therapist Practice, Volume I: A Description of Patient Management* in the August 1995 issue of *Physical Therapy*.[2] The process was refined with adoption of the conceptual framework of Volume I and passage of RC 32-95 by the APTA House of Delegates, which provided for the process to develop Volume II.

Volume II was designed to describe the preferred patterns of practice for patient/client groupings commonly referred for physical therapy. The process for completion of Volume II was by expert consensus and included a Project Advisory Group, a

Board Oversight Committee, and four Panels. Volume II also was intended to reflect current APTA standards, policies, and guidelines. Membership review was provided throughout the development with more than 600 individual field reviewers and general input at various APTA-sponsored forums.[1] In 1997, Volume I and Volume II became Part One and Part Two of the *Guide*. Part One was refined to reflect information obtained in the development of Part Two with the House of Delegates approving the conceptual framework of Part Two in June 1997. The first edition of the *Guide* was published in the November 1997 issue of *Physical Therapy*.[3]

The *Guide* was developed with the understanding that it is an evolving document that will need to be updated to reflect changes that occur in the base of knowledge for physical therapists.[3] Since publication in November 1997, the *Guide* has been formally revised two times to reflect membership input and changes in APTA policies by the House of Delegates.[4,5] In addition, the *Guide* is evolving through further description of practice. In 1998, APTA initiated Part Three and Part Four of the *Guide* to catalog the specific tests and measures used by physical therapists in four system areas and the areas of outcomes, health-related quality of life, and patient/client (this term is used throughout this chapter to conform with the specifications of the *Guide*) satisfaction. An additional goal was to develop standardized documentation forms that incorporated the patient/client management process. This further development of the *Guide* also involved expert task force members, field reviews, and membership input at APTA forums. Documentation templates for inpatient and outpatient settings were developed and published in Appendix 6 of the *Guide*.[1] During this time, APTA also developed a patient/client satisfaction instrument which is available as Appendix 7 of the *Guide*.[1]

During 1999 to 2001, work continued on reviewing tests and measures. Part Four was incorporated into Part Three with the result being a listing of tests and measures that were used in Chapter Two of the *Guide*. Part Three contains reference literature describing the tests and provides available data regarding each test's reliability and validity. Part Three is available only on CD-ROM. This part is searchable and linked to Chapter Two, as well as to specific patterns. The CD-ROM includes the entire *Guide* (ie, Parts One through Three). During 1999 and 2000, the *Guide* was revised further to reflect input from membership, leadership, Part Three revisions, and changes in House policies. This revision resulted in the publication of the *Guide to Physical Therapist Practice, Second Edition* in the January 2001 issue of *Physical Therapy*.[1]

The *Guide* is intended to describe the practice of the physical therapist to those within the physical therapy community and to those outside physical therapy, including policy makers, regulators, payers, administrators, and other professionals. The *Guide* does this through a general description of physical therapist practice that is based on:

- The disablement model
- A description of the physical therapist's role in prevention, health/wellness and fitness, and in primary, secondary, and tertiary care
- Standardization of terminology
- Delineation of tests and measures and interventions
- Delineation of preferred practice patterns[1]

The *Guide* also states what it is not intended to do:

- The *Guide* does not provide specific protocols for treatments, nor are the practice patterns contained in the *Guide* intended to serve as clinical guidelines
- The *Guide* is not intended to set forth the standard of care for which a physical therapist may be legally responsible in any specific case[1]

ORGANIZATION OF THE *GUIDE*

The *Guide* is available in print format (which does not include Part Three) and CD-ROM (which includes all Parts). The *Guide* is organized in three parts with an introduction, appendices, and indices. The Introduction addresses the concepts, development, and content overview of the *Guide*.

Part One: A Description of Patient/Client Management

This section provides the foundation for practice. Chapter One is an overview of who physical therapists are and what they do and includes a description of the five elements of patient/client management. Chapter Two is a description of the 24 tests and measures categories. Chapter Three is a description of the 11 intervention categories.

Part Two: Preferred Practice Patterns

This section contains four chapters of practice patterns, which describe the patient/client management process grouped by body system. These chapters are:
- Chapter Four: Musculoskeletal
- Chapter Five: Neuromuscular
- Chapter Six: Cardiovascular/Pulmonary
- Chapter Seven: Integumentary

Part Three

This section is a catalog of specific tests and measures used by physical therapists with citations of related literature on the reliability and validity of each tool.[6] The specific tests and measures are linked through Chapter Two and through the Patterns.

Appendices

- A glossary of terms used in the *Guide*
- APTA Standards of Practice, Ethics documents, and Documentation Guidelines
- APTA Documentation Template for Inpatient and Outpatient Settings
- Patient/Client Satisfaction Questionnaire

The Indices include a numerical and alphabetical index to ICD-9-CM Codes

CONCEPTS OF THE *GUIDE*

The *Guide* has three key concepts on which it is based. These concepts include the disablement model, a continuum of service that goes across all settings, and the five elements of patient/client management.

Disablement Model

The first concept is the disablement model that serves as the basis for physical therapist practice. The disablement model provides a structure for physical therapist practice. Disablement is a process that addresses the consequences of the pathology/pathophysiology for the person and the role the person has in society.

TABLE 7-1

Definitions Used in the *Guide**

Pathology/Pathophysiology (Disease, Disorder, Condition)

An abnormality characterized by a particular cluster of signs and symptoms and recognized by either the patient/client or practitioner as "abnormal." It is primarily identified at the cellular level.

Impairment

A loss or abnormality of anatomical, physiological, mental, or psychological structure or function.

Functional Limitation

The restriction of the ability to perform, at the level of the whole person, a physical action, task, or activity in an efficient, typically expected, or competent manner.

Disability

The inability to perform or a limitation in the performance of actions, tasks, and activities usually expected in specific social roles that are customary for the individual or expected for the person's status or role in a specific sociocultural context and physical environment. In the *Guide*, the categories of roles are self-care, home management, work (job/school/play), and community/leisure.

* Appendix 1: Glossary Guide to Physical Therapist Practice. 2nd ed. Phys Ther. 2001;81:S677-S683.

Several models of disablement have been developed.[7-9] The concept first was proposed by Nagi,[7,10,11] a sociologist, next by the World Health Organization (WHO),[8,12] and, finally, by the National Center for Medical Rehabilitation and Research (NCMRR).[9] The models all vary in the terminology used to describe the process of disablement, however, the concepts of the process are consistent. The *Guide* provides an overview and comparison of these models on pages S19-S21.[1] The *Guide* uses the terminology based on Nagi's model, and the concepts of the disablement process serve as the basis for physical therapy practice (Table 7-1).

The disablement process incorporates four components: pathology, impairment, functional limitation, and disability (Figure 7-1). Disablement is not unidirectional. It cannot be assumed that pathology leads to impairments, that impairments lead to functional limitations, or that functional limitations lead to disability. There are many factors that can impact the process and change the relationship of the four components. These factors include those of the individual and those of the environment. Individual factors include the following:

- Those inherent to the individual (eg, biological, demographic)
- Those in which the individual makes choices (eg, health habits, personal behaviors, lifestyles)
- The psychological attributes of the individual (eg, motivation, coping, social support)

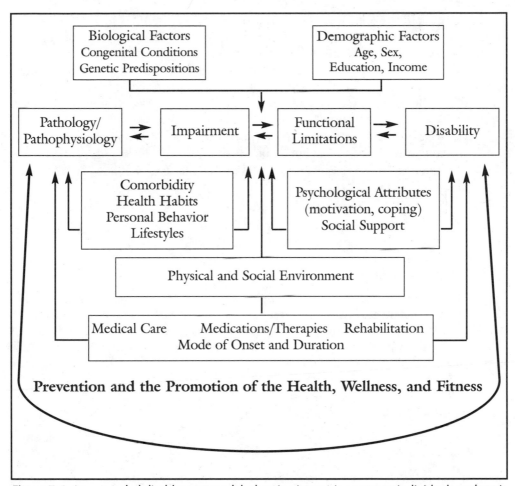

Figure 7-1. An expanded disablement model, showing interactions among individuals and environmental factors, prevention, and the promotion of health, wellness, and fitness (reprinted with permission from the American Physical Therapy Association from *Guide to Physical Therapist Practice*. 2nd ed. *Phys Ther.* 2001;81:S24, as adapted from Guccione AA. Arthritis and the process of disablement. *Phys Ther.* 1994:74;410).

- The individual's social support (eg, social interactions, relationships)

Environmental factors include:

- Available health care
- Physical therapy services
- Medications
- Other therapies
- The physical and social environment[1]

The Institute of Medicine (IOM) introduced the concept of prevention being a factor that could impact the disablement model in 1991.[13] In this model of disablement, prevention is the act of providing intervention, before or within the disablement process, at the level of the components (ie, pathology, impairment, functional limitation, disability) or at the level of risk factors to positively impact the individual. This concept of impacting the process of disablement was expanded further by IOM in 1997 to include rehabilitation as a method of preventing disability, thereby resulting in "enabling" the individual and removing disability from the process.[14]

The disablement model is the model the physical therapist uses to view how an individual interacts with the environment and how that impacts the individual's sense of well-being or health-related quality of life.[15-23] As a primary resource for physical therapist practice, the *Guide* incorporates the concepts of disablement through:

1. The four main components of the disablement process (pathology/pathophysiology, impairment, functional limitation, disability)
2. Individual factors (risk reduction/prevention; health, wellness, and fitness; patient/client satisfaction)
3. Environmental factors (societal resources)

These factors are addressed throughout the continuum of service within the patient/client management model, concluding in the global outcomes.

Continuum of Service

The second concept of the *Guide* is that "physical therapist practice addresses the needs of patients/clients through a continuum of service across all delivery settings."[1] The continuum of service requires that the physical therapist address the health-related quality of life for all patients/clients. This is done by addressing the four components of disablement and all the factors (individual and environmental) that impact these components. These factors include:

- Risk reduction/prevention (primary, secondary, tertiary)
- Promotion of health, wellness, and fitness
- Acute care
- Habilitation
- Rehabilitation
- Chronic care
- Specialized maintenance

The delivery setting is the location in which the patient/client is present, for example, in the home/residence, community/leisure setting, or at work (job/school/play).

The *Guide* incorporates the continuum of service in the wide range of patient/client diagnostic classifications of the preferred practice patterns (primary prevention) and within the preferred practice patterns throughout the patient/client management process.

Five Elements of Patient/Client Management

The third concept is that physical therapist practice includes the patient/client management model. This model includes the five essential elements of examination, evaluation, diagnosis, prognosis, and intervention that result in optimal outcomes. Figure 7-2 illustrates the patient/client management process with a brief explanation of the five elements. The patient/client management process is dynamic and allows the physical therapist to progress the patient/client in the process, return to an earlier element for further analysis, or exit the patient/client from the process when the needs of the patient/client cannot be addressed by the physical therapist.

DIAGNOSIS

Both the process and the end result of evaluating examination data, which the physical therapist organizes into defined clusters, syndromes, or categories to help determine the prognosis (including the plan of care) and the most appropriate intervention strategies.

EVALUATION

A dynamic process in which the physical therapist makes clinical judgments based on data gathered during the examination. This process also may identify possible problems that require consultation with or referral to another provider.

PROGNOSIS

Determination of the level of optimal improvement that may be attained through intervention and the amount of time required to reach that level. The plan of care specifies the interventions to be used and their timing and frequency.

EXAMINATION

The process of obtaining a history, performing a systems review, and selecting and administering tests and measures to gather data about the patient/client. The initial examination is a comprehensive screening and specific testing process that leads to a diagnosis classification. The examination process also may identify possible problems that require consultation with or referral to another provider.

INTERVENTION

Purposeful and skilled interaction of the physical therapist with the patient and, if appropriate, with other individuals involved in care of the patient, using various physical therapy methods and techniques to produce changes in the condition that are consistent with the diagnosis and prognosis. The physical therapist conducts a reexamination to determine changes in patient status and to modify or redirect intervention. The decision to reexamine may be based on new clinical findings or on lack of patient progress. The process of reexamination also may identify the need for consultation with or referral to another provider.

OUTCOMES

Results of patient management, which include the impact of physical therapy interventions in the following domains: pathology/pathophysiology (disease, disorder, or condition); impairments, functional limitations, and disabilities; risk reduction/prevention; health, wellness, and fitness; societal resources; and patient satisfaction.

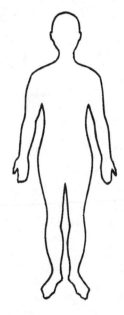

Figure 7-2. The elements of patient management leading to optimal outcomes (reprinted with permission from the American Physical Therapy Association from *Guide to Physical Therapist Practice.* 2nd ed. *Phys Ther.* 2001;81:S35).

The patient/client management process incorporates the disablement model through-out the five elements and outcomes and is to be used throughout the continuum of service in all settings. This is the physical therapist's clinical decision-making model.

The *Guide* provides a description of the elements of patient/client management in Part One, Chapter One. The preferred practice patterns in Part Two are organized by these five elements of patient/client management. Appendix 6 of the *Guide* is the documentation template of the patient/client management for inpatient and outpatient settings developed by APTA.[1]

APPLICATION OF THE *GUIDE* TO CLINICAL PRACTICE

The *Guide* can be applied in a number of ways. We will explain an application of the *Guide*, *Second Edition*, by looking at the structure of the preferred patterns in Part Two. You will need the *Guide*, *Second Edition*, to follow the examples. We will show you how the patient/client management process and the disablement model are incorporated into Parts One, Two, and Three. We then will show you specific applications of the *Guide* for three of the case studies described in Chapter 6.

For a more detailed explanation of the *Guide*, the reader is encouraged to read the *Guide*, *Second Edition*, and related articles.[1,6,24]

For the purpose of application we will use, as an example, Chapter 5: Neuromuscular Table of Contents (p. S305) and Pattern 5D: Impaired Motor Function and Sensory Integrity Associated with Nonprogressive Disorders of the Central Nervous System–Acquired in Adolescence or Adulthood (pp. S357-S374).

Table of Contents

This page, S305, identifies the patterns included in this chapter on the neuromuscular system. While the patterns are grouped by four body systems, the physical therapist will need to address the "whole" patient/client to determine the system in which the primary impairment(s) that drive the intervention are located. The physical therapist should not assume that the patient/client automatically will be classified in the system of associated pathology or condition. For example, in a patient/client with a pathology diagnosis of cardiovascular accident, the system of origin of the pathology is the cardiovascular system. The system of primary impact of the pathology is the neuromuscular system. The system of secondary or tertiary impact may be the musculoskeletal, cardiovascular/pulmonary, or integumentary system.

Title Page

The title page (p. S357) identifies the title and the patient/client diagnostic classification characteristics for this specific pattern. The title is the diagnostic classification or the diagnosis by the physical therapist for patient/clients grouped in this pattern. The titles are based on the impairment or group of impairments that drive the intervention for that patient/client grouping. Patterns may or may not have a condition or pathology/pathophysiology associated with them. When there is only an impairment(s) listed in the title, the patient/client can be included with or without an associated condition or pathology/pathophysiology. It is up to the physical therapist to decide if the condition or pathology/pathophysiology significantly alters the patient/client management from that described in the pattern and whether to make the decision to include the patient/client. In the *Guide*, physical therapists need to classify/diagnose the patient/client by the impairment(s) that is driving the intervention, **not** the associated condition or pathology/pathophysiology. The title also may specify an age range. If an age is not specified, the pattern applies to all ages.

Patient/Client Diagnostic Classification

This section (p. S357) is a description of examination findings that may support the inclusion, exclusion, or classification in multiple patterns. The findings are organized into two categories:

- Risk Factors or Consequences of Pathology/Pathophysiology (Disease, Disorder, or Condition)
- Impairments, Functional Limitations, or Disabilities

All patterns include a "Note" which addresses risk factors or consequences of pathology/pathophysiology that may require modification of the pattern or exclusion of the patient/client. The examples listed in the pattern are specific to that pattern.

ICD-9-CM Codes

This section (p. S358) is provided as an example of codes that relate to the patient/client diagnostic grouping for the pattern. This is not an inclusive or exclusive list. Patient/clients may be placed in the pattern if their primary impairments are consistent with the pattern, regardless if their assigned ICD-9-CM code is or is not listed.

Examination

The examination (p. S359) is required for all patient/clients and is performed prior to the initial intervention. The three components of the examination are delineated in each pattern. *Patient/Client History* (p. S359) is a complete list of the types of data that may be generated from the patient/client history and is found in every pattern. It also is found on page S36, in Chapter One. The *System Review* (p. S360) contains a complete list of what the system review may include. The components of the system review are listed in every pattern and also can be found on pages S34-S35 of Chapter One. Pages S360-S362 identify the *Tests and Measures* categories and bullets that are specific to the pattern. Chapter Two describes the tests and measures categories in detail including:

- A general definition and purpose
- Clinical indications
- Tests and measures methods and techniques
- Tools used for gathering data
- The data generated

The clinical indications provided in each test and measure are examples of specific findings of the history and system review which may indicate the need for use of that specific test and measures category (see p. S48). Clinical indications are provided in the following disablement areas: pathology/pathophysiology (disease, disorder, or condition); impairments; functional limitations; disability; risk factors; and health, wellness, and fitness. Part Three of the *Guide* provides a catalog of specific tests and measures with citations to related literature on the psychometric properties of each tool. You will be able to access the information on a specific test multiple ways. The tests are linked from the bullets listed under the Tests and Measures category (p. S49) in each of the 24 categories. This will give you an entire list of tests and measures appropriate for that test category. The tests also are linked in the patterns through the tests and measures bullets, however, these tests are specific to that pattern. By clicking through Part Three, you will be able to locate specific tests and the literature that relates to that tool. Thus, a tool that is appropriate to your specific patient/client can be selected. (Note: The tests and measures and literature are only accurate and current as of the date stated in the CD-ROM.)

Evaluation, Diagnosis, and Prognosis (Including the Plan of Care)

These sections (p. S363) are grouped together on one page in each pattern. The page includes an explanation of the evaluation and diagnostic process and the factors that may impact the process. During the *Evaluation*, examination data are analyzed, taking into consideration the patient's/client's expectations and patient's/client's potential for remediation or accommodation. The physical therapist identifies the primary impairments that are impacting the patient's/client's functional abilities. The patient's/client's *Diagnosis* is determined at this point in the patient/client management process. The pattern title is the diagnostic classification for the pattern. You need to determine your specific patient's/client's diagnosis, identifying the primary impairments that will drive the interventions. You then determine if your patient/client can be managed in this pattern with or without modifications, if another pattern is needed in addition to this pattern, or if a different pattern is more appropriate. Page S363 includes a *Prognosis* statement that identifies the optimal level of improvement in impairments and functional abilities as well as the amount of time needed. For patterns that include patients/clients with lifelong conditions, the prognosis statement provides for improvement "within the context of the impairments, functional limitations, and disabilities"[1] as the patient/client always will have some level of impairment that may impact the level of function. The prognosis also includes a column identifying the expected range of number of visits per episode of care. The range is based on following the patient/client throughout the continuum of service across all settings. It is anticipated that 20% of patients/clients who are appropriate for this pattern will be outside this range for each episode of care. The column "Factors That May Require New Episode of Care or That May Modify Frequency of Visits/Duration of Care"[1] provides a listing of individual and environmental factors that are specific to that pattern. The prognosis also has a "Note" section in those patterns where the patient/client may require multiple episodes of care. This section also lists factors that, in addition to those in the factor column, may impact this pattern.

The three components of *Intervention* are delineated in each pattern. The first two: *coordination, communication, and documentation* and *patient/client-related instruction* are required for all patients/clients. The third components; the nine *procedural intervention* categories, selected for the specific pattern.

Pages S364-S373 list the intervention categories, bullets, and anticipated goals/expected outcomes specific for the pattern. Chapter Three describes the interventions categories in detail including general definitions, clinical considerations, interventions, and anticipated goals and expected outcomes. For coordination, communication, and documentation and patient/client-related instruction, the examples of the clinical considerations that may direct that intervention and the anticipated goals and expected outcomes related to that intervention are listed, but are not grouped by disablement areas. For the nine procedural intervention categories, the clinical considerations provided in intervention are examples of "examination findings that direct the type and specificity of"[1] that intervention and are grouped in the following disablement areas:

- Pathology/pathophysiology (disease, disorder, or condition)
- History of medical/surgical conditions or signs and symptoms
- Impairments
- Functional limitations
- Disability
- Risk reduction/prevention
- Health, wellness, and fitness needs (see p. S104)

Examples of anticipated goals and expected outcomes related to that intervention are grouped in the following disablement areas: pathology/pathophysiology; impairment; functional limitation; disability; risk reduction/prevention; health, wellness, and fitness; societal resources; and patient/client satisfaction.

The final page of this pattern, page S374, includes Reexamination, Global Outcomes for Patient/clients in This Pattern and Criteria for Termination of Physical Therapy Services.

Reexamination can be performed at any time, after the initial examination, in the episode of care. It may result in:

- Modification of the anticipated goals, expected outcomes frequency, or duration of care
- Reclassification of the patient/client to a different pattern, addition of another pattern, or termination of the physical therapy service

Global Outcomes for Patients/Clients in This Pattern are measured at the end of the episode of care and measure the impact of physical therapy service in the domains of:

- Pathology/pathophysiology
- Impairment
- Functional limitation
- Disability
- Risk reduction/prevention
- Health, wellness, and fitness
- Societal resources
- Patient/Client satisfaction

These are the same domains for the anticipated goals and expected outcomes identified in the interventions. The ***Guide*** defines anticipated goals and expected outcomes as the "intended results of patient/client management and indicate changes in impairments, functional limitations, and disabilities and the changes in health, wellness, and fitness needs that are expected as the result of implementing the plan of care."[1] Goals and outcomes need to be meaningful to the patient/client, measurable, and time specific.

The two processes of ***Termination of Physical Therapy Service*** are discharge and discontinuation. Discharge occurs when the anticipated goals and expected outcomes have been achieved. Discontinuation occurs when services are ended but the anticipated goals and expected outcomes have not been met. This may occur at the request of the patient/client or guardian. In other instances, the patient/client is unable to make progress toward outcomes due to individual or environmental/economical factors, or the physical therapist determines the patient/client will no longer benefit from the current episode of care.[1]

Three of the five case studies have been selected to illustrate various applications of the *Guide*.

CASE STUDY #1
Jane Smith

- *Age: 74 years*
- *Medical Diagnosis: Right hemiplegia, secondary to left CVA*
- *Status: 6 months post onset*
- *Practice Pattern 5D: Impaired Motor Function and Sensory Integrity Associated with Nonprogressive Disorders of the Central Nervous System—Acquired in Adolescence or Adulthood*

This case is used as an example of applying all of the categories of the *Guide* to patient/client management.

How does the patient/client management model help you determine what is wrong with Mrs. Smith, and what do you do? During the examination, how did you know which specific tests and measures to use? How did you know how to place Mrs. Smith in Practice Pattern 5D?

EXAMINATION

History

The first information you received about Mrs. Smith was from her history. You reviewed her previous medical information, physical therapy chart/notes, and information provided to you on her intake form. You proceed to interview Mrs. Smith and her husband to complete the information from the history section of the examination. Based on the information in her history, you begin to form a picture of what her concerns are and what impairments may be impacting her ability to do what she wants to do. You now have an overview of her medical status and how that may impact your examination today, as well as how it may impact Mrs. Smith's prognosis and plan of care. The history may include the following elements.

- General Demographics—Mrs. Smith is a 74-year-old English-speaking woman.
- Social History—She is married and lives with her husband who is the primary caregiver. She has two grown sons and four grandchildren.
- Employment/Work (Job/School/Play)—She is retired.
- Growth and Development—Normal.
- Living Environment—She lives in a split-level home. She has to go upstairs to bedrooms and downstairs to the laundry area. There are three steps to enter her home and to reach the mailbox. She has to go down a small incline to the driveway.

- General Health Status—(Self-Report, Family Report, Caregiver Report)
  - Perception—Status of prior health reported to be excellent until a few months ago.
  - Physical Function—Normal for age prior to onset of hemiparesis.
  - Psychological Function—Normal prior to current episode.
  - Role—Mother, grandmother, wife.
  - Social Function—Her hobbies include gardening, sewing, and bowling.
- Social/Health Habits (Past and Current)—She doesn't smoke or drink.
- Family History—Noncontributory.

Medical/Surgical

Mrs. Smith has a medical history of hypertension, peripheral vascular disease, and bilateral endarterectomies. Six months ago, Mrs. Smith woke up in the morning with a right hemiparesis and marked aphasia. Her husband brought her into the emergency room of the local hospital where she received medical treatment.

Four days following onset of her cerebrovascular accident (CVA), physical therapists, occupational therapists, and speech/language pathologists evaluated Mrs. Smith. The initial physical therapy examination noted that she was oriented and cooperative, but with severe expressive aphasia. She could say "yes" and "no," but her responses were unreliable. Her right upper extremity was flaccid; she had adductor and extensor stiffness in the right lower extremity. She needed maximal assistance to roll and complete all transfers and activities of daily living (ADLs), and she could not stand and bear weight on the right leg. Her sitting balance was fair and she had poor sensation on the right side of her body. Her occupational and speech therapy examinations indicated that her apraxia interfered with performance on language and ADL tasks. She had severe verbal apraxia with moderate to marked aphasia. Verbal production was limited to isolated episodes of automatic speech.

Two weeks following onset, Mrs. Smith was transferred to the rehabilitation unit in another facility. The physical therapy examination at that time indicated Grade 2 strength in the right hip and knee musculature with muscles around the ankle and foot at Grade 1. Rolling to the right could be accomplished with minimal assistance and to the left with moderate assistance of one adult. Mrs. Smith needed assistance in pivot transfers, coming from sit to stand, balancing in standing, and with maneuvering her wheelchair. She required frequent verbal cues because of severe neglect of the right side. A hinged ankle foot orthosis (AFO) was ordered for her right lower extremity. She also demonstrated preservation in dressing and difficulty with sequencing tasks. Reading comprehension was good, but she was only able to use gestures and automatic speech to communicate.

Current Conditions/Chief Complaint

Mrs. Smith is not ambulating safely. She continues to have difficulty with speech, and transfers are difficult. Currently she is receiving physical therapy and occupational therapy twice each month, as well as weekly speech therapy. She wants to be able to transfer and ambulate safely in the home.

Functional Status and Activity Level

She ambulates using a hemi-walker and an AFO. She needs assistance with ADLs and instrumental activities of daily living (IADLs).

Medications

Current information should be documented including name of medication(s), dose, frequency, what they are being taken for, side effects, and the use of herbal or over-the-counter drugs.

Systems Review

You next complete a review of Mrs. Smith's systems by observing her symmetry and movement as she transitions from the waiting room area to the examination area (sitting posture, sit to stand, walking, maneuvering through doors and hallways, stand to sit in examination area), asking her to perform or imitate basic movements (reach overhead, behind back), visually inspecting her skin (skin color, nail color, swelling), taking basic measurements (heart rate, blood pressure, respiratory rate, height, and weight), and noting her awareness and responses to her environment and situation and her ability to follow directions and communicate.

The systems review may include the following:

- Anatomical and Physiological status
- Cardiovascular
    - Blood Pressure—145/84
    - Edema—None noted
    - Heart Rate—80 bpm
    - Respiratory Rate—18 bpm
- Integumentary
    - Presence of Scar Formation—N/A
    - Skin Color—Good
    - Skin Integrity—Good
- Musculoskeletal
    - Gross Range of Motion—Gross range of motion is within normal limits; mild limitation of ankle dorsiflexion on right
    - Gross Strength—Weakness or difficulty recruiting the appropriate muscle groups is present in the right extremities, as well as in the trunk. Mrs. Smith does not always move through the range of motion available to her.
    - Gross Symmetry
    - Height—5 feet 3 inches
    - Weight—120 pounds
- Neuromuscular
    - Gross Coordinated Movements—Mrs. Smith has poor balance when transferring and standing. She walks short distances with a hemi-walker. She wears an AFO on right foot.
    - Communication, Affect, Cognition, Language, and Learning Style—She is oriented to time, person, and place. She has aphasia but is able to make her needs known via facial expressions and gestures. She learns by demonstration, pictures, and verbal instructions.

Tests and Measures

Based on the findings of the history and system review, you determine which specific tests and measures you will use. The history and system review will identify clinical indicators for pathology/pathophysiology, impairments, functional limitations, disability, risk factors, health/wellness, and prevention needs that will assist you in ruling in or ruling out specific tests and measures for Mrs. Smith.

You can use the *Guide* to assist in identifying tests and measures categories, as well as specific tests and measures. Based on Mrs. Smith's findings, you select tests and measures from the following categories

Tests and measures for this pattern may include those that characterize or quantify the following:

- Aerobic Capacity/Endurance
- Anthropometrics Characteristics
- Arousal, Attention, and Cognition—Mrs. Smith continues to demonstrate severe verbal apraxia with moderate aphasia. She is 85% accurate with "yes" and "no" to complex questions and 50% accurate to two-step verbal commands. She can sing familiar tunes, but cannot use sentences. She communicates via facial expressions and gestures. She demonstrates some impulsivity during treatment, is often frustrated, and occasionally will throw things. Deficits in response selection (making decisions) and response programming during motor tasks are evident. Mrs. Smith has poor balance, especially during transfers and in standing. She has a decreased awareness of her balance problems and poor appreciation of safety factors.
- Assistive and Adaptive Devices—Mrs. Smith uses a hemi-walker.
- Circulation
- Cranial and Peripheral Nerve Integrity
- Environmental, Home, and Work—Functional barriers in the home are decreased balance and decreased awareness of safety which make transfers to chairs, the bathtub, and toilet difficult. She is unable to safely stand to dress. She also needs assistance to cook and do housework.
- Ergonomics and Body Mechanics
- Gait, Locomotion Balance—Mrs. Smith is ambulating in the parallel bars and approximately 30 feet with a hemi-walker. She has active hip flexion, but poor right foot placement. Mrs. Smith lacks knee flexion during gait, circumducting the right leg. She tends to lead with the left side with the right side of her pelvis retracted. Step length on the right is decreased. Mrs. Smith continues to wear a hinged AFO on the right foot.
- Integumentary Integrity
- Joint Integrity and Mobility
- Motor Function (Motor Control and Motor Learning)—Mrs. Smith has difficulty combining limb synergies within and between the upper and lower extremities. She cannot vary her speed and tends to move slowly. She has poor reciprocal extremity movement (eg, flexion/extension of elbow). A flexion synergy often is observed in the right upper extremity, especially when she is physically or emotionally stressed. She has voluntary hand grasp with poor release. She is independent in feeding.

- Muscle Performance—Weakness or difficulty recruiting the appropriate muscle group(s) is present in the right lower and upper extremities, as well as in the trunk. Mrs. Smith does not always move through the range of motion available to her.
- Neuromotor Development and Sensory Integration
  - Orthotic, Protective, and Supportive Devices—Mrs. Smith wears a hinged AFO on right her lower extremity. It fits appropriately and helps to improve her gait pattern, making her safer.
  - Pain—None reported.
  - Posture—She has asymmetrical body alignment (leaning to the left both in sitting and standing). She is only able to partially bear weight on the right hip during sitting and the right leg during standing.
  - Prosthetic Requirements—N/A
  - Range of Motion—Passive range of motion is within normal limits in all joints with the exception of limited ankle dorsiflexion on the right, associated with tightness in the gastrocnemius muscle.
  - Reflex Integrity
  - Self-Care and Home Management—Mrs. Smith needs standby assistance to shower. She is unable to prepare meals or do housework. Her husband does the laundry and shopping. She is able to assist in dressing.
  - Sensory Integrity—Generally poor sensory appreciation of the right extremities is present to tactile and somatosensory input. She reports that her right side feels numb and tends to neglect the right extremities and the right side of space. She has a right visual field deficit. Auditory perception appears intact.
  - Ventilation and Respiration/Gas Exchange
  - Work (Job/School/Play), Community, and Leisure Integration or Reintegration—She is able to visit children and grandchildren and occasionally visits friends with help from her family.

EVALUATION (CLINICAL JUDGMENT)

You now organize the data from the examination to determine which impairments are impacting Mrs. Smith's functional abilities. You determine if her expectations for therapy are realistic, establish a diagnosis and a prognosis, and develop a plan of care.

Mrs. Smith has impairments of decreased motor function, weakness, decreased balance, and poor sensory appreciation on the right side. She has some right-sided neglect and right side visual field cut. This has resulted in functional deficits of decreased ability to transfer and ambulate safely with or without an assistive device. She is not a community ambulator. She is unable to cook or do housework. She needs assistance to exit her home and to go up- and downstairs.

DIAGNOSIS

Based on the evaluation, you determine that deficits in motor function and sensory integrity are the primary impairments and problems with balance. In addition, muscle performance is the secondary impairment that is interfering with Mrs. Smith's functional abilities. You review the patterns and see that these impairments are addressed most appropriately in 5D.

The data collected helped determine the primary dysfunction that will drive the interventions. Mrs. Smith was placed in the practice pattern of 5D Impaired Motor Function and Sensory Integrity Associated with Nonprogressive Disorders of the Central Nervous System—Acquired in Adolescence or Adulthood.

PROGNOSIS

Using pattern 5D, you review the prognosis statement, expected range of visits, and factors that may modify frequency of visits and duration of care. Then you develop a prognosis for Mrs. Smith that addresses her expectations with an agreed frequency and duration. As part of the Plan of Care, you determine the anticipated goals and expected outcomes with Mrs. Smith.

Over the course of 12 months, Mrs. Smith will demonstrate optimal motor function, sensory integrity, and the highest level of function in the home and community within the context of her impairments, functional limitations, and disability. She is to receive physical and occupational therapy two times per month and weekly speech therapy for 3 months with patient/client and family education on a home program. After that, she will be placed on a prevention program and be rechecked in 6 months or sooner if problems arise. During the episode of care, Mrs. Smith will achieve the anticipated goals, expected outcomes, and the global outcomes. The patient/client and family have agreed to the program, and the informed consent is signed. Mrs. Smith will be discharged from physical therapy when her anticipated goals and expected outcomes have been met.

INTERVENTIONS (FOR CLINICAL CONSIDERATIONS)

Using the anticipated goals and expected outcomes you developed as part of the Plan of Care, you review the interventions to determine which interventions will be appropriate. We have provided an example only for the two required interventions of coordination, communication, and documentation and patient/client-related instruction. You will need to select procedural interventions to complete her plan of care.

Coordination, Communication, and Documentation

- Interventions—Coordination and communication with occupational and speech therapy.
- Anticipated Goals and Expected Outcomes—Family and caregivers demonstrate enhanced decision making regarding Mrs. Smith's health and good use of resources.

Patient/Client-Related Instruction

- Interventions—The patient/client and family will receive instruction and education in a home program and updates. They will receive information on when it is appropriate to seek additional services or to call 911.

- Anticipated Goals and Expected Outcomes—Mrs. Smith and her husband will have increased understanding of goals and outcomes and demonstrate her home program independently.

Procedural Interventions

You will need to select additional interventions from the nine procedural interventions to complete Mrs. Smith's plan of care. Use the information presented in the pattern under the categories of "Interventions" and "Anticipated Goals and Expected Outcomes" and the information in Chapter Three to assist in determining appropriate interventions and anticipated goals and expected outcomes for Mrs. Smith. The following are examples of interventions:

- Therapeutic exercise
- Self-care and home management
- Functional training in work (job/school/play), community, and leisure integration or reintegration
- Manual therapy techniques
- Prescription, application, and as appropriate, fabrication of devices and equipment
- Airway clearance techniques
- Integumentary repair and protection techniques
- Electrotherapeutic modalities
- Physical agents and mechanical modalities
- Reexamination
- Global outcomes for patient/clients—At the end of episode of care, the global outcomes of physical therapy services are measured by impact of the interventions in the following areas:
  - Pathology/pathophysiology (disease, disorder, or condition)
  - Impairments
  - Functional outcomes
  - Disabilities
  - Risk reduction/prevention
  - Health, wellness, and fitness
  - Societal resources
  - Patient/Client satisfaction

Criteria for Termination of Physical Therapy Services

- Discharge—End physical therapy services for this episode of care when anticipated goals and expected outcomes have been achieved.
- Discontinuation—End physical therapy for episode of care when there is a decline in performance, Mrs. Smith is unable to progress, or Mrs. Smith will no longer benefit from this physical therapy episode of care.

CASE STUDY #3
Shirley Teal

- *Age: 21 years*
- *Medical Diagnosis: Traumatic brain injury*
- *Status: 4 months post injury*
- *Practice Pattern 5D: Impaired Motor Function and Sensory Integrity Associated with Nonprogressive Disorders of the Central Nervous System—Acquired in Adolescence or Adulthood*

This case is an example of using the *Guide* for reexamination and modifying the plan of care.

REEXAMINATION

Summary of History and Systems Review from Initial Examination

- General Demographics—Ms. Teal is a 21-year-old woman 4 months post motor vehicle accident (MVA). She has a high school education and training as a beautician.
- Social History—She is a single parent with a 2-year-old child.
- Employment/Work (Job/School/Play)—Shirley worked at a beauty salon.
- Living Environment—She has been in an extended care facility since 2 months post MVA. Her plans are to live with her parents and young child in the next 2 months. They live in a second-floor apartment.
- General Health Status
  - Perception—Stated prior health was excellent.
  - Role—Daughter, mother, employee.

Medical/Surgical

At the time of admission to the hospital following the MVA, Ms. Teal was decerebrate, had intracranial bleeding in the right occipital horn, and was diagnosed with traumatic brain injury (TBI). She was comatose and received a tracheotomy and a gastrostomy immediately after admission to the hospital. At 2 months post trauma, she was transferred to an extended care facility. At that time, she was able to open her eyes to verbal and tactile stimuli, but was unable to visually track an object. She was able to move her upper and lower extremities spontaneously, but not on command. The initial physical therapy examination noted that she had mild to moderate resistance to passive movement in both upper extremities (right greater than the left) and severe stiffness in her lower extremities. She was limited in passive range of motion in right elbow extension (-30 degrees), right knee extension (-15 degrees), and right hip extension (-15 degrees). Other joint range of motion was passively within normal limits. She exhibited bilateral ankle clonus (right greater than left) when minimal stretch was applied. She exhibited poor head and trunk control when supported sitting was attempted.

Current Conditions/Chief Complaint

Currently, Ms. Teal is being seen to improve her functional status in areas of self-care, locomotion, and transfers. She is receiving physical and occupational therapy at the extended care facility twice a day. Her goal is to return home to help care for her daughter.

Tests and Measures

Arousal, Attention, and Cognition

Ms. Teal continues to demonstrate problems with cognition. She has difficulty with maintenance of concentration and demonstrates an inability to switch attention between tasks or objects within the environment. She is able to follow simple instructions but occasionally forgets what is asked of her.

Assistive and Adaptive Devices

Ms. Teal has a manual wheelchair on loan.

Gait, Locomotion Balance

She tends to lose her balance easily if she moves quickly. She also demonstrates positional dizziness due to benign paroxysmal positional nystamus (BPPN) and vertigo. She is able to perform pivot transfers and stands in the parallel bars for 5 minutes with minimal assistance. She does not initiate ambulation on her own. She is independent in a wheelchair by using the left arm for pushing and her left leg for pulling.

Motor Function (Motor Control and Motor Learning)

Ms. Teal has good head control in all positions. She is able to sit independently, although she lists to the left. She is able to come to sitting by rolling to the side and with minimal assistance from the therapist. She requires supervision and occasional minimal assistance from the therapist.

She is able to move her right wrist, fingers, elbow, and shoulder free of synergistic patterns, but with decreased strength and coordination. Additionally, her coordination patterns in the left upper extremity are impaired. She is unable to reach with her left arm directly to an object that is held out to her. She has foot placement problems with the left leg in sitting and in standing.

Muscle Performance

Ms. Teal continues to demonstrate increased stiffness bilaterally (right greater than left) in both upper and lower extremities. Her strength is decreased in the right lower extremity and she is unable to sustain right knee extension during stance.

Neuromotor Development and Sensory Integration

Ms. Teal is aware of sensory input to all extremities. However, she is unable to discriminate common objects that are placed in her hands. She has an excessive dependence on vision for her balance control in sitting and standing. Auditory perception appears intact. She has BPPN and vertigo.

Posture

In sitting, she has difficulty in maintaining weight equally on both buttocks. She tends to list to the left side while placing weight primarily on her left buttock. She is able to stand in parallel bars but has to be reminded to place weight on her right lower extremity.

Range of Motion

She has decreased range of motion in the right lower extremity, including a 40-degree plantarflexion contracture and–10 degrees of hip and knee extension. She has full range of motion actively in the left extremities.

Self-Care and Home Management

Ms. Teal plans to live with her parents and young child in a second-floor apartment. Her parents report that they do not have an elevator, and their daughter will have to walk up and down the stairs to access apartment. At this time, Ms. Teal is able only to stand using handrails on both sides with minimal support of one other adult and is unable to initiate lifting either foot for placement on step. Ms. Teal's balance and motor skills limit her ability to perform ADLs. She is currently receiving occupational therapy to work on specific ADL skills. Supervision is required for safety. Ms. Teal is dependent for all IADLs and requires assistance and supervision to access the community.

EVALUATION (CLINICAL JUDGMENT)

Ms. Teal is 4 months post injury. She has made progress, but is becoming more difficult in therapy sessions, being agitated and combative. She continues to have problems with cognition. She is able to follow simple commands but does forget what is asked. There are contractures in her right lower extremity and general decreased strength. She is able to sit but leans to the left. She needs assistance to transfer and stand. She is unable to ambulate or climb stairs. She is mobile using a wheelchair within a controlled environment. She is dependent for most of her ADLs and all of her IADLs. She requires supervision for safety.

Primary impairments include areas of behavior, cognition, motor function, sensory integrity, and balance. Secondary impairments include areas of range of motion, muscle performance, and posture. Functional limitations include activities of self-care, home management, and community/leisure. Disability includes inability to complete roles of daughter, mother, and beautician. Risk reduction/prevention needs include falls, contractures, and skin break down.

DIAGNOSIS

The primary impairments that impact Ms. Teal's functional abilities continue to be consistent with Pattern 5D: Impaired Motor Function and Sensory Integrity Associated with Nonprogressive Disorders of the Central Nervous System—Acquired in Adolescence or Adulthood.

PROGNOSIS

Ms. Teal will demonstrate optimal motor function and sensory integrity and the highest level of functioning in the home and community within the context of her impairments, functional limitations, and disabilities. At this time, Ms. Teal's rate of progress has been limited due to her combative behavior and inability to participate effectively during therapy. Current behavior modification programs have not been effective in improving her behavior.

How can you use the *Guide* to help you determine how to progress with Ms. Teal? The first step is to review the Factors column on the prognosis page (pp. S363). This list provides factors that you can use to modify the frequency of visits or duration of care. For Ms. Teal, factors that you may use include: adherence to the intervention program, cognitive status, and psychological factors. The next step is to review the anticipated goals and expected outcomes within the intervention pages (pp. S364–S373). These lists identify anticipated goals and expected outcomes at various levels of patient performance. You may decide to select goals and outcomes that focus on educating the patient and family as to realistic expectations and understanding of goals and objectives. You may also include training of family and caregivers in physical management of the patient throughout her daily routine for improved safety and decreased risk of secondary impairments, in addition to or rather than, those goals and outcomes focusing on improving her impairments.

CASE STUDY # 5
Robert Anderson

- *Age: 38 years*
- *Medical Diagnosis: Incomplete T9-10 spinal cord injury with left radial nerve damage*
- *Status: 6 months post injury*
- *Practice Pattern 5H: Impaired Motor Function, Peripheral Nerve*
- *Integrity, and Sensory Integrity Associated with Nonprogressive Disorders of the Spinal Cord*

EXAMINATION

History

- General Demographics—Mr. Anderson is a 38-year-old man with an incomplete T9-10 spinal cord injury and residual nerve damage resulting from a upper extremity fracture.
- Social History—He has a large extended family who lives in the area. He is married with two young children (5 and 8 years of age). His wife works as a teacher.

- Employment/Work (Job/School/Play)—Mr. Anderson is a banker and has returned to work part-time.
- Living Environment—He lives in an older two-story house with bedrooms and bath on the upper level.
- General Health Status (Self-Report, Family Report, Caregiver Report)
  - Perception—Mr. Anderson was in good health prior to the accident.
  - Physical Function—He has mobility using a wheelchair.
  - Psychological Function—He is motivated to improve.
  - Role—Husband, father, and employee.
  - Social Function—Recreational activities included running and motorcycle racing.
- Social/Health Habits (Past and Current)—He doesn't smoke or drink.
- Family History—There are no known family health risks.

Medical/Surgical

Six months ago, Mr. Anderson lost control of his motorcycle on a slippery road and sustained an incomplete T9-10 spinal cord injury. He had fractures of the right femur and left radius with residual damage to the left radial nerve. He was in an inpatient rehabilitation facility for 4 months. He reports that prior to the accident, he was in generally good health.

Current Conditions/Chief Complaint

Mr. Anderson continues to have difficulty transferring and has limited ambulation. He received physical therapy as an inpatient after the accident for 4 months, and then was discharged to home. He is receiving physical therapy two times a week as an outpatient at the local hospital.

Functional Status and Activity Level

He is independent in ADLs (dressing, bowel and bladder care). He uses a wheelchair and drives a car that has hand controls. He has returned to work part-time.

Medications

List drug, dose, how taken, and side effects, include herbal and over-the-counter drugs.

Other Clinical Findings

Hospital and clinic records were reviewed. Mr. Anderson has had problems with sacral skin breakdown. For a short time, he was in diagnostic pattern of 7B: Impaired Integumentary Integrity Associated with Superficial Skin Involvement due to superficial skin involvement.

SYSTEMS REVIEWS

The systems review may include the following:

Anatomical and Physiological Status

- Cardiovascular
  - Blood Pressure—136/84
  - Edema—None noted
  - Heart Rate—80 bpm
  - Respiratory Rate—18 bpm
- Integumentary
  - Presence of Scar Formation—There are scars as a result of the accident. They are healed, and examination shows no need for intervention at this time.
  - Skin Color—Good
  - Skin Integrity—Sacral area is healed. The patient has a good understanding of prevention and is being monitored.
- Musculoskeletal
  - Gross Range of Motion—Mr. Anderson's range of motion is within functional limits.
  - Gross Strength—Mr. Anderson has flaccid paralysis of lower extremities with some increased tone and with some weakness in left arm.
  - Gross Symmetry
  - Height—6-feet 1 inch
  - Weight—164 pounds.
- Neuromuscular
  - Gross Coordinated Movements—He is able to sit without upper extremity support. He cannot stand independently but needs walker or forearm crutches, long leg braces with pelvic support, and knee-ankle-foot orthoses (KAFOs).
- Communication, Affect, Cognition, Language, and Learning Style—He is oriented and knowledgeable about his condition.
- Tests and Measures—may include Aerobic Capacity/Endurance
- Anthropometric Characteristics
- Arousal, Attention, and Cognition—Mr. Anderson is a very cooperative and motivated patient who is anxious to return to work full-time and to achieve full independence. He has no cognitive deficits.
- Assistive and Adaptive Devices—Walker or forearm crutches, lower leg bracing with pelvic support, lightweight wheelchair, and modified car.
- Circulation
- Cranial and Peripheral Nerve Integrity
- Environmental, Home, and Work
- Ergonomics and Body Mechanics
- Gait, Locomotion Balance—Mr. Anderson is able to sit independently without upper extremity support and sustain minor balance disturbances in all directions.

He cannot stand independently, but must use a walker or forearm crutches and lower leg bracing with pelvic support (ie, KAFO). For household ambulation, Mr. Anderson occasionally walks with a swing through gait using his braces and forearm crutches. He does not have the endurance to use this method for community ambulation. He uses an ultralight manual wheelchair during his daily routine. He is currently driving a car that has been modified with hand controls.

- Integumentary Integrity
- Joint Integrity and Mobility
- Motor Function (Motor Control and Motor Learning)—He is independent in self-care (eg, dressing, bowel and bladder care). He has some difficulty with transfers, including sit to stand with KAFOs and to the bed, floor, bath, car, and his wheelchair.
- Muscle Performance—Initially, Mr. Anderson had a flaccid paralysis of the lower extremities, but has had increasing stiffness (tone). His right upper extremity strength is normal, but he has some weakness in the left arm due to the radial nerve damage.
- Neuromotor Development and Sensory Integration
- Orthotic, Protective, and Supportive Devices
- Pain
- Posture—No difficulties or abnormal postures are noted.
- Prosthetic Requirements
- Range of Motion—Normal passive range of motion is present at all joints. Mr. Anderson notes occasional muscle spasms in his lower extremities.
- Reflex Integrity
- Self-Care and Home Management—He is independent in dressing and bowel and bladder care.
- Sensory Integrity—Loss of sensation is noted associated with the spinal cord injury and the residual nerve injury. Intermittent problems with sacral breakdown have occurred.
- Ventilation and Respiration/Gas Exchange
- Work (Job/School/Play), Community, and Leisure Integration or Reintegration

EVALUATION (CLINICAL JUDGMENT)

- Pathology/Pathophysiology (Disease, Disorder, or Condition)—Spinal cord injury at T9-10 and residual radial nerve damage.
- Impairments—Impaired motor function in lower extremities, impaired muscle performance.
- Functional Limitations—Difficulty accessing the community.
- Disabilities—Inability to keep up with peers.
- Risk Reduction/Prevention—Monitor for sacral skin breakdown.
- Health, Wellness, and Fitness—Mr. Anderson plans to play on a wheelchair basketball team.
- Societal Resources
- Patient Satisfaction

DIAGNOSIS

Pattern 5H: Impaired Motor Function, Peripheral Nerve Integrity, and Sensory Integrity Associated with Nonprogressive Disorders of the Spinal Cord.

REEXAMINATION SUMMARY

Mr. Anderson has a new complaint of increased pain in his left shoulder with decreased ROM and strength that is affecting his ability to transfer, wheel his wheelchair, and ambulate. Diagnostic results from his physician state that he has inflammation in the left shoulder due to overuse.

A complete reexamination is performed by the physical therapist, including the left shoulder. Primary impairments impacting Mr. Anderson's functional abilities are limited joint mobility, pain, and impaired muscle performance of the left shoulder. Secondary impairments include deficits in motor function and sensory integrity.

How does the *Guide* help you in determining what to do with Mr. Anderson following the reexamination? Patients are placed in the patterns based on diagnosis of the primary impairments that are driving the intervention. Mr. Anderson was originally placed in Pattern 5H: Impaired Motor Function, Peripheral Nerve Integrity, and Sensory Integrity Associated with Nonprogressive Disorders of the Spinal Cord because the primary impairments driving the interventions were lack of motor function and impaired sensory integrity associated with his spinal cord injury. At the reexamination, new primary impairments of left shoulder joint immobility, pain, inadequate muscle performance, and limited range of motion would now drive the interventions. You reclassify Mr. Anderson into musculoskeletal pattern of 4E: Impaired Joint Mobility, Motor Function, Muscle Performance, and Range of Motion Associated with Localized Inflammation. This is the pattern that addresses management of these impairments and also provides for resumption of functional skills. Reexaminations will determine when it is appropriate to reclassify Mr. Anderson back to Pattern 5H. Note: For the remaining chapters in the text, Mr. Anderson will be classified in Pattern 5H.

REFERENCES

1. APTA. Guide to physical therapist practice. 2nd ed. *Phys Ther.* 2001;81:9-744.
2. APTA. Guide to physical therapist practice. Vol I: a description of patient management. *Phys Ther.* 1995;75:707-764.
3. APTA. Guide to physical therapist practice. *Phys Ther.* 1997;77:1163-1650.
4. APTA. Guide to physical therapist practice. Revisions. *Phys Ther.* 1999;81:623-629.
5. APTA. Guide to Physical Therapist Practice. Revisions. *Phys Ther.* 1999;81:1078-1081.
6. Bernhardt-Bainbridge D. What's new: guide to physical therapist practice. 2nd ed. *PT Magazine.* 2001;9:34-37.
7. Nagi S. Some conceptual issues in disability and rehabilitation. In: Sussman M, ed. *Sociology and Rehabilitation.* Washington, DC: American Sociological Association; 1965:100-113.
8. ICIDH. *International Classification of Impairments, Disabilities, and Handicaps.* Geneva, Switzerland: World Health Organization; 1980.

9. National Advisory Board on Medical Rehabilitation Research. *Draft V: Report and Plan for Medical Rehabilitation Research*. Bethesda, Md: National Institutes of Health; 1992.

10. Nagi S. *Disability and Rehabilitation*. Columbus, Ohio: Ohio State University Press; 1969.

11. Nagi S. Disability concepts revisited: implications for prevention. In: *Disability in America: Toward a National Agenda for Prevention*. Washington, DC: Institute of Medicine, National Academy Press; 1991.

12. *ICIDH-2: International Classification of Functioning, Disability, and Health*. Geneva, Switzerland: World Health Organization; 2000.

13. *Disability in America: Toward a National Agenda for Prevention*. Washington, DC: Institute of Medicine, National Academy Press; 1991.

14. Brandt EN Jr, Pope AM, eds. *Enabling America: Assessing the Role of Rehabilitation Science and Engineering*. Washington, DC: American Sociological Association; 1965:100-113.

15. Guccione AA. Physical therapy diagnosis and the relationship between impairments and function. *Phys Ther.* 1991;71:499-504.

16. Jette AM. Using health-related quality of life measures in physical therapy outcomes research. *Phys Ther*. 1993;73:528-537.

17. Jette AM. Physical disablement concepts for physical therapy research and practice. *Phys Ther.* 1994;74:380-386.

18. Craik RL. Disability following hip fracture. *Phys Ther.* 1994;74:387-398.

19. Duncan PW. Stroke disability. *Phys Ther.* 1994;74:399-407.

20. Guccione AA. Arthritis and the process of disablement. *Phys Ther.* 1994;74:408-414.

21. Rimmer JH. Health promotion for people with disabilities: the emerging paradigm shift from disability prevention to prevention of secondary conditions. *Phys Ther.* 1999;79:495-502.

22. Gill-Body KM, Beninato M, Krebs DE. Relationship among balance impairments, functional performance, and disability in people with peripheral vestibular hypofunction. *Phys Ther.* 2000;80:748-758.

23. Hermann KM, Reese CS. Relationships among selected measures of impairment, functional limitation, and disability in patients with cervical spine disorders. *Phys Ther.* 2001;81:903-914.

24. Giallonardo L. Guide in action: patient with total hip replacement. *PT Magazine.* 2000;8:76-86.

CHAPTER 8

Examination and Evaluation of Motor Control

Mitzi B. Zeno, PT, MS, NCS
Patricia Leahy, PT, MS, NCS

INTRODUCTION

The examination of individuals with motor control impairments is the foundation for the other elements of patient management leading to optimal outcomes. The physical therapy evaluation, diagnosis, prognosis, and intervention are based on the therapist's expertise in performing a thorough and accurate examination. According to the ***Guide to Physical Therapist Practice***, an examination of motor control consists of three parts: history, systems review, and tests and measurements.[1]

While taking a history, the physical therapist gathers data from both the past and present that is relevant to the patient's need for physical therapy services. The history should include written information from the patient's chart or other records, as well as an interview with the patient, patient's family and caregivers, and other individuals interested in contributing to the patient's welfare, such as teachers, vocational counselors, and employers. Relevant data to be gathered by the physical therapist may include medical/surgical history, chief complaints, medications, social and family history, education or work status, living environment, past and current social and health habits, functional level, and perhaps, most importantly, the patient's own goals. Individuals contributing to the history should feel comfortable in expressing thoughts and opinions without worrying about a possible bias that the examiner may have regarding factors such as culture, social status, or religious beliefs. When gathering a history, the physical therapist should be an active listener.

The history may guide the physical therapist in choosing certain tests and measurements to perform in conjunction with the systems review, which is the second component to a motor control examination. A systems review is a brief screening of the patient's cardiopulmonary, integumentary, musculoskeletal, and neuromuscular systems, as well the patient's orientation, communication, and cognition. For the patient with motor control deficits, a quick review will likely lead to more specific and detailed testing, particularly of the musculoskeletal, neuromuscular, and cognition/communication systems.

Tests and measurements, the third component of the examination process, have become critically important in today's health care which places emphasis on evidence-based practice. More than ever before, physical therapists are being asked by funding agencies, case managers, and other health practitioners to supply evidence in the form of published, peer-reviewed research that suggests treatment interventions are cost-effective and beneficial to the patient. It is no longer acceptable for a therapist to say that something works simply because he or she has observed it over a long period of time or because he or she has always done it that way. Given the number of factors that contribute to motor control, ranging from psychological to physiological states, and given the complexity of each of these factors, it is not surprising that the evaluation of motor control is a challenge.

If tests and measurements are important in identifying impairments and functional limitations to determine physical therapy prognoses, diagnoses, and especially interventions, we should begin by describing the difference between tests and measurements. Tests are procedures used to determine reactions or the presence or absence of responses. Some tests, such as urinalysis, are easy to interpret while others, such as those used to assess pain responses, are not. Measurements are assigned dimensions or values used to describe something we feel, see, or hear. Measurements are used to determine the cadence or step length of gait, to assess range of motion of the shoulder, or quantify the amount of assistance required to perform functional activities.

Tests and measurements that are considered objective, valid, and reliable are most acceptable in today's practice. For example, in 1995 when the United States Department of Health and Human Services published the ***Clinical Practice Guidelines on Post-Stroke Rehabilitation: Assessment, Referral, and Patient Management***, the use of standardized testing instruments was recommended. Several assessments currently being used were listed along with their major strengths and weaknesses.[2] However, some variables, such as spasticity, are difficult to define let alone measure (see Chapter 12). One must remember that physical therapy is both a science and an art which sometimes relies on the judgments of professionals without the use of a specific measurement tool.

When examining the strengths and weaknesses of various tools, the issues of reliability and validity need to be addressed. If a test measures what it is supposed to measure, it is said to be ***valid***. A valid test provides the therapist with meaningful information. Three types of validity may be described when discussing measurement instruments. ***Construct validity*** refers to concepts or ideas supporting the measure. Strength, which will be discussed in detail later, is a construct that is poorly understood because it may have many different meanings. ***Content validity*** measures how thoroughly or accurately a test represents a person's status. Content validity is typically determined by knowledgeable peers. ***Predictive*** and ***concurrent validity*** are two subcategories of ***criterion validity*** which compare one measure to another. Predictive validity is used to predict future status and concurrent validity refers to how a test compares to other tests proven to measure similar items. Concurrent validity frequently is used to validate a new test by comparing it with a previously validated test.

There are two types of reliability or consistency. Because patients with motor control deficits often display great variability in motivation and performance, it may be difficult to determine the reliability of tests and measurements. *Intrarater reliability* refers to the same person using the same test on different occasions and obtaining the same results. *Interrater reliability* refers to different people using the same test to measure the same thing and obtaining the same results.

Many therapists assume that the tests and measurements they have always used in the clinic are valid and reliable. Unfortunately, there may not be research to support these assumptions. Whenever possible, the issues of validity and reliability will be addressed as part of the discussion of the different types of tests and measurements most commonly used in the examination of motor control by physical therapists.

COMMUNICATION, AFFECT, AND COGNITION

Because many of the tools used in the examination of motor control require the patient's understanding and cooperation, a more in-depth examination of the patient's cognitive functioning, communication abilities, and affect may be needed. Much of this information can be determined during the interview process while taking the history. However, some patients will need more thorough testing due to impaired cognition and/or communication skills. Reviewing the speech pathologist's report, if available, may be helpful in determining more effective ways in which to communicate with the patient who has dysarthria or aphasia. Sometimes it is useful to ask a family member to act as an intermediary when the patient speaks a different language or appears to respond better to those more familiar to him or her. Simple questions can be used to determine the patient's orientation to person, place, and time. Response time to questions or instructions should be noted as it will affect the patient's motor control and motor learning abilities. Occasionally a measurement tool such as the Glasgow Coma Scale or Rancho Los Amigos Levels of Cognitive Function (Table 8-1) may be needed for patients with more extensive brain damage. Physical therapists may also enlist the aid of a neuropsychologist if more formal testing is required.

RANGE OF MOTION

The examination of range of motion (ROM) is very important to any motor control evaluation because adequate ROM must be present to allow functional excursions of muscles and normal biomechanical alignment. Adequate ROM is also necessary to prevent the development of secondary deficits that result from immobilization. The ROM at particular joints varies considerably among individuals and may be affected by age, gender, and other factors such as disease or pathology. Average ranges of motion for the joints of the body may be found in the handbook of the American Academy of Orthopaedic Surgeons[3] and a variety of other texts.[4,5] A summary table is found in Norkin and White.[6] However, these averages should be used with caution because the populations from which the averages were derived are undefined, and the specific test positions and types of instruments that were used are not always identified.

TABLE 8-1

Rancho Los Amigos Hospital Levels of Cognitive Function*

I.	No response—total assistance
II.	Generalized response—total assistance
III.	Localized response—total assistance
IV.	Confused—agitated—maximal assistance
V.	Confused—inappropriate—nonagitated—maximal assistance
VI.	Confused—appropriate—moderate assistance
VII.	Automatic—appropriate—minimal assistance
VIII.	Purposeful—appropriate—standby assistance
IX.	Purposeful—appropriate—standby assistance on request
X.	Purposeful—appropriate—modified independent

The Rancho Levels of Cognitive Functioning have been revised and expanded from 8 to 10 levels by Chris Hagan, PhD, 1998, Rancho Los Amigos National Rehabilitation Center, Department of Communication Disorders, Harriman Building, 7601 E. Imperial Highway, Downey, Calif, 90242.

Range of motion should be assessed both actively (without assistance from the examiner) and passively (without assistance from the individual). Normally, passive range of motion (PROM) is *slightly* greater than active range of motion (AROM) because each joint has a small amount of available motion (joint play) that is not under voluntary control. The additional PROM that is available at the end of the normal AROM helps to protect joint structures, because it allows the joint to absorb extrinsic forces.

Testing PROM provides information about the integrity of the articular surfaces and the extensibility of the joint capsule, associated ligaments, and muscles. The extent of PROM is determined by the unique structure of the joint capsules being tested. Some joints are structured so the joint capsules limit the end of ROM in a particular direction, while other joints are structured so ligaments limit the end of a particular ROM. Other limitations to motion include contact of joint surfaces (eg, metacarpophalangeal joint flexion), muscle tension (eg, dorsiflexion with knee extension), and soft tissue approximation (eg, hip flexion).[6] Each specific structure that serves to limit a ROM has a characteristic feel to it, which may be detected by the examiner who is performing PROM. This feeling, which is experienced by the examiner as resistance to further motion at the end of a PROM, is called the *end-feel*. End-feels may be considered normal (physiologic) or abnormal (pathologic). Clinical decisions regarding interventions often are based not only on the amount of ROM present, but also on the end-feel. End-feels are usually classified as soft, firm, hard, or empty. The first three types may be either normal or abnormal, depending on where they occur. An empty end-feel is never normal. It describes the situation in which the patient experiences pain before the examiner experiences an end-feel.

In addition to testing the amount of motion and end-feels, PROM can give the therapist information about muscle tone. Muscle tone has been defined as the amount of tension in a muscle.[7] Several factors contribute to the amount of tension in a muscle including intrinsic elasticity and neural components. While subjective, the clinician can detect variations in the normal resting tone of a muscle during passive movement. These variations will be discussed further under the category of muscle tone.

Testing AROM provides additional information about muscle strength, motor control, and coordination when compared to PROM. The patient's ability to use available PROM for active movement is vital in performing simple, as well as complex functional activities. Both the quantity and quality of active movement should be included in the examination of range of motion. The use of abnormal synergy (groups of muscles working together) patterns in which the patient is unable to isolate specific movements should be noted either individually or as part of an overall evaluation of functional abilities. The patient typically has little or no control over the stereotypical movement patterns seen with abnormal synergies (see Chapters 11 and 12).

The most common method of measuring the degree of ROM is *goniometry*, a measurement of the angles of joints. This word was derived from two Greek words, *gonia*, meaning angle, and *metron*, meaning measure. Several studies have been published regarding the reliability and validity of goniometry for the various joints.[8-10] Electrogoniometers are very similar to their manual counterparts, but instead of a scale that is read by the examiner, there is an electrical potentiometer attached to a fulcrum. An output signal representing the joint angle is available and can be read by the therapist or fed into a computer for data reduction.

MUSCLE PERFORMANCE

Muscle Strength

Although *strength* is one of the most widely used terms in physical therapy, it remains poorly understood. Strength typically refers to force production. Usually force is measured in one of two ways, the ability to produce a movement or the ability to resist a movement. Both manual muscle testing (MMT) and dynamometry have used these two approaches to document strength. Some authors have chosen to differentiate between strength and power, with the latter referring to the ability to produce force through a ROM in a particular time. Only isokinetic testing allows the clinician to assess power (see Chapter 5). It should be noted that the controversy over strength training in patients with central nervous system (CNS) pathology or spasticity is being resolved in favor of incorporating strengthening in treatment programs (see Chapter 12).

In 1916, orthopedic surgeon Robert Lovett[11] developed a grading scale of normal (N), good (G), fair (F), poor (P), trace (T), and totally paralyzed (0) to measure strength. Henry and Florence Kendall et al[12] introduced the use of percentages in the 1930s which correlated to the letter system developed by Lovett. In 1947, Daniels et al[13] included positions for testing various muscles, including gravity-resisted and gravity-lessened positions. Pluses and minuses have been added to increase the sensitivity of the tool. Others have suggested using numbers rather than letters and pluses or minuses. Table 8-2 illustrates a comparison of the various classification methods.

One of the most important concepts in MMT is the effect of gravity in grading. While gravity has little effect on some muscles (eg, fingers, toes, supinators, and pronators), from a clinical perspective, it may have a major influence on the strength of other muscles. A patient typically is asked to first actively move a body part through a full ROM against gravity to determine whether the muscle is better or worse than a grade of fair (3/5). If the patient is able to complete this task, varying amounts of resistance

TABLE 8-2
Manual Muscle Testing Grades

Kendall's Percent		Lovett's Letters		
Percent	Abbreviation	Word	Letter	Numerals
100	10	Normal	N	5
95	–	Normal minus	N-	5-
90	9	Good plus	G+	4+
80	8	Good	G	4
70	7	Good minus	G-	4-
60	6	Fair plus	F+	3+
50	5	Fair	F	3
40	4	Fair minus	F-	3-
30	3	Poor plus	P+	2+
20	2	Poor	P	2
10	–	Poor minus	P-	2-
5	1	Trace	T	1
0	0	Zero	0	0

are added for grades of good (4/5) or normal (5/5). During a "break" test, the examiner applies increasing isometric resistance until the patient's ability to resist has been overcome or until maximal resistance has been applied.[14,15] While the "make" test is sometimes mentioned in the literature, the "break" test is most often used in the clinic. The "make" test involves giving the patient isotonic resistance throughout the range.

If the patient is unable to actively complete a movement through the full ROM against gravity, the movement then is attempted in gravity-lessened positions for grades of fair minus (3-), poor (2), trace (1), or zero (0). For very weak muscles, palpation of a contraction is critical.

It may be difficult to follow the standard MMT procedures for young children, especially those under the age of 5 years because they are unwilling to cooperate with instructions or do not understand what they are supposed to do.[16] Connolly[17] and others have provided guidelines for grading a muscle test for infants and small children.[18]

Another important concept in muscle testing is substitution. When a muscle or muscle group is used to compensate for the lack of function by a weak muscle, the result is substitution. For accurate muscle testing, substitutions should not be permitted. Abnormal synergy patterns have been described as a type of substitution.

Several studies have been done on the reliability and validity of MMT. Wadsworth et al.[19] in 1987 studied intrarater reliability and reported test-retest coefficients of r=.63 for the knee flexors, r=.74 for the hip flexors and r=.98 for the shoulder abductors. In 1992, Florence et al[20] reported on the intrarater reliability of testing done by physical therapists. Using Cohen's kappa, the scores ranged from r=.65 to .93. In 1995, in a somewhat similar study, Brandsma et al[21] showed a range from r = .71 to .96 for intrarater and r=.72 to .93 for interrater reliability. Although the reliability of MMT tends to vary (particularly for grades of good and above), more consistent results can be obtained by using a standardized method which ensures the patient is positioned appropriately, the proximal segment is stabilized securely, and, in most cases, resistance is applied using a short lever arm.

Studies by Lazar et al[22] and Brown et al[23] have shown that MMT has predictive validity. Other studies such as those done by Bohannon[24] and Schwartz et al[25] compared MMT to handheld dynamometers and/or strain gauges, demonstrating that manual testing is a valid method of measuring muscle strength particularly for muscles with grades of good minus and below.

To quantify the evaluation of muscle strength, a number of devices have been developed to measure the force exerted by the body on an external object. Such devices, called *force transducers*, give electrical signals proportional to the applied force. There are many kinds available, ranging from simple to elaborate.

Dynamometers are instruments used to measure mechanical force. Handheld dynamometers can be incorporated into MMT procedures (Figure 8-1). Instead of the examiner estimating the amount of pressure required to "break" the patient's hold on a position, the instrument provides a readout of force. In more sophisticated systems, the handheld device is attached to a computer which provides a reading in Newtons. This type of testing is limited to cases in which the examiner can overcome the strength of the muscle group being tested. It also requires the examiner to be aware of and prevent substitutions. Limited studies on the validity of handheld dynamometers currently exist. A review of the studies done on the reliability of handheld dynamometry was done by Soderberg.[26]

HANDHELD DYNAMOMETER

Larger and more sophisticated dynamometers have been incorporated into isokinetic testing devices. As mentioned previously, these devices offer the major advantage of allowing the assessment of force production at varying speeds. In isokinetic testing, the amount of resistance changes throughout the patient's muscle contraction to match exactly the force applied by the patient. Because of this accommodation, it allows for maximal dynamic loading throughout the ROM. As opposed to isotonic testing, where the resistance is set and the patient determines the speed, isokinetic testing sets the speed, and the patient must perform at that speed to produce force. This is important because it allows examination of the patient's ability to produce force at high speeds, as is required for most functional activities. Although often used when evaluating patients with musculoskeletal deficits, isokinetic equipment is equally useful for the assessment of patients with neurologically based movement disorders. The inability to generate force quickly, maintain the force as desired, and terminate the force are all common motor control deficits that can be evaluated on isokinetic equipment. Equipment allows for testing of the ability to produce movement (isotonic and isokinetic tests), as well as the ability to resist movement (isometric and eccentric tests).

Kinesiological Electromyography

During a muscle contraction, the force twitches produced by the active motor units summate to produce the force output of the muscle. We cannot measure directly the force twitches or the muscle force. We can only measure the resultant torque generated by the forces acting on a joint. Current methods of measuring torque (ie, isokinetics,

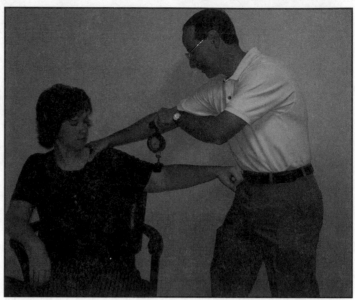

182   Chapter 8

Figure 8-1. Handheld dynamometer.

strain gauges) require relatively constrained movement, and cannot isolate individual muscle contributions to the torque production.

Electromyography (EMG) is a graphical representation of the electrical activity within skeletal muscle (Figure 8-2). The EMG signal originates after a nerve action potential has been transmitted along the axon of a motoneuron and its branches to activate the muscle fibers associated with the motor unit. The fiber action potential then propagates in both directions toward the ends of the muscle fiber. The algebraic summation of these fiber action potentials produces the motor unit action potential, which is recorded during EMG.[27]

Two types of electrodes are used clinically: surface electrodes and indwelling electrodes. Diagnostic EMG requires the use of in-dwelling electrodes. The invasive nature of in-dwelling electrodes, however, restricts their use primarily to diagnostic purposes, with limited clinical and research applications. Surface electrodes are easily applied and noninvasive, but they have a large pickup area and only can be used with superficial muscles. With any type of electrode, proper placement is critical to avoid crosstalk from other muscles and to avoid distortion of the EMG signal. Electrodes should be placed on the belly of the muscle, and then placement should be checked by asking the patient to perform a functional test to isolate the muscle, if possible.

Due to the nature of the EMG signal, it contains information about the numbers of active motor units and their frequency of firing. This information represents the commands from the nervous system, so the EMG can serve as a means of monitoring the neural control of movement. The amplitude of the individual MUAP is influenced by the number of muscle fibers in the motor unit and their diameters, as well as by the degree of synchronization in the summation of single fiber action potentials.[27]

Because EMG provides a qualitative and quantitative record of muscle activation, it has the potential to enhance the evaluation of patients who are neurologically involved. It gives information about which muscle activity is responsible for a muscle movement

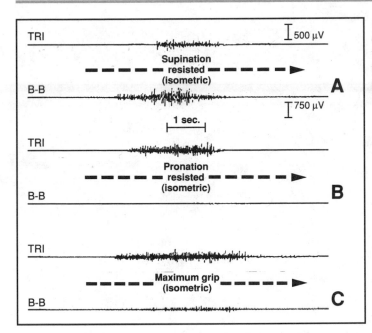

Figure 8-2. Example of electromyography records for synergistic actions of the triceps brachii (TRI) and biceps-brachialis (B-B) muscles.

and whether antagonistic activity is taking place. In attempting to assess motor control, the addition of EMG provides broader and more detailed information on which to base decisions.

REFLEX INTEGRITY

Muscle Tone/Tension

Muscle tone has been used by a variety of people to mean a variety of things. The Bobaths described normal muscle tone as being high enough to hold the body part against gravity, but low enough to permit movement.[28] Others have defined it simply as the amount of resistance to passive stretch. Muscle tone that is abnormally high (hypertonicity) has been described as resistance to passive movement, while abnormally low tone (hypotonicity) has been described as exaggerated assistance to passive movement. Regardless of the definition, a wide variation exists in the amount of muscle tone that may be present. Two types of hypertonicity are *spasticity* and *rigidity*. Spasticity (an imbalance in tone between an agonist and antagonist, sometimes called stiffness) is common to patients after a cerebrovascular accident (CVA). Spasticity appears to be more velocity-dependent than the second type of hypertonicity which is rigidity. Rigidity (an exaggerated co-contraction of both agonist and antagonist) is commonly seen with Parkinson's disease and in patients recovering from brain injuries. Flaccidity indicates a significant decrease in muscle tone and may be seen after a CVA or spinal cord injury.

In recent years, controversy has risen over the clinical significance of examining and documenting muscle tone (see Chapter 12). The relationship between muscle tone and abnormal movement is not yet clearly understood. Studies on patients after a dorsal rhizotomy have shown that, although the amount of spasticity may be greatly reduced fol-

TABLE 8-3

Modified Ashworth Scale*

Grade	Description
0	No increase in muscle tone.
1	Slight increase in muscle tone, manifested by a catch and release or by minimal resistance at the end of the ROM when the affected part(s) is moved in flexion or extension.
1+	Slight increase in muscle tone, manifested by a catch followed by minimal resistance throughout the remainder (less than half) or the ROM.
2	More marked increase in muscle tone through most of the ROM, but affected part(s) easily moved.
3	Considerable increase in muscle tone; passive movement difficult.
4	Affected part(s) rigid in flexion or extension.

*Reprinted with permission of the American Physical Therapy Association from Bohannon R, Smith M. Interrater reliability of a modified Ashworth scale of muscle spasticity. Phys Ther. 1987;67:207.

lowing surgical ablation of selected sensory nerve roots, abnormal movement patterns that existed prior to the surgery persist.[29,30] Jackson[31] described two distinct types of symptoms resulting from neurologic lesions: negative and positive. Negative symptoms were defined as deficits of normal motor behavior such as the inability to move. Positive symptoms were viewed as release phenomena, such as spasticity, and clasp knife phenomena. Jackson concluded that positive and negative symptoms were two distinct entities that may be related but that do not have a cause-effect relationship. Sahrmann and Norton[32] suggested that motor deficits in patients with hemiplegia are due to limited and prolonged recruitment of the agonist and delayed cessation of the agonist contraction at the end of movement, or a "shortening" response deficit. McLellan[33] demonstrated that the response of a spastic muscle to stretch is not the same during passive motion as during active movement. Other studies have suggested that deficits in normal movement may be caused by biomechanical factors such as crossbridge stiffness or the inability to organize movement patterns due to abnormal sequencing or timing.[34,35]

These and other studies may indicate that clinicians should concentrate more on facilitating normal active motor control through the performance of functional activities rather than passively inhibiting spasticity.[36] Nevertheless, there are therapists who may continue to assess the amount of spasticity by subjectively determining muscle resistance to passive stretch using various velocities of stretching, as well as positions. More objective measurements such as the Modified Ashworth (Table 8-3) and the Oswestry[37] scales attempt to quantify the amount of spasticity. Bohannon et al[38] reported the interrater reliability of the Modified Ashworth Scale to be r= .86 when testing elbow flexor spasticity. Gregson et al,[39] also using the Modified Ashworth Scale, reported interrater (kappa = .84) and intrarater (kappa = .83) reliabilities on patients following a CVA. The pendulum or drop test, originally described by Boczko et al[40] (Figure 8-3) also has

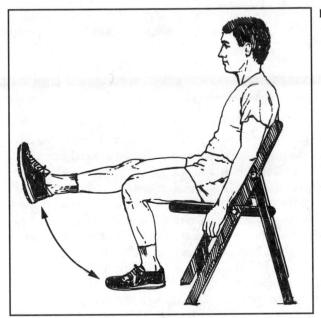

Figure 8-3. Pendulum test.

been used to assess the response of the quadriceps to a sudden passive stretch by dropping the leg from a horizontal position.

In neurologically intact subjects and patients with hypotonia, the leg will oscillate freely for a brief time after suddenly being dropped. In patients with spastic quadriceps, there will typically be a delay in how quickly the leg drops.[41] The results of this test can be quantified by using isokinetic equipment such as the Cybex (Cybex Division of Luxex, Inc, Ronlonloma, NY) or KINCOM (Chattecx Corp, Chattanooga, Tenn). Bohannon[42] reported a reliability of r = .96 between the pendulum test and the Cybex when testing the quadriceps muscle.

Deep Tendon, Pathological, and Primitive Reflexes

Deep tendon reflexes (DTRs) sometimes are used to assess the state of the CNS. An increased or hyperactive DTR is indicative of disinhibition of the stretch reflex mechanism and may be seen in patients with hypertonicity. In patients with spasticity, there is an increased amplitude and decreased threshold to a DTR. However, in certain neurological diagnoses such as Parkinson's disease, the patient exhibits hypertonic muscles, but not hyperactive DTRs. A decreased or hypoactive DTR indicates either interruption of the monosynaptic reflex arc or a generalized excitability of the motoneuron pool (eg, spinal shock following a spinal cord injury) exhibiting a decreased amplitude and increased threshold. DTR responses are subjectively graded from 0, being no response to stretch, to 4, which indicates a hyperactive response to stretch. An electrodynamic hammer can be used to vary the speed and force while an EMG can be used to record the muscle's responses. Instead of a tendon tap, an H-reflex is an electrically elicited tendon jerk sometimes used to stimulate large diameter Ia afferents.

Clonus of the ankles and/or wrists also may be elicited or observed as an additional method of examining hyperactivity of the CNS. Testing and observation of pathological reflexes, such as a Babinski, as well as primitive reflexes, such as an asymmetrical tonic neck reflex or positive supporting reflex, may lend further information to the overall state of the CNS.

POSTURE

Posture refers to the maintenance of an upright position against the forces of gravity. Ideal posture involves a minimal amount of stress which is conducive to maximal efficiency in the use of the body. Static posture is evaluated by comparing skeletal alignment of the individual to an ideal posture. Usually, this is done by using a plumb line to determine whether the points of reference of the individual being tested are in the same alignment as the corresponding points in the standard posture. For testing, the subject steps up to a suspended plumb line and is viewed from the front, back, and both sides. In the back and front views, he or she stands so the feet are equidistant from the line and in a side view, so the point just in front of the lateral malleolus is in line with the plumb line. In ideal alignment, viewed from the side, the plumb line will fall in alignment with the lobe of the ear, the shoulder joint, the midline of the trunk, the greater trochanter of the femur, slightly anterior to the midline of the knee, and slightly anterior to the lateral malleolus.[12] By comparing this ideal alignment with the actual alignment of the individual, faulty posture is identified.[43]

In patients with motor control deficits, the examination of postural alignment may need significant modification. Many patients are unable to maintain a standing position. Nevertheless, the principles remain the same and alignment should be evaluated in sitting. Some patients with even more significant deficits may not be able to maintain an upright position in sitting. For these individuals, the ideal alignment should be considered when designing adaptive seating systems. The ideal posture is one that requires minimal muscular activity to maintain and allows for maximal movement efficiency. Therefore, patients with severe motor control deficits should be provided with an advantageous posture so that they can relearn control of movement.

SENSORY INTEGRITY/PERCEPTION

Sensory deficits are a major factor in motor control impairments caused by CNS deficits. For example, patients who have proprioceptive loss around the ankles exhibit balance impairments and subsequently must learn to compensate by using other sensory information (such as vision) and different movement strategies when standing and walking. Similarly, patients who are tactily defensive may respond adversely when the therapist asks them to perform certain motor tasks that require touching different surfaces such as walking barefoot on cool, tile floors during a gait analysis. Following a right CVA, some patients may exhibit various perceptual deficits (such as agnosia) where sensory information is processed or interpreted incorrectly. Finally, incoordination may result from deficits of the visual and vestibular systems. However, not every person needs detailed testing of every sensation. The therapist's job is to determine which tests need to be performed and to objectify those results whenever possible. Most clinicians document the number or percentage of correct responses out of the total for the various tests of proprioception, touch, and pain/temperature. Dermatome or other anatomical charts may assist the therapist in organizing the information. Specialized tests for two-point discrimination, stereognosis, and graphesthesia also may be included (see Chapter 9).

MOTOR FUNCTION

Coordination

Coordination has been defined as "smooth, accurate, purposeful movement brought about by the integrated action of many muscles, superimposed upon a base of efficient postural activity, monitored primarily by sensory input."[44] Gross motor coordination involves large muscle groups of an extremity whereas fine motor coordination primarily involves small muscle groups, especially those of the hands, where the manipulation of objects is the major goal. Several variables must be considered in the examination of coordination including speed, control, steadiness, response orientation, and reaction time.[45] Coordinated movement includes the ability to stop and start, as well as change the range, direction, and speed of a movement. Quantification is achieved by noting the number of repetitions that the person can complete in a given time frame (eg, six repetitions in 10 seconds) or the number/percentage of successes out of a given number of attempts (eg, four successes out of five attempts). Qualitative examination includes an observation and description of dysmetria, dysdiadochokinesia, and/or dyssynergia.

The following are a few of the simple coordination tests commonly administered. The patient is asked to:

1. Touch his nose, then touch the examiner's finger alternately
2. Alternately supinate and pronate his forearms
3. Rapidly oppose each finger to his thumb
4. Slide the heel of one foot up and down the opposite shin
5. Touch the index fingers of opposing hands in midline from a position of 90 degrees of shoulder abduction
6. Perform jumping jacks in supine and/or standing
7. Walk heel to toe on a line

Efforts to increase the reliability of coordination testing have led to the development of standardized assessments that allow for specific functions to be performed under specific conditions. A sample of these standardized tests include:

- Purdue Pegboard Test—a timed test of finger dexterity where the patient is asked to place pins in the holes of a standardized board. The test has been validated and has found to be reliable but not appropriate for patients with severe motor control deficits.[46]
- The Tufts Assessment of Motor Performance (TAMP)—evaluates fine motor skills such as grasp, release, and object manipulation. The TAMP also can be used to assess other activities of daily living (see Functional Activities Section). It has been shown to have good interrater reliability.[47]
- The 9-Hole Peg Test—a timed finger dexterity test requiring the patient to place nine pegs into a board and then remove them individually with one hand. Normative data have been established.[48]

- Jebsen Hand Function Test—the patient is asked to perform seven functional activities such as writing, stacking, and card turning. Normative data have been established for age, gender, maximum time, and hand dominance.[49]
- Sensory Integration and Praxis Tests (SIPT)—these tests are used to detect and determine the nature of sensory integrative impairments in children. Tests of eye-hand coordination, tactile functions, and various forms of praxis, such as postural, oral, and constructional praxis, are included. Normative data for children between 4 to 8 years of age are available, as well as information on reliability and validity.[50]
- Bruininks-Oseretsky Test of Motor Proficiency (BOTMP)—the BOTMP is used to assess gross and fine motor skills in children between the ages of 4.5 and 14.5 years. Tests for bilateral coordination, upper limb speed and dexterity, response speed, and visual motor control are included. Reliability and validity data have been obtained.[51]

Technology has been developed for more formal and objective testing of coordination using computers and EMG equipment. Not only is it possible to test both upper and lower extremities, but also eye and head movement can be tested.[52,53] Problems with cognitive reaction time can be differentiated from an abnormally long motor reaction time due to physical impairments.[54]

Atypical Movements/Dysfunctional Postures

The presence of atypical (eg, involuntary) movements and dysfunctional postures should be noted during the examination process. Clinical observation is the major examination tool used for impairments such as tremors, dystonia, athetosis, ataxia, and other similar signs of CNS pathology.

CRANIAL NERVE INTEGRITY

For some individuals with motor control impairments, additional testing of the cranial nerves may be necessary. Persons with deficits in cranial nerve VIII, for example, may have difficulty hearing the examiner's questions during a history or may have difficulty complying with balance testing due to vestibular involvement. Safety issues also may need to be addressed through more specific testing when an individual appears to have a visual field loss or diminished acuity from cranial nerve II dysfunction. Occasionally, a referral to another health practitioner may be warranted when a cranial nerve deficit is discovered by the physical therapist. Patients with traumatic brain injuries or vascular lesions in the brainstem are likely to exhibit deficits in function requiring more thorough testing of individual cranial nerves. If detailed testing is required, the sensory, motor, and autonomic functions should be considered and tested appropriately (see Chapter 9).

ACTIVITIES OF DAILY LIVING AND INSTRUMENTAL ACTIVITIES OF DAILY LIVING

The usual reason an individual with motor control deficits seeks medical and rehabilitative care is because he is faced with a functional limitation. The ***Guide to Physical***

Therapist Practice differentiates between activities of daily living (ADL) and instrumental activities of daily living (IADL).[1] An ADL is classified as an activity basic to self-care and hygiene such as bed mobility and transfers, toileting, grooming, eating, and dressing. An IADL is an activity the individual performs within the home or community involving work, school, or play such as cooking and other household chores, driving a car, or negotiating school environments.

When evaluating an individual for the purpose of setting goals and creating an intervention, physical therapists often develop functional measurements that are designed to meet the specific needs of that individual. These functional measurements can supplement information from standardized tests and describe the person's ability or inability to perform a specific functional activity. Examples are rolling in bed; transferring from supine to sitting, bed to wheelchair, or sitting to standing; propelling a wheelchair; negotiating curbs and inclines; walking up and down stairs; and ambulating. The amount of assistance needed during a task also should be noted and a key provided given the subjectivity of these terms. What is "maximal" assistance to one therapist may be "moderate" assistance to another. Table 8-4 presents the possible notations that one might use in describing the amount of assistance needed. Charts listing the dates and specific activities tested may be included in the examination to assist in detailing and organizing the information.

A large number of measurement tools have been developed to quantify the performance of functional activities. Two of these, the TAMP and Berg Balance Scale, have previously been discussed in other sections. Other tools that may be used include:

- The Barthel Index is a measure of a person's ability to function independently in 10 self-care and ability skills including feeding, hygiene, dressing, transfers, and locomotion.[55] The score for each item is based on the time required to perform the task and the amount of assistance needed by the patient. A moderate level of interrater reliability was reported, and the Barthel Index was found to have a strong level of content predictive validity.[56]

- The Kenny Self-Care Evaluation is a measure of a person's ability to perform 17 basic daily living skills, divided into six major categories of bed mobility, transfers, locomotion, dressing, personal hygiene, and feeding.[57] Each area is given a grade of 0 to 4 ranging from completely dependent to independent. Reliability and validity studies are not available.

- The Acute Care Index of Function (ACIF) is a standardized measurement of the functional status of patients in an acute care setting. It consists of 20 items that are divided into four subsets: 1. mental status, 2. bed mobility, 3. transfers, and 4. mobility.[58] Reliability data ranged from r=.60 to .98 using Kappa values and validity was reported as r=.81, p <.01 using the Spearman rank-order correlation coefficient.

- Functional Independence Measure (FIM) consists of 18 tasks that are designed to measure the degree of disability that a patient experiences. Although one of the purposes of the tool was to assess adults in rehabilitation centers more reliably, data to support this assumption have not been forthcoming.[59] A pediatric version of the FIM called the WeeFIM also has been developed.[60]

- The Pediatric Evaluation of Disability Inventory (PEDI) is a standardized assessment that uses parental reporting to determine a child's comprehensive level of function. Part one consists of the broad categories of self-care, mobility, and social

TABLE 8-4

Grades of Assistance Required During Functional Activities*

Amount of Assistance	Numerical Value	Descriptor #1	Descriptor #2
Independent	7/7	The patient can safely perform the activity with no assistance.	The patient needs no verbal assistance or supervision.
Standby Assistance	6/7	The patient can perform the activity without assitance, but may need verbal cues or someone nearby as a precaution.	The patient needs verbal cues or someone to watch him to ensure he is safe and independent.
Minimal Assistance	5/7	The patient requires physical assistance of approximately 25% to perform the activity safely.	One person needs to touch the patient for balane or for safety purposes during the activity.
Moderate Assistance	4/7	The patient requires physical assistance of approximately 50% to perform the activity safely.	One person is helping to a greater extent and may have to physically move a body part for the patient.
Maximal Assistance	3/7	The patient requires physical assistance of approximately 75% to 100% to perform the activity safely.	One person is providing 100% of the effort to assist the patient in carrying out the activity.
Moderate Assist X2	2/7		One person's effort is insufficient to help this patient, therefore, two people are required.
Maximal Assist X2	1/7 ·		Two people are maximally helping (almost 100%) to get the patient to complete the activity.
Unable	0/7		The patient is unable to do the activity at all.

*Adapted from Documenting Quality Care, Inc, PO Box 33978, Washington, DC 20033-0978.

function, with each item evaluated on a scale of 1 to 5. This part of the test indicates those items that the child is able or unable to perform, with or without assistance. In part two, the same categories are evaluated based on the level of assistance and modifications the child typically needs to function on a daily basis. Reliability and validity information are included in the *Pediatric Evaluation of Disability Inventory Development, Standardization, and Administration Manual.*[61,62]

TABLE 8-5
Functional Balance Grades

Normal: Patient is able to maintain balance without support, actively weight shift in all directions, and accept outside challenges from all directions without loss of balance.

Good: Patient is able to maintain balance without support, actively weight shift in all directions, and accept outside challenges although there may be an occasional loss of balance.

Fair: Patient is able to maintain balance without support, cannot maintain balance while weight shifting, and cannot tolerate outside challenges.

Poor: Patient requires assistance to maintain balance.

Zero: Patient requires total support to maintain balance.

GAIT, LOCOMOTION, AND BALANCE

Balance

Balance refers to the maintenance of the center of mass over the base of support (see Chapter 11). Patients should be observed for the presence or absence of protective extension responses and equilibrium reactions. Beyond observation, many tests have been developed in the last several years to examine balance. The simplest tests involve examining the individual's ability to remain upright with or without support, to tolerate challenges to the upright position, and to move within the upright position so that postural control is examined in both static and dynamic situations. The nudge/push test is one such tool. Grading, while subjective, should be accompanied by a key such as the one in Table 8-5.

The Romberg Test is another simple tool used to evaluate the influence of proprioceptive, visual, and vestibular input on balance. It is performed by having the person stand with his feet together and arms crossed over his chest with the eyes open, then closed for four trials of 60 seconds per trial. The amount of sway is subjectively measured by the examiner. The Sharpened Romberg (Figures 8-4a and 8-4b) is a variation where the person is asked to stand with his feet in tandem. It has not been found to be predictive of falls, but interrater reliability was reported as r=.99.[63] The use of computerized force plates provides more objective measurements of postural sway. Newer, more sophisticated systems with movable platforms and visual screens measure response latency, symmetry of weight distribution, amplitude of response in relation to the amplitude of perturbation, and patterns of muscle activation used in the balance response. Although these systems are quite expensive, they are becoming more common in research centers and clinics where large numbers of patients with neurologic impairments including balance problems are treated.

Figure 8-4a. Sharpened Romberg Test— start position.

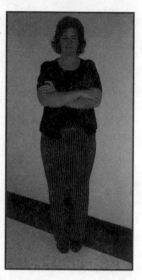

Figure 8-4b. Sharpened Romberg Test— end position.

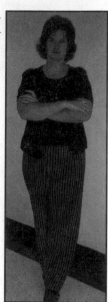

Other balance tests are mentioned here as part of the overall examination of motor control, but more detailed information and additional tests are provided in Chapter 11.

- Functional Reach—the individual stands next to a yardstick with the shoulder flexed to 90 degrees and the elbow fully extended (Figures 8-5a and 8-5b). Measurements are taken from the head of the third metacarpal before and after the person reaches as far forward as possible without taking a step. Three attempts are given following two practice trials. Norm values have been established for persons ages 20 to 40, 41 to 69, and 70 to 87 years. Interrater reliability of r = .98, intrarater reliability of r = .92, and criterion validity of r = .71 have been reported.[64]

- Berg Balance Scale—the individual is asked to perform 14 common functional activities such as moving from sitting to standing, standing on one leg, and turning 360 degrees. Each activity is rated from 0 to 4; best total score would be 56. Interrater reliability of .99 and test-retest reliability of .98 have been reported, as well as construct validity compared to the Barthel Index and Fugl-Meyer Evaluation.[65]

- Timed Up and Go—the individual is asked to stand from an armchair, walk 10 meters, turn around, and return to sitting by scooting to the back of the chair. The patient is given one practice run, followed by three trials which are averaged and then compared to score categories. Interrater reliability values of r=.99, test-retest reliability of r=.98, and concurrent validity of r=.81 when compared to the Berg have been reported.[66]

- Fugl-Meyer Balance Sub-Test—the individual is asked to perform seven items including sitting/standing without support and standing on one leg. Activities are rated from 0 to 2; best total score would be 14. The Fugl-Meyer has been validated for patients who are post-CVA with reported interrater reliability of r=.93 and test-retest reliability of r=.89-.98.[67]

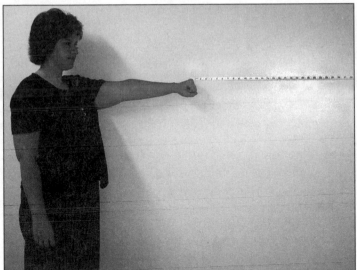

Figure 8-5a. Functional Reach Test—start position.

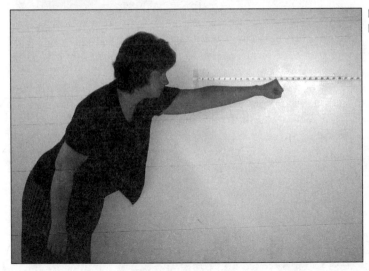

Figure 8-5b. Functional Reach Test—end position.

Gait

Almost all patients with motor control impairments will have the ability to ambulate as one of their physical therapy goals. Because gait is a complex process requiring efficient and coordinated motor control, its analysis can be challenging (see Chapter 13). In certain situations only a superficial examination of gait is indicated. Such an examination would include a description of variables, such as a subjective grading of the amount of assistance the patient requires, the use of assistive devices, the gait pattern used, the distance the patient can traverse, the speed with which he does so, and a brief description of any gait deviations. This type of examination is used most often in settings where function is the primary objective and time does not allow a thorough quantitative analysis of the patient's gait. Efforts to quantify functional gait include the use of such tools as the Functional Ambulation Profile, the Locomotion Scale of the

Functional Independence Measure, and the GaitGrid developed by EFI Medical Systems/Total Gym.[68-70]

In all clinical gait analyses, the energy costs of ambulation should be considered. Efficiency is important if an individual will be able to return to functional activities. Energy cost is most accurately assessed by measurement of oxygen consumption, carbon dioxide production, and pulmonary ventilation used during ambulation. Although accurate, these measures are not commonly available in clinical situations. The monitoring of heart rate before and after ambulation, with continued monitoring until the heart rate returns to baseline, gives an indication of energy consumption and is highly recommended. Winter[43] identified four major causes of inefficiency and excessive energy consumption commonly seen in patients with motor control deficits. These include inappropriate co-contraction, isometric contractions against gravity, jerky movements, and generation of energy at one joint with simultaneous absorption of energy at another.

There are times when gait analysis is a primary concern and more sophisticated evaluation is indicated. In these instances, the type of gait analysis that is selected depends on the purpose of the analysis, the type of equipment that is available, and the knowledge and skill level of the examiner. The purpose of a gait analysis may be to determine what deviations are present in order to develop a treatment intervention to eliminate or minimize them, to compare gait with different orthoses, to compare gait following different interventions, or to describe normal values for a particular group.

The most commonly used gait tool today is the *observational gait analysis*. This involves systematic observation of each segment of the body during each phase of gait. To assist the therapist in performing an observational gait analysis, there are a number of published protocols that outline the necessary observations and provide methods of describing what is observed, such as the Rancho Los Amigos Observational Gait Analysis.[71] The use of a videotape can assist the therapist by providing multiple observations without making the person walk repeatedly. However, standard videotaping for this purpose has its limitations. Unless a special setup allows the camera to move as the individual does, the examiner quickly loses the direct side view as the individual moves forward and the camera position remains unchanged. Studies of intertester reliability during observational gait analysis have yielded only moderate levels of reliability, even when experienced therapists have used this tool.[72,73]

The GAITRite (CIR Systems, Inc, Clifton, NJ) is a computerized gait analysis system which has been compared to video-based and paper and pencil methods. It measures spatial and temporal parameters of gait, including cadence, velocity, step and stride lengths, and step times. Reliability and validity results are available.[74]

Limitations of Motor Control Examination Tools

A number of motor control examination tools have been discussed in this chapter. There are many tools that have been developed for specific patient populations that have not been presented such as the Kurtzke Scale used for patient with multiple sclerosis,[75] Brunnstrom Motor Assessment in Hemiplegia,[76] Alberta Infant Motor Scale (AIMS),[77] and the Unified Parkinson's Disease Rating Scale (UPDRS).[78] Several measurement tools have been developed specifically for the pediatric population. In determining motor control in children, physical therapists have the additional dimension of motor development to consider. While adults may have difficulty with acquired motor deficits that result from injury or disease, children may not have experienced normal motor control that occurs by achieving normal motor milestones. Adults then are evaluated in terms of what they are no longer able to do, while children with developmental disabilities must be considered in terms of what they have not been able to do. For a thorough review of pediatric tests and measures, the reader is referred to Chapter 2 in ***Therapeutic Exercise in Developmental Disabilities***.[79]

The most important consideration of motor control is a tool's usefulness in a given situation. Many of the tools discussed in this chapter were developed to provide quantitative methods to measure motor function. This is desirable when attempting to use statistical analysis to assess change. There are times, however, when qualitative information may be more useful. It is important to remember that most of the tools described measure performance outcome only. In evaluating individuals for the purpose of planning an intervention, it is often the manner in which the movement evolves that interests us. For example, in an individual with motor planning impairments, it may be more useful to describe his performance under varying conditions than to administer a standardized assessment. It may be that problems with planning can more easily be differentiated from problems with execution using qualitative observation rather than quantitative examination tools. Factors contributing to the qualitative aspects of motor control and resulting movement patterns along with strategies for examination, evaluation, and intervention are presented in Chapter 12.

Motor control is very complex and multi-faceted. As movement scientists, physical therapists hope to improve individuals' abilities in this area. In order to assess effectiveness of intervention, valid and reliable tools are needed to measure performance. Much more research is needed to determine the validity, reliability, and value of examination tools.

CASE STUDY #1
Jane Smith

- *Age: 74 years*
- *Medical Diagnosis: Right hemiplegia, secondary to left CVA*
- *Status: 6 months post onset*
- *Practice Pattern 5D: Impaired Motor Function and Sensory Integrity Associated with Nonprogressive Disorders of the Central Nervous System—Acquired In Adolescence or Adulthood*

EXAMINATION AND EVALUATION

Given Mrs. Smith's medical history of hypertension, peripheral vascular disease, and bilateral endarterectomies, her vital signs should be taken and recorded on a regular basis. One or more of her therapists made a home visit prior to her discharge to determine what problems she might encounter with ADLs and IADLs due to architectural barriers.

Sensory Integrity/Perception

Mrs. Smith should be observed for additional perceptual deficits and/or more formal testing procedures should be instituted to monitor her changes. She is at risk for falling/injury due to impaired safety awareness, and safety will be an issue in the home environment.

Flexibility/Range of Motion

Because Mrs. Smith is at risk for a frozen shoulder, additional goniometric measurements of the proximal right upper extremity should be taken and recorded.

Muscle Performance/Strength

More detailed information regarding Mrs. Smith's strength in her extremities and trunk is needed to measure her progress. A dynamometer may be employed to measure her grip strength on the right, particularly if that is her dominant hand.

Motor Function/ADL/IADL

The Barthel Index or Kenny Self-Care Evaluation may be used to quantify her ability to function independently since terms such as *minimal* or *moderate assistance* do not clearly indicate what kind(s) of assistance is required. The Barthel Index may be more helpful for Mrs. Smith since it has been found to have predictive validity.

Balance

If a computerized balance system is not available, the Fugl-Meyer Balance Subtest would be appropriate for quantifying Mrs. Smith's balance responses since it has been validated for patients who are post-CVA.

Gait/Locomotion

Since ambulation appears to be one of the goals for Mrs. Smith, more formalized testing procedures would be helpful in documenting her progress. If a GAITRite or Gait Grid are not available, the Rancho Los Amigos Observational Gait Analysis could be used. Videotaping her would allow the therapist(s) to review Mrs. Smith's progress periodically.

CASE STUDY #2
Daniel Johnson

- *Age: 59 years*
- *Medical Diagnosis: Parkinson's disease*
- *Status: 4 years post initial diagnosis*
- *Practice Pattern 5E: Impaired Motor Function and Sensory Integrity Associated with Progressive Disorders of the Central Nervous System*

EXAMINATION AND EVALUATION

Muscle Performance/Strength

It has been noted that Mr. Johnson has decreased endurance. Therefore, a record of the number of required rest breaks or length of exercise sessions he is able to tolerate should be included. Other types of cardiopulmonary testing, such as incentive spirometry, also would be helpful.

Motor Function/ADL/IADL

Mr. Johnson exhibits difficulty initiating movement and bradykinesia. Timed tests for the performance of ADLs and IADLs would document progress. The UPDRS should be administered periodically and a record kept with the rest of the documentation on him.

Balance

A computerized balance testing system would be helpful for measuring Mr. Johnson's impairments. If one is not available, the Timed Up and Go could be administered because he is still ambulatory, but is displaying difficulties with stopping and turning.

Gait/Locomotion

Videotaping Mr. Johnson's gait pattern would provide additional information with which to set future goals. At some point in time, gait may no longer be a reasonable method of locomotion due to safety concerns. Videotaping Mr. Johnson's gait during different sessions over time may help family members deal more effectively with the difficult decisions that will have to be made regarding the progression of his disease.

C A S E   S T U D Y   # 3
Shirley Teal

- *Age: 21 years*
- *Medical Diagnosis: Traumatic brain injury*
- *Status: 4 months post injury*
- *Practice Pattern 5D: Impaired Motor Function and Sensory Integrity Associated with Nonprogressive Disorders of the central nervous system (CNS)—Acquired in Adolescence or Adulthood*

Examination and Evaluation

Arousal, Attention, Cognition, and Communication

Because Ms. Teal has cognitive and behavioral impairments, it would be beneficial to seek additional testing by a qualified neuropsychologist who has experience working with persons with traumatic brain injury. Although Ms. Teal also could be assigned to a cognitive level based on the Revised Rancho Los Amigos Scale, a neuropsychological evaluation would provide the therapist(s) and family members with better information to effectively plan for her discharge to home. Vocational rehabilitation testing also would be beneficial if she has plans to start working again.

Sensory Integrity/Perception

Ms. Teal has obvious impairments in balance as well as benign paroxysmal positional nystagmus (BPPN) and vertigo. Therefore, more definitive testing may need to be done on other cranial nerves as well. Vital signs should be taken and recorded, at least on a periodic basis. Clinical observations for additional perceptual deficits should continue until discharge.

Flexibility/Range of Motion

Detailed goniometric measurements should be taken and recorded due to existing limitations and the possibility of future ambulation.

Muscle Performance/Strength/Tone

In addition to documenting ROM measurements, more specific MMT results should be recorded. A measurement tool such as the Modified Ashworth Scale may be helpful in quantifying her problems with stiffness/spasticity.

Motor Function

Ms. Teal exhibits coordination impairments in the right upper and lower extremities. In order to document progress, timed tests to measure upper extremity coordination should be performed or tools such as the TAMP should be administered. Fine motor coordination should be assessed using the Jebsen Hand Function Test or similar tool, especially if she is right hand dominant and hopes to return to her job as a beautician.

Balance

Traditional balance testing may be somewhat limited by Ms. Teal's ability to fully bear weight on both lower extremities. The Fugl-Meyer Balance Sub-Test may be used to determine her baseline abilities even though it has only been validated for patients who are post-CVA. A sophisticated system using a computer, movable forceplates, and visual screens could be used to provide more objective and accurate information.

Posture

Further testing should be done to determine the cause of Ms. Teal's listing to the left in sitting. Is the impairment due to lack of strength, midline orientation deficits, or some other factor?

ADL/IADL/Gait/Locomotion

A tool such as the FIM may be helpful in determining and documenting Ms. Teal's functional abilities as well as planning for discharge.

CASE STUDY #4
Shawna Wells

- *Age: 4 years*
- *Medical Diagnosis: Cerebral palsy, spastic quadriparesis, and mild mental retardation*
- *Status: Onset at birth*
- *Practice Pattern 5C: Impaired Motor Function and Sensory Integrity Associated with Nonprogressive Disorders of the Central Nervous System—Congenital Origin or Acquired in Infancy or Childhood*

EXAMINATION AND EVALUATION

Sensory Integrity/Perception

Shawna has tactile hypersensitivity, avoidance reactions, and gravitational insecurity. These impairments may be measured by using tools such as the Infant/Toddler Sensory Profile[80] comparing her to a 36-month-old child and then readministered using the Sensory Profile[81] when she reaches the age of 5 years.

Flexibility/Range of Motion

In addition to keeping records of her extremity ROM, Shawna should be monitored for scoliosis as she ages, particularly if she begins sitting in a wheelchair for prolonged periods and reduces the time she spends using other forms of locomotion.

Motor Function

A tool such as the Gross Motor Function Measure (GMFM)[82] may be used for Shawna because it has been normed for children with cerebral palsy. The PEDI may be helpful for determining her ADL abilities in a home or preschool setting.

Reflex Integrity

Because Shawna displays atypical movement patterns such as "bunny-hopping," a more detailed examination of reflex integrity also may be warranted.

Posture/ADL/IADL

Shawna should be assessed carefully to determine her needs for adaptive seating and possibly a wheelchair (eg, manual versus power). Additionally, her ability to propel a wheelchair should be assessed.

Gait/Locomotion

A Gait Grid, or possibly a GAITRite could be useful in examining the parameters of Shawna's gait and determining a baseline by which improvement could be documented.

CASE STUDY # 5
Robert Anderson

- *Age: 38 years*
- *Medical Diagnosis: Incomplete T9-10 spinal cord injury with left radial nerve damage*
- *Status: 6 months post spinal cord injury*
- *Practice Pattern 5H: Impaired Motor Function, Peripheral Nerve Integrity, and Sensory Integrity Associated with Nonprogressive Disorders of the Spinal Cord*

EXAMINATION AND EVALUATION

Sensory Integrity/Perception

The loss of sensation following Mr. Anderson's spinal cord injury should be carefully documented using a dermatome or anatomical chart/figure. His intermittent problems with sacral skin breakdown should be carefully noted, assessing the shape and size of skin involvement, as well as the continuity of skin color. Most importantly, identification of aggravating activities or positions, effectiveness of his current wheelchair cushion, and his knowledge of pressure relief skills should be addressed.

Muscle Performance/Strength/Tone

Detailed results of Mr. Anderson's MMT should be documented, especially of his left upper extremity. A chart containing key muscle groups with innervation levels would assist in keeping the information organized. Because his lower extremity stiffness (tone) is continuing to increase, some type of rating scale may be helpful, particularly if the stiffness begins to interfere with his functional activities.

Motor Function

Mr. Anderson is continuing to receive outpatient physical therapy twice a week. His difficulty with various types of transfers should be quantified by listing each type separately and using a rating scale.

Gait/Locomotion

Mr. Anderson should be observed performing advanced wheelchair skills such as going up and down curbs and ramps and performing lateral shifts. His ability to perform each activity should be rated and documented appropriately. Measures of endurance, such as vital signs, measuring the distance walked or propelled, or counting the frequency of rests required in a certain amount of time should be documented.

REFERENCES

1. APTA. Guide to physical therapist practice. 2nd ed. *Phys Ther.* 2001;81:S34-S121.

2. Gresham GE, Duncan PW, Stason WB, et al. *Post-Stroke Rehabilitation: Assessment, Referral, and Patient Management. Clinical Practice Guideline. Quick Reference Guide for Clinicians.* Rockville, Md: U.S. Department of Health and Human Services, Public Health Service, Agency for Health Care Policy and Research; 1995:8-11.

3. American Academy of Orthopaedic Surgeons. *Joint Motion: Method of Measuring and Recording.* Chicago, Ill: American Academy of Orthopaedic Surgeons; 1965.

4. Hoppenfeld S. *Physical Examination of the Spine and Extremities.* New York, NY: Appleton-Century-Crofts; 1976.

5. Kapandji IA. *Physiology of the Joints, Vol 1.* 2nd ed. London, England, Churchill-Livingstone; 1970.

6. Norkin CC, White DJ. *Measurement of Joint Motion: A Guide to Goniometry.* Philadelphia, Pa: FA Davis; 1985:221-223.

7. Gordon J, Ghez C. Muscle receptors and spinal reflexes: the stretch reflex. In: Kandel ER, Schwartz JH, Jessell TM eds. *Principles of Neural Science.* 3rd ed. Norwalk, Conn: Appleton & Lange; 1991:564-580.

8. Boone DC. Reliability of goniometric measurements. *Phys Ther.* 1978;68:1355-1360.

9. Gajdosik RL, Bohannon RW. Clinical measurement of range of motion: review of goniometry emphasizing reliability and validity. *Phys Ther.* 1987;67:1867-1872.

10. Riddle DL, Rothstein JM, Lamb RL. Goniometric reliability in a clinical setting: shoulder measurements. *Phys Ther.* 1987;67:668-673.

11. Legg AT. Physical therapy in infantile paralysis. In: Mock, ed. *Principles and Practice of Physical Therapy, Vol II.* Hagerstown, Md: WF Prior Co; 1932:45.

12. Kendall FP, McCreary EK. *Muscles: Testing and Function.* 3rd ed. Baltimore, Md: Williams & Wilkins; 1983:10-13, 270-278.

13. Daniels L, Worthingham C. *Muscle Testing: Techniques of Manual Examination.* Philadelphia, Pa: WB Saunders Co; 1986:2-7.

14. Bohannon RW. Make tests and break tests of elbow flexor strength. *Phys Ther.* 1988;68(2):193-194.

15. Smidt GL, Rogers MW. Factors contributing to the regulation and clinical assessment of muscular strength. *Phys Ther.* 1982;62(9):1283-1290.

16. Alexander J, Molnar GE. Muscular strength in children: preliminary report on objective standards. *Arch Phys Med Rehabil.* 1973;54:424.

17. Connolly BC. Testing in infants and children. In: Hislop HJ, Montgomery J, eds. *Daniels and Worthingham's Muscle Testing.* Philadelphia, Pa: WB Saunders Co; 1995:236-260.

18. Lovelace-Chandler V. Techniques of pediatric muscle testing. In: Reese NB. *Muscle and Sensory Testing.* Philadelphia, Pa: WB Saunders Co; 1999:338-376.

19. Wadsworth CT, Krishnan R, Sear M, et al. Intrarater reliability of manual muscle testing and handheld dynametric muscle testing. *Phys Ther.* 1987;67(9):1342-1347.

20. Florence JM, Pandya S, King WM, et al. Intrarater reliability of manual muscle test (Medical Research Council scale) grades in Duchenne's muscular dystrophy. *Phys Ther.* 1992;72(2):115-126.

21. Brandsma JW, Schreuders TAR, Birke JA, et al. Manual muscle strength testing: Intraobserver and interobserver reliabilities for the intrinsic muscles of the hand. *J Hand Ther.* 1995;8:185-190.

22. Lazar RB, Yarkony GM, Ortolano D, et al. Prediction of functional outcome by motor capability after spinal cord injury. *Arch Phys Med Rehabil.* 1989;70:819-822.

23. Brown PJ, Marino RJ, Herbison GJ, et al. The 72-hour examination as a predictor of recovery in motor complete quadriplegia. *Arch Phys Med Rehabil.* 1991;72:546-548.

24. Bohannon RW. Manual muscle test scores and dynamometer test scores of knee extension strength. *Arch Phys Med Rehabil.* 1986;67:390-392.

25. Schwartz S, Cohen ME, Herbison GJ, et al. Relationship between two measures of upper extremity strength: manual muscle test compared to handheld myometry. *Arch Phys Med Rehabil.* 1992;73:1063-1068.

26. Soderberg GL. Handheld dynamometry for muscle testing. In: Reese NB. *Muscle and Sensory Testing.* Philadelphia, Pa: WB Saunders Co; 1999:377-389.

27. Brown WF. *The Physiological and Technical Basis of EMG.* Stoneham, Mass: Butterworth; 1984.

28. Bobath B. *Adult Hemiplegia: Evaluation and Treatment.* 2nd ed. London, England: William Heinemann Medical Books Limited; 1978:5.

29. Chambers HG. The surgical treatment of spasticity. *Muscle and Nerve.* 1997;6:S121-S128.

30. Giuliani CA. Dorsal rhizotomy for children with cerebral palsy: support for concepts of motor control. *Phys Ther.* 1991;71:248-259.

31. Jackson JH. *Selected Writings of John Hughlings Jackson.* In: Taylor J, ed. London, England: Hodder & Stoughton; 1932.

32. Sahrmann SA, Norton BS. The relationship of voluntary movement to spasticity in the upper motoneuron syndrome. *Ann Neurol.* 1977;2:460-465.

33. McLellan DL. Co-contraction and stretch reflex in spasticity during treatment with baclofen. *Neurol Neurosurg Psych.* 1977;40:30-38.

34. Badke MB, DiFabio RP. Balance deficits in patients with hemiplegia: considerations for assessment and treatment. In: Duncan P, ed. *Balance: Proceedings of the APTA Forum.* Alexandria, Va: APTA; 1990:73-78.

35. Shumway-Cook A, Woollacott M. Postural control in the Down syndrome child. *Phys Ther.* 1985b;9:211-235.

36. Duncan PW, Badke MB. *Stroke Rehabilitation: The Recovery of Motor Control.* Chicago, Ill: Yearbook; 1987:172-175.

37. Goff B. Grading of spasticity and its effect on voluntary movement. *Physiotherapy.* 1976;62:358-361.

38. Bohannon RW, Smith MB. Interrater reliability of a modified Ashworth scale of muscle spasticity. *Phys Ther.* 1987;67:206-207.

39. Gregson JM, Leathley M, Moor AP, et al. Reliability of the tone assessment scale and the modified Ashworth scale as clinical tools for assessing poststroke spasticity. *Arch Phys Med Rehabil.* 1999;80:1013-1016.

40. Boczko M, Mumenthaler M. Modified pendulous test to assess tonus of thigh muscles in spasticity. *Neurology.* 1954;8:846-851.

41. Dimitrijevic MM, Dimitrijevic MR, Sherwood AM, et al. Clinical neurophysiological techniques in the assessment of spasticity. In: Davis R, Kondraske GV, et al, eds. *Quantifying Neurologic Performance*. Philadelphia, Pa: Hanley & Belfus; 1989.

42. Bohannon RW. Variability and reliability of Pendulum test for spasticity using the Cybex isokinetic dynamometer. *Phys Ther.* 1987;67:659-661.

43. Winter DA. *Biomechanics of Human Movement*. New York, NY: Wiley & Sons; 1979.

44. New England Rehabilitation Hospital, Physical Therapy Department. *Protocol for the evaluation and documentation of coordination*. Adapted from Occupational Therapy Department, Schwab Rehabilitation Hospital, 1981.

45. O'Sullivan S, Cullen, Schmitz T. *Physical Rehabilitation: Evaluation and Treatment Procedures*. Philadelphia, Pa: FA Davis; 1981:28.

46. Tiffin J, Asher EJ. The Purdue pegboard: norms and studies of reliability and validity. *J Applied Psych*. 1948;32:234-247.

47. Gans BM, Haley SM, Hallenborg SC, et al. Description and interobserver reliability of the Tufts assessment of motor performance. *Am J Phys Med Rehabil*. 1988;88:202-210.

48. Kellor M, Frost J, et al. Hand strength and dexterity. **Am J Occup Ther.** 1971;25:77-83.

49. Jebsen RH, Taylor N, Trieschmann RB, et al. Objective and standardized test of hand function. *Arch Phys Med Rehabil*. 1969;50:311-319.

50. Ayres AJ. **Sensory Integration and Praxis Test Manual.** Los Angeles, Calif: Western Psychological Services; 1988.

51. Bruininks RH. *Bruininks Oseretsky Test of Motor Proficienc: Examiner's Manual*. Circle Pines, Minn: American Guidance Service; 1978.

52. Eckhouse RH, Maulucci RA. Assessment of eye-head-hand coordination. In: Davis R, Kondraske GV, Tourtellotte WW, et al, eds. *Quantifying Neurologic Performance*. Philadelphia, Pa: Hanley & Belfus; 1989.

53. Bizzi E. The coordination of eye-head movement. *Scientific American*. 1974;231:100-106.

54. Maulucci RA, Eckhouse RH. A workshop for quantifying perceptuo-motor behavior. In: Davis R, Kondraske GV, Tourtellotte WW, et al. *Quantifying Neurologic Performance*. Philadelphia, Pa: Hanley & Belfus; 1989.

55. Mahoney FI, Barthel DW. Functional evaluation: the Barthel index. *Maryland State Medical J.* 1965;14:61-65.

56. Loewen SC, Anderson BA. Reliability of the Modified Motor Assessment Scale and the Barthel Index. *Phys Ther.* 1988;68(7):1077-1081.

57. Schoening H, Iversen I. Numerical scoring of self-care status: a study of the Kenny self-care evaluation. *Arch Phys Med Rehabil*. 1968;49:221-229.

58. Van Dillen LR, Roach KE. Reliability and validity of the Acute Care Index of Function for patients with neurologic impairment. *Phys Ther.* 1988;68:1098-1108.

59. *Guide for the Uniform Data Set for Medical Rehabilitation (Adult FIM), Version 4.0.* Buffalo, New York. State University of New York at Buffalo; 1993.

60. Msall ME, Roseberg S, DiGuadio KM, et al. Pilot test for the WeeFIM for children with motor impairments (abstract). *Dev Med & Child Neurol*. 1990;32(9 suppl 62):41.

61. Haley SM, Coster WJ, Ludlow LH, et al. *Pediatric Evaluation of Disability Inventory (PEDI), Development, Standardization and Administration Manual, version 1.0*. Boston, Mass: New England Medical Center Publications; 1992:61-67.

62. Feldman AB, Haley SM, Coryell J. Concurrent and construct validity of the Pediatric Evaluation of Disability Inventory. *Phys Ther.* 1990;70:602-610.

63. Heitmann Dk, Gossman MR, Birch R, et al. Balance performance among noninstitutionalized elderly women. *Phys Ther.* 1989;69:748-756.

64. Duncan PW, Weiner DK, Chandler J, et al. Functional reach: a new clinical measure of balance. *J Gerontol.* 1990;45:M192-M197.

65. Berg KO, Wood-Dauphine SI, Williams JL, et al. Measuring balance in the elderly: Validation of an instrument. *Can J Pub Health.* 1992;S2:S7-S11.

66. Podsiadlo D, Richardson S. The timed "Up and Go": a test of basic functional mobility for frail elderly persons. *JAGS.* 1991;9:142-148.

67. Duncan PW, Propst M, Nelson SG. Reliability of Fugl-Meyer assessment of sensorimotor recovery after CVA. *Phys Ther.* 1983;63:1606-1610.

68. Nelson AJ. Functional ambulation profile. *Phys Ther.* 1974;54:1059-1065.

69. Morton T. Uniform data system for rehab begins: first tool measures dependence level. *Progress Report, APTA.* 1986;15:14.

70. Waagfijord J, Levangie PK, Certo C. Effects of treadmill training on gait in a hemiparetic patient. *Phys Ther.* 1990;70:548-558.

71. Gronley JK, Perry J. Gait analysis techniques. Rancho Los Amigos Hospital Gait Laboratory. *Phys Ther.* 1984;64:1831-1838.

72. Goodkin R, Diller L. Reliability among physical therapists in diagnosis and treatment of gait deviations in hemiplegics. *Percept Mot Skills.* 1973;37:727-731.

73. Krebs D, Edelstein J, Fishman S. Observational gait analysis reliability in disabled children. *Phys Ther (Abstract).* 1984;64:741.

74. McDonough AL, Batavia M, Chen FC, et al. The validity and reliability of the GAITRite system's measurements: a preliminary evaluation. *Arch Phys Med Rehabil.* 2001;82:419-425.

75. Kurtzke JF. On the evaluation of disability in multiple sclerosis. *Neurology.* 1961;11:688.

76. Brunnstrom S. Motor testing procedures in hemiplegia: based on sequential recovery stages. *Phys Ther.* 1966;46:357-375.

77. Piper MC, Darrah J. *Motor Assessment of the Developing Infant.* Philadelphia, Pa: WB Saunders Co; 1994:26-181.

78. Richards M, Marder K, Cote L, Mayeux R. Interrater reliability of the Unified Parkinson's Disease Rating Scale motor examination. *Mov Disord.* 1994;9:89.

79. Connolly BH, Montgomery P. *Therapeutic Exercise in Developmental Disabilities.* 2nd ed. Thorofare, NJ; SLACK Incorporated; 1993:15–33.

80. Dunn W, Daniels DB. *Infant/Toddler Sensory Profile.* New York, NY: The Psychological Corporation; 2000.

81. Dunn W. *Sensory Profile.* New York, NY: The Psychological Corporation; 1999

82. Russell D, Rosenbaum P, Gowland C, et al. *Gross Motor Function Measure Manual.* Hamilton, Ontario: McMaster University; 1993.

Sensory and Perceptual Issues Related to Motor Control

Audrey Zucker-Levin, PT, MS, GCS

INTRODUCTION

The environment as we know it is created in our brain from information received through our senses. In turn, our behaviors, including motor functions, are produced in relationship to environmental stimuli.[1] These stimuli are perceived, organized, integrated, and interpreted by the nervous system to produce an appropriate response, which is often a motor action. A person with a deficit in the nervous system that interferes with interpreting environmental stimuli will likely produce an inefficient movement if asked to perform a motor task.[2]

Motor control, "the control of both movement and posture,"[3] depends on continuous input from our environment through sensory receptors. Sensory receptors inform the central nervous system (CNS) where objects are in space and what the body's position is in relationship to these objects. Somatosensory receptors, located on the body surface, inform the CNS of texture, temperature, and painful stimuli while receptors in muscles and joints inform the CNS about the length and tension of muscles, joint angles, and the body's position in space. Special sense organs, the eyes, ears, and vestibular apparatus, provide visual and auditory information about the environment, as well as information about balance and movement of the head. The nose and mouth also possess special sensory organs, including taste buds and the olfactory bulbs; however, these play a relatively minor role in motor control. The integration of all sensory information is required for planning movements and altering movements already in progress.[1]

The purpose of this chapter is to discuss how our senses and perception of the environment influence motor control and to describe examination procedures for the evaluation of sensory processing issues.

SENSORY PROCESSING

How much of the nervous system is devoted to sensory processing? Hundreds of years of neuroanatomic study cannot answer this question. In fact, the answer to this question will change throughout the life span as the CNS matures and ages. A large portion of the CNS must assist in sensory processing as a relatively simple behavior recruits activity of many sensory systems.[4] For example, sitting in a restaurant while waiting for a friend requires the visual system to scan the environment for your friend, the auditory system to detect environmental sounds and possibly the sound of your friend's voice, the somatosensory system to detect the pressure from the chair in which you are sitting, and the vestibular system to maintain the body upright. In addition, you will be receiving information about the aroma of the restaurant and the taste of something you may be eating. All of this information must be processed appropriately by the nervous system to maintain your position and produce the appropriate response when your friend arrives. Each system (somatosensory, visual, auditory, and vestibular) will activate many neurons that traverse through pathways to target different areas of the CNS (see Chapter 3).

Somatosensory reception begins in the periphery with a large number of receptors that perceive three different somatosensory modalities: discriminative touch, pain and temperature, and proprioception. Discriminative touch includes the perception of pressure, vibration, and texture and is perceived by neurons with encapsulated endings such as Paccinian corpuscles, Ruffini's corpuscles, Meissner's corpuscles, and Merkel's disks. These encapsulated endings are located at different depths in the skin.[5] Pain and temperature are perceived by nonencapsulated free nerve endings located throughout the skin, muscle, bone, and connective tissue. Proprioception relies on stimulation of golgi tendon organs (GTOs) and muscle spindle receptors. The GTOs measures stress and forces about the tendons and joints, the muscle spindle receptors detects stretch and changing muscle length. In addition to somatosensory information, visual information is detected by specialized photoreceptors (rods and cones) located in the retina. Auditory information is detected by vibrations of the tympanic membrane and vestibular information is received by a pair of three semicircular canals: the *utricle* and the *saccule.*

Impulses from the stimulation of any sensory receptor is brought into (afferent) the CNS via action potential propagation along peripheral or cranial nerves. The CNS processes the afferent information in a series of relays that project in an orderly pattern from the pathway to the thalamus (except olfaction), then to the primary and secondary sensory cortices for perception of the sensation.[3] Interpretation occurs in higher level sensory processing areas in the parietal, occipital, and temporal lobes, as well as in the amygdala, hippocampus, cerebellum, and basal ganglia. In many respects, the nervous system remains a mystery because the exact function of each structure is unknown; however, structures located throughout the nervous system are required for integration and interpretation of sensory input. Because of the myriad of receptors, pathways, and subcortical and cortical structures responsible for sensory processing, we can assume a large proportion of the nervous system is devoted to sensory processing.

AGE-RELATED CHANGES IN SENSORY PROCESSING

Accurate interpretation of the environment requires maturation of nervous system structures. A newborn human has an immature nervous system that undergoes profound changes throughout the life span.[6] These specific changes are under investigation using modern technology such as magnetic resonance imaging (MRI), computer-assisted tomography (CT), and evoked potential recordings (EP). Historically, examination of the nervous system could only be performed posthumously, leading to conclusions that recently have been proven false. New technologies have enabled researchers in vivo examination of the maturation and plasticity of the nervous system throughout the life span in health and disease. One example of maturation is the finding that the cortical surface of the brain of an infant is different than the highly gyrified cortical surface of the adult brain.[7-9] Magnotta[7] described the formation of sulcal and gyral patterns in the brain as genetically programmed with possible modification by environmental influences, such as general health, nutrition, and injury. The highly gyrified human cortex, when compared with other species, is needed to increase surface area in response to functional demands that require an increase in the number of neurons without increasing intracranial size.[4,7] Major sulci, such as the Sylvian fissure (lateral sulcus) and the central sulcus, form during the sixth and seventh months of fetal life and continue to develop throughout gestation and after birth.[7,8] The Sylvian fissure defines the superior surface of two sensory cortices, the *primary auditory*, and the *auditory association cortex*. The central sulcus is a significant landmark as it defines the anterior surface of the primary somatosensory cortex and the posterior surface of the primary motor cortex. The continued development of these fissures after birth indicates that these cortices and their function in sensory interpretation are immature at birth. That leads the reader to the question: When does nervous system maturation occur? The answer to this question is still under investigation with present research reporting that the different senses mature at different times during development.

Geidd et al,[10] through a longitudinal MRI study of brain development, determined that gray matter (cell bodies) reached maximal volume at approximately 12 years of age in the frontal lobe, but not until 16 years of age in the temporal lobes. The frontal lobe contains areas responsible for abstract thinking, decision making, social behavior, and anticipation of the consequences of a particular course of action. The temporal lobe contains the primary auditory cortex and areas responsible for processing language.

MRI study is a valuable tool in the detection of brain development as is EP. Kraemer et al[11] tested 20 healthy infants to determine a relationship between visual evoked potential development and visual development. An evoked potential is a wave form recorded from active electrodes placed over specific areas of the spine and scalp. A visual evoked potential (VEP) is a wave form recorded from active electrodes placed over the scalp, corresponding to the primary visual and visual association cortex. Kraemer et al measured VEPs on the day of birth and weeks and months after birth. At approximately 5 weeks of age, changes in the VEP were simultaneous with the development of responsive smiling, indicating that the motor response, a smile, was a result of recognizing a visual stimulus. This finding does not indicate that the visual pathway is fully mature at 6 months; however, it indicates that the pathway is maturing, probably through myelination.

Just as VEPs can be recorded and measured, sensory evoked potentials (SEPs) also can be recorded and measured. A SEP is a wave form recorded from active electrodes placed over the scalp corresponding to the primary somatosensory and the sensory association cortex. Fagan et al[12] described the somatosensory system as the most immature sensory system at birth and found variation in the SEP rate of maturation until 3 to 8 years of age. They also found that the SEP remains constant between 10 and 49 years of age with slowing after 49 years of age. This is an excellent study of the maturation and subsequent slowing of a sensory system. In a similar study, Pasman et al[13] tested auditory evoked potentials (AEP) in a cross-sectional study of infants born at 36 to 41 weeks gestation through children age 16 years and compared their wave form to adults. AEPs are recorded from electrodes placed over the scalp corresponding to the primary auditory and auditory association cortex. They found a transitional (developing) period of the wave form between 4 and 6 years of age with a second transition to the adult wave form between 14 and 16 years of age. As a whole, these studies provide insight into the maturation of the nervous system, specifically areas associated with sensory perception.

In addition to changes noted in the maturation of the cortex, cortical changes in thickness, brain volume, and ventricle size are present in both normal and pathological aging.[7,14-17] Recent research supports the presence of brain atrophy, as indicated by decreased brain weight, with increasing age and to a greater extent in the presence of Alzheimer's or Parkinson's disease.[14-22] There is evidence to support that large neurons shrink with aging, resulting in a larger proportion of small neurons.[6,14] Mueller et al[14] performed quantifiable volumetric MRI annually for 5 years on 46 healthy subjects, 65 years of age and older, who had maintained cognitive health. They found a small constant rate of brain volume loss with healthy aging with the healthy oldest "old" subjects not showing greater rates of brain loss when compared with younger elderly. In a similar study, Bartzokis et al[6] examined brain volume and structure changes in 75 healthy men ages 19 to 76 years. They found significant age-related decreases in gray matter, with increased white matter in the temporal and frontal lobes into the fifth decade of life; however, the proportion of change did not affect the total volume size. After the fifth decade of life, both gray and white matter decline is evident in the temporal and frontal lobes. In a similar study, Sandor et al[15] performed CT scans on 64 healthy men between 31 and 87 years of age and found atrophy of the left primary somatosensory cortex and the right somatosensory association cortex in the older subjects. Unlike studies performed on postmortem specimens that revealed marked brain atrophy with increasing age, contemporary in vivo sampling (as described collectively) documents a slight decrease in cortical mass with healthy aging.

In addition to a normal decreased brain mass, a progressive increase in ventricle size occurs with aging.[2] This occurs at a constant rate up to the seventh decade, with marked increases noted during the eighth and ninth decade of life. The combination of decreased brain weight and ventricular enlargement suggests loss of neurons in the normally aging brain. This leads the reader to the question: How does this neuron loss affect sensory interpretation? Not surprisingly, the answer to this question is under investigation. As described earlier, Sandor et al[15] reported atrophy in the left primary somatosensory and the right somatosensory association cortex in older subjects. The reader may deduce that atrophy in these areas may produce a somatosensory loss; however, this correlation is not described in the current literature. It is generally accepted that sensory integrity, including somatosensory, visual, auditory, and vestibular, declines with aging[2]; however, the exact relationship between brain atrophy and sensory decline is not known.

AFFERENT SENSORY PATHWAYS

Direct examination of the structures of sensory systems is not possible in the clinical setting. For this reason, tests and measures have been established to determine the function of sensory system structures, as well as to allow the examiner to localize pathology within a sensory system. A working knowledge of neuroanatomy is required to perform a sensory exam, allowing the examiner the ability to localize the source of a sensory problem. To begin, a brief review of the basic sensory pathways is presented.

Somatosensation

Somatosensation can be conscious or unconscious. Conscious sensation provides the individual with the ability to recognize the exact location of a stimulus, as well as the ability to define the stimulus. The target for conscious sensation is the cerebral cortex, specifically the primary somatosensory cortex located in the postcentral gyrus. Unconscious sensation is not used for recognition of a stimulus, but instead is necessary for smooth motor control. The target for unconscious sensation is the cerebellum. Both conscious and unconscious sensation reflect information from the external world (exteroceptive) and from within the body (proprioceptive).

Somatosensations are categorized into three groups: discriminative touch, pain and temperature, and unconscious proprioception. Discriminative touch is a conscious modality that includes light touch, pressure, vibration perception, and conscious proprioception. The peripheral receptors that are responsible for the reception of discriminative touch are Paccinian corpuscles, Ruffini's corpuscles, Meissner's corpuscles, Merkel's disks, hair follicles, free nerve endings, GTOs, and muscle spindle receptors. These receptors are located throughout the body in the skin, connective tissue, muscle, and tendon.[5,23] Discriminative touch enables us to describe the shape and texture of an object without seeing it. The second category, pain and temperature, includes the sensations "itch" and "tickle" and is perceived by activation of nociceptors (pain) and thermoreceptors (temperature) located throughout the skin, muscle, bone, connective tissue, and viscera. Pain and temperature reception enables us to detect stimuli that may be damaging to the tissues of the body.[23,24] The third sensory modality, unconscious proprioception, is perceived by activation of the GTOs and muscle spindle receptors located in muscles and joints. Proprioception enables us to determine the location of where our body is in space and the relationship of body parts to each other.[23,25]

Each somatosensory modality (discriminative touch, pain and temperature, unconscious proprioception) is carried via a different path to reach its target. The pathways include the dorsal column/medial lemniscus, the anterolateral spinothalamic (ALS) path, and the spinocerebellar path. A path is the route traveled by the signal, from the peripheral receptor to the target. Along the conscious pathways (the dorsal column/medial lemniscus, ALS), the signal will synapse twice and cross to the contralateral side of the spinal cord prior to reaching the cerebral cortex. Along the unconscious pathway (spinocerebellar), the impulse will synapse once and remain ipsilateral prior to reaching the cerebellum.

Discriminative Touch

The dorsal column/medial lemniscal path is the primary "road" that carries discriminative touch information from stimulated sensory receptors located in the body to the primary somatosensory cortex. Discriminative touch information, sent by action potential propagation, enters the spinal cord through the dorsal root and ascends the spinal cord within the dorsal column.[5,23] The dorsal column can be divided into two distinct paths: the *gracile fasciculus* and the *cuneate fasciculus*. Discriminative touch information from receptors of the legs is carried to the medulla in the gracile fasciculus, while discriminative touch information from receptors of the arms is carried to the medulla in the cuneate fasciculus. Once in the medulla, impulses from the legs will synapse in the gracile nucleus, while impulses from the arms will synapse in the cuneate nucleus. After synapsing in the appropriate nucleus, the impulse crosses to the opposite side of the spinal cord and ascends through the brainstem via the medial lemniscus to a second synapse in the ventroposterior lateral nucleus (VPL) of the thalamus. After synapsing in the VPL, the impulse travels through the internal capsule to its target, the *primary somatosensory cortex*.[5,23] The impulse, as it enters the spinal cord and progresses to its final destination, is maintained in a very topographically organized manner. Stimuli from the foot ascends medially along the pathway and more proximal impulses from the leg and thigh are layered laterally. This layered organization is maintained through the entire pathway and within the primary somatosensory cortex. In the primary somatosensory cortex, this organization is referred to as a homonculus where small areas of the cortex are designated to represent specific parts of the body. From the primary somatosensory cortex, the impulse proceeds to the secondary somatosensory cortex with interpretation at higher levels of the cortex.[5,23]

Impulses conveying discriminative touch information from receptors of the face follow a slightly different path than information from the body. Facial discriminative touch sensation is propagated over the trigeminal lemniscal pathway synapsing in the ventroposterior medial nucleus (VPM) of the thalamus. After synapsing in the VPM, impulses travel through the internal capsule to the region of the primary somatosensory cortex designated for facial sensation. Both pathways, the dorsal column/medial lemniscal and the trigeminal lemniscal, transmit precise, highly organized discriminative touch information that can be precisely localized and graded in intensity from its original location. Pathology anywhere along either pathway, from the receptor to the primary somatosensory cortex, results in an impairment of discriminative touch sensation.

Pain and Temperature

The second sensory modality, pain and temperature, is carried within the ALS.[23,24] In addition to pain and temperature information, the ALS makes a small contribution to our perception of coarse (nonlocalized) touch and provides a gross secondary source of touch sensation. In general, the ALS is much less organized than the dorsal column/medial lemniscal pathway, which is why the touch perception is nonlocalized. The signal from stimulated thermoreceptors and nociceptors enter the spinal cord through the dorsal root. The action potential may synapse immediately on entering the spinal cord or travel one or two segments up or down the cord in Lissauer's tract before entering and synapsing in the dorsal horn. The dorsal horn is a multilayered structure. The thin outermost layer is the posterior marginalis layer, the second layer is the substantia gelatinosa, and the deepest layer is the nucleus proprius.[23,24,26,27]

This layering is responsible for organizing the progression of two different types of pain impulses. Fast localized pain impulses are propagated along A fibers, while slow, achy pain impulses are propagated along C fibers, each entering different layers of the dorsal horn. Type A fibers enter the posterior marginalis and the nucleus proprius layers where the impulse synapses on a second set of neurons. After synapsing, the impulse crosses to the opposite side of the spinal cord before ascending to the VPL of the thalamus via the lateral spinothalamic tract. The impulse then is propagated to the primary somatosensory cortex via thalamocortical neurons allowing localization of pain or temperature to a specific area of the body. This is a direct route bringing fast, sharp pain information to the cerebral cortex, which in turn, allows a quick motor response to the stimulus.[23,24]

The type C fibers propagating the impulse of dull, achy, throbbing pain do not traverse the same direct route as the type A fibers. Instead, the type C fibers enter the substantia gelatinosa and synapse on interneurons (neurons that do not project out of the immediate area) which then carry the signal to synapse in either the posterior marginalis or the nucleus proprius layer. After synapsing, the impulses cross to the contralateral side of the spinal cord and then ascend through the spinomesencephalic tract or the spinoreticular tract.[28] Impulses carried in these pathways eventually reach the basal ganglia, the thalamus, the reticular formation, the amygdala, and parts of the cerebral cortex involved with emotions, sensory integration, personality, and movement.[24,26-29] To complicate matters, some impulses traveling in the spinothalamic tract do not cross, but instead ascend ipsilaterally.[23,24,26-29] This nonspecific, circuitous route of dull, achy pain projecting through multiple synapses and pathways provides the emotion associated with pain. The dull, achy pain pathway does not provide the CNS with the ability to decipher the precise location of the pain. For example, if you break your third metatarsal, you will have immediate pain via type A fibers alerting your cerebral cortex via the primary somatosensory and secondary association cortices that you have injured your foot, specifically, your third metatarsal. However, when the acute pain subsides and a dull ache persists, the C fibers continue to send impulses from nociceptors and thermoreceptors in your foot. However, this sensation will not localize the pain to the third metatarsal and instead, your entire foot will ache.

In the same manner that discriminative touch sensation from the face is not projected over the dorsal column/medial lemniscal system, pain from the face is not projected through the ALS. Pain and temperature sensations from the face are carried into the pons through the trigeminal nerve over the trigeminothalamic tract. Once in the pons, the impulses travel down the brainstem through the spinal tract of cranial nerve (CN) V until reaching the caudal medulla where it synapses in the spinal nucleus of CN V. After synapsing, the impulse crosses to the contralateral side and joins the spinothalamic tract on its way to the VPM of the thalamus.[24,28]

Unconscious Proprioception

The third somatosensory modality, unconscious proprioception, is carried via the spinocerebellar tract.[25] Clinically, this tract cannot be isolated from the dorsal column/medial lemniscal pathway during clinical testing, however, the presence of this tract emphasizes the importance of the sense of proprioception. Proprioception is so important to motor control that duplicate information is carried over two tracts, one to the cerebellum and one to the primary somatosensory cortex. When GTOs and muscle spindles are stimulated, impulses are carried along the dorsal column/medial lemniscal pathway to provide conscious proprioception. During the ascent in the dorsal column, duplicate impulses are projected from the gracile fasciculus (legs) to synapse in the nucleus dorsalis (Clarke's nucleus), and the cuneate fasciculus (arms) to synapse in the external (lateral) cuneate nucleus. From the nucleus dorsalis and the external cuneate nucleus, the impulse travels along the posterior spinocerebellar tract and the cuneocerebellar tract respectively.[29] Both tracts then enter the cerebellum through the inferior cerebellar peduncle. A unique difference between the spinocerebellar tract and the other two somatosensory tracts (dorsal column/medial lemniscus and the ALS) is that the information reaching the cerebellum is primarily ipsilateral. Most information does not cross before reaching its target.[29]

The three main pathways: dorsal column/medial lemniscus, ALS, and spinocerebellar, have been specifically described, however, there is a fair amount of mixing that goes on between the tracts. As described, some touch information travels in the spinothalamic tract, so that lesions in the dorsal columns will not completely abolish sensation. Proprioception is propagated along two pathways, the dorsal column/medial lemniscus and the spinocerebellar path. Pain and temperature impulses ascend to multiple targets, including the primary and secondary somatosensory cortex, the amygdala, reticular activating system, and limbic system.

Somatosensory processing provides information from the environment and from within the body to allow us to investigate the environment, to move accurately, or to have memories of movement for future reference. Additionally, some sensory information will produce an immediate motor response (ie, a reflex). A reflex is "an involuntary response to a stimulus."[30] The deep tendon reflex (DTR) is also known as the phasic stretch reflex or muscle stretch reflex. The DTR is an example of how a sensory stimulus (quick stretch) can produce a motor response. The DTR is produced when the muscle spindle receptor is stimulated producing an action potential propagated along type 1a primary afferents to the spinal cord where it synapses with the α (alpha) motoneuron of the same muscle resulting in contraction. This single synapse causes a motor action in response to a sensory stimulus; however, to prevent contraction of the activated muscle from producing a similar response in the antagonist muscle, an additional spinal connection is required. This additional spinal connection between the 1a primary afferent and an interneuron acting to inhibit contraction in the antagonist muscle is known as *reciprocal inhibition.* For a more detailed description of the muscle spindle, please refer to the recommended reading list. If reciprocal inhibition did not occur, a quick stretch of a muscle would alternately trigger a quick stretch response of the antagonist muscle. Clinically, loss of reciprocal inhibition in the ankle dorsiflexors can produce ankle clonus in response to a quick stretch of the gastroc/soleus complex.

Another automatic response to a sensory stimulus is the response of the GTO. The GTO is sensitive to muscle tension from contraction or excessive stretch of the muscle.[31] When the GTO is overly stimulated, there is reflex inhibition to the stimulated muscle. For example, if you were carrying a large rock that was too heavy for you, the GTOs in your biceps may send impulses to the spinal cord, which contact an inhibitory interneuron resulting in relaxation of the biceps and you drop the rock. In general, the GTO acts to protect the body as too much tension exerted over a muscle may lead to avulsion.

In addition to the reflexive response of the muscle spindle and GTO, superficial cutaneous reflexes may be elicited by the introduction of specific somatosensory stimuli. Superficial cutaneous reflexes are produced when specific surfaces on the body are stimulated by tickle or noxious stimuli. An example is the Babinski reflex when the toes are observed to assume a specific posture with stimulation of the lateral border of the foot.

SPECIAL SENSORY PATHWAYS

Visual

The visual system is primarily responsible for receiving information about the environment including the location of objects in space. The visual system also provides proprioceptive information about where our body is in space and the spatial relationship between body parts. Like somatosensation, a specific pathway is necessary for sensing, perceiving, and interpreting visual stimuli. Light enters the eyes and is converted into action potentials by photoreceptors (rods and cones) located in the retina. These impulses progress through the optic nerve, partially cross in the optic chiasm, and proceed along the optic tract to the lateral geniculate nucleus (LGN) of the thalamus. After synapsing in the LGN, the signal proceeds along the optic radiations to its target, the primary visual cortex in the occipital lobe.[32] From here, impulses are propagated to higher level cortices in the temporal and parietal lobes where integration of somatosensory and visual information is achieved. This integration allows for spatial orientation.[33]

Auditory

The auditory system functions to provide conscious recognition of sounds, to orient the eyes and head toward a sound, and to increase activity levels throughout the nervous system. Sound waves are picked up by the outer ear and funneled toward the tympanic membrane where vibration moves the ossicles that are connected to a membrane at the opening of the upper chamber of the cochlea. Within the cochlea, the organ of Corti converts the vibration into neural signals conveyed by the auditory nerve to the cochlear nuclei. From the cochlear nuclei, auditory information is transmitted to the reticular formation, the inferior colliculus, and the medial geniculate body. It is through the reticular formation that sound activates the CNS. An example of this activation is the startle that may occur in response to a loud noise. Stimulation of the inferior colliculus integrates information from both ears to determine the location of sound. The inferior colliculus sends impulses to the superior colliculus which elicits movement in the muscles of the eyes and face to turn toward the sound.[34] The medial geniculate nucleus is part of the thalamus that relays the neural signal to the primary auditory cortex which allows for conscious awareness of the sound. It is through this pathway that motor response to a loud noise may precede the recognition of the sound. For example, the sound of a car backfiring may produce the response of turning the head and eyes to the sound before the sound is identified.

Vestibular

The vestibular system provides sensory information about head movement and head position relative to gravity and postural adjustments, thereby allowing the eyes to maintain focus on an object when the head moves. The receptors for converting head position and motion are located within the inner ear, specifically in the semicircular canals and the otolith organs (utricle and saccule). Three semicircular canals are located within each inner ear and are responsible for detecting rotational acceleration or deceleration of the head in all three planes. The canals are fluid filled and situated at right angles to each other allowing at least one canal to detect planar rotation of the head with oblique head rotation detected by more than one semicircular canal. When the head moves, the fluid in the semicircular canals shifts, stimulating sensory hair cells which results in either excitation or inhibition of the vestibular nerve. Pairing of the semicircular canals (two ears) results in stimulation of sensory hair cells in paired canals, causing excitation of one vestibular nerve with inhibition of the other. Loss of reciprocal inhibition of paired semi-circular canals results in nausea and difficulty in controlling posture and eye movements.[34]

The utricle and saccule are sensitive to head position relative to gravity, linear acceleration, and deceleration of the head. The sensory hair cells, located within the utricle and saccule, are stimulated by movement during change of head position. The impulse then is transmitted through the vestibular nerve. The vestibular nerve conveys the signal to the vestibular nuclei which have multiple reciprocal connections to the spinal cord, reticular formation, superior colliculus, nucleus of CN XI, and the cerebellum. Through these reciprocal connections, postural adjustments, head and eye movements, and consciousness are influenced.[34]

EXAMINATION AND EVALUATION PROCEDURES

Sensory integrity, "the ability to organize and use sensory information"[26] depends on one's ability to receive, organize, integrate, and interpret environmental stimuli. Aging, injury, disease, and maturation of the nervous system will impact perception of a sensory stimulus.[35] Sensory integrity testing, as presented in The *Guide to Physical Therapist Practice,*[36] includes testing the modalities of proprioception, pallesthesia, stereognosis, and topognosis. *Proprioception* is the reception of stimuli from within the body, including position sense (awareness of joint position) and kinesthesia (awareness of movement).[36] *Pallesthesia* is the ability to sense mechanical vibration.[36] *Stereognosis* is the ability to perceive, recognize, and name familiar objects.[36] *Topognosis* is the ability to localize exactly a cutaneous sensation.[36]

Testing the integrity of the above modalities allows an examiner to gather information about a patient's ability to receive and interpret information from the environment.[26] A number of tests can be used, however, to perform all tests would be time consuming, expensive, and unnecessary. Only the most appropriate tests and measures should be performed based on the patient history and signs and symptoms revealed in the systems review. If during history-taking, the patient reports a loss (numbness) or change (tingling) of sensation in the leg, then somatosensory testing should begin in the leg, with comparison made to the identical regions on the opposite leg. If the patient does not or is unable to report a loss or change in sensation, the sensory exam should be guided by signs and symptoms revealed in the systems review. For example, if your patient has a flaccid right lower extremity due to a cerebrovascular accident, yet states that he "feels everything" in the right leg, it would be appropriate to perform a somatosensory exam beginning by examining the right leg with comparison to the left leg.

To obtain accurate data, the examiner must appropriately prepare the room as well as the patient. Room preparation includes adequate lighting, moderate temperature, and minimal noise. The room should have an armchair and a plinth for positioning to examine the patient in sitting, prone, and supine. Sensation cannot be adequately tested through clothing; therefore, the patient should wear a hospital gown or clothing that maintains modesty while allowing easy access to all areas for testing. The examiner should have all tools for performing the sensory exam readily accessible to facilitate the exam process. Basic testing tools include a wisp of cotton, a safety pin, a 128-Hz tuning fork, and calipers. Additional tools required for special sensory testing may be required and will be covered later in this chapter.

Prior to testing, the patient should be told the purpose of the sensory exam and instructed not to guess if uncertain of the correct response.[26] An accurate and complete sensory examination can be done only with an actively cooperative patient. Prior to testing each modality, it is necessary for the patient to watch you demonstrate the technique and instruments used for testing in an area where sensation is intact, allowing the patient the opportunity to understand what the sensation will feel like, as well as to provide a reference against which sensation in impaired areas can be compared. This preparation allows the patient to be comfortable with the testing tool, procedure, and appropriate response for each stimulus.

Once the patient is comfortable, vision should be occluded for testing. If the patient is unable to maintain closed eyes, a blindfold or towel can be used to occlude vision. If vision is not occluded, the patient may respond to the stimulus because he can see that you are touching him, not because he feels he is being touched. This will lead to collection and interpretation of inaccurate data.

The examination begins in an area where sensation is impaired and progresses to areas where sensation is intact,[37] with the results recorded on a dermatome or peripheral nerve chart to facilitate interpretation. A dermatome chart represents the cutaneous area that corresponds to the spinal segment providing its somatosensory innervation.[26] A peripheral nerve chart represents the specific peripheral nerve providing somatosensory innervation. Selection of the appropriate chart will depend on the patient's medical diagnosis and expected findings. For example, for a patient with a herniated lumbar disk, a dermatome chart would be selected. For a patient with polyneuropathy, a peripheral nerve chart would be selected.

There are several common mistakes that are noted during somatosensory examinations by inexperienced therapists or other professionals. These are noted in Table 9-1.

It is imperative that the examiner practice the somatosensory exam in order to be comfortable with the testing procedure thus obtaining accurate information for interpretation and subsequent treatment. Additionally, practicing the exam on normal subjects will allow the examiner to note individual variations in the normal somatosensory exam. Individual variations may include decreased perception of a modality in a small area, especially in the presence of dermatologic conditions such as scar tissue, tattoos, or calluses. Hypersensitivity to a modality may be present in situations of anxiety.

IMPAIRMENTS/SPECIFIC TESTS AND MEASURES

Impairments are defined as a loss or abnormality of anatomical, physiological, mental, or psychological structure or function and are indicated by signs and symptoms.[36] Impairments are usually the result of pathology that causes underlying changes in the normal state and may include loss of range of motion (ROM), decreased muscle strength, loss of sensation, and loss of reflexes. Sensory and perceptual impairments typically are measured using noninvasive procedures and may predict risk for functional limitation or disability.[36]

Discriminative touch, including light touch, proprioception, two point discrimination, pain, temperature, pallesthesia, visual, auditory, and vestibular examinations can be performed in the clinic.

TABLE 9-1

Common Mistakes in Somatosensory Examinations

1. Failure to test the anterior and posterior aspects of the body segment.
2. Repeatedly stimulating an area where no response was elicited in the hopes of obtaining a response.
3. Verbally cuing the patient with "do you feel that?" during the examination process.
4. Assuming an entire dermatome or peripheral nerve distribution is impaired if an abnormal response is obtained from testing only one area in the distribution.
5. Failure to test the corresponding area on the opposite extremity.
6. Application of the stimulus in a predictable manner.
7. Failure to allow the patient adequate time to respond to the stimulus prior to introducing the next stimulus.
8. Not performing a sensory exam based on a verbal statement from the patient that he cannot feel anything in a specific area.
9. Continuing to test for sensation when the patient appears confused or is giving inappropriate responses during the exam. In this case, the examiner should return to an area where sensation is intact and reintroduce the sensation as well as the appropriate response.

Touch Sensation

To test touch sensation, the patient is asked to respond with "now" or "yes" whenever he feels the stimulus. Testing is done with a wisp of cotton applied with equal force to all areas tested. The cotton should not be wiped on the skin as this may produce a tickle or be perceived as pain. Testing should begin in the area where a loss of sensation is suspected. If the patient fails to respond to a stimulus that has been presented in the same location twice, document this as an area of impaired sensation.

An additional component of this test includes comparing perceived touch sensation to the corresponding area on the opposite side of the body. During this component of the testing, the patient is asked to respond with "same" or "different." The reported sensation should be documented on a dermatome or peripheral nerve chart.

The use of a touch test monofilament (Figure 9-1) is a valuable tool for testing the threshold of touch sensation. This is particularly valuable in people who are at risk for skin ulceration due to loss of sensation.[38,39] The monofilaments are available in different thicknesses and are graded to bend under a specific amount of pressure. Patients who cannot feel the 5.07-mm sensory filament (a filament designed to bend under 10 g of force) have a loss of protective sensation and are at risk for ulceration.[38] Using the monofilaments, the examiner can obtain objective measures of sensation. For example, if on initial evaluation the smallest filament felt by a patient is the 3.61-mm filament at the base of the first metatarsal, but on reevaluation, the smallest filament that the patient can feel is the 4.31-mm filament in the same location, a progression of sensory loss is suspected.

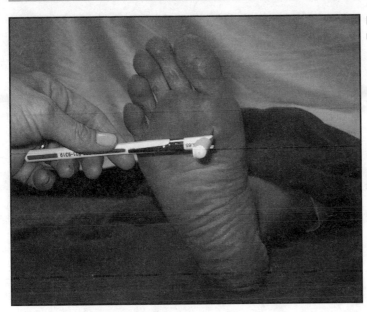

Figure 9-1. Touch test monofilament.

Two-Point Discriminative Touch

In two-point discriminative touch, the patient must distinguish between two non-noxious, light touch stimuli applied simultaneously to closely adjacent areas of skin.[40] Blunt calipers or commercially available instruments such as the Disk Criminator (Mackinnon-Dellon, Baltimore, Md) (Figure 9-2) can be used to perform the test. During testing, the patient is asked to to respond with "one" or "two" whenever he feels the stimulus. The test begins with two points that are set apart at the limits of normal[40-42] (Table 9-2). When applying two points, they must make simultaneous contact with the skin, applied with just enough pressure to depress the skin no more than 1 mm. Depression greater than 1 mm may be perceived as a painful stimulus.[40-42] If the patient fails to perceive the two points, the test is performed in the same area with two points that are further apart. If the patient perceives this as two points, note the distance on the dermatome or peripheral nerve chart. The results should be compared to corresponding areas on the contralateral side of the body.

Position Sense: Proprioception

In testing proprioception, the patient is asked to respond with "up" or "down" whenever he feels the digit stop moving. The sides of the finger or toe are grasped with uniform pressure and passively moved. By grasping the sides, as opposed to the top and bottom, any influence pressure perception may have when moving the digit is eliminated. For example, if you are moving a patient's index finger into extension with pressure applied to the pad of the finger, the pressure may be perceived, thus cuing him to say "up" in response to the pressure, rather than to proprioception. A patient with intact position sense should be able to detect a change of two degrees in either direction when testing one phalanx at a time.

Testing proprioception of an entire extremity can be performed by placing the extremity into a position and asking the patient to match the position with the opposite

Figure 9-2. Disk Criminator (Mackinnon-Dellon, Baltimore, Md).

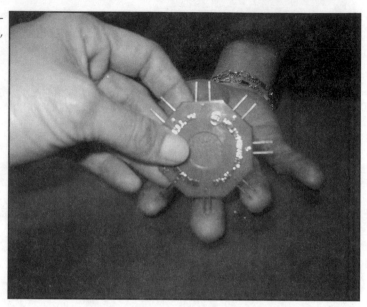

TABLE 9-2

Two-Point Discrimination Limits of 20- to 24-Year-Olds[40-42]

Palmar surface distal phalanx, 3rd digit, thumb	2.6 (0.7) mm
Palmar surface distal phalanx, 5th digit	2.5 (0.7) mm
Medial forearm	31.5 (8.9) mm
Lateral forearm	35.9 (11.6) mm
Mid-posterior thigh	42.2 (15.9) mm
Distal-anterior thigh	23.2 (9.3) mm
Tip of great toe	6.6 (1.8) mm
Lateral neck	35.2 (9.8) mm
Iliac crest	44.9 (10.1) mm
Lateral to umbilicus	36.4 (7.3) mm

extremity. For example, if you passively place the left shoulder in 90 degrees of flexion, the elbow in 45 degrees flexion, and the wrist in neutral, this position should be matched by the right upper extremity. To accurately perform this test, normal motor function in the extremity the patient is moving must be present.

An additional test of proprioception is the rhomberg test which is used to determine if standing balance is compromised due to a proprioceptive or a cerebellar lesion (see Chapter 8). During testing, the examiner stands near the patient as a sudden, unanticipated loss of balance may result. The patient is asked to stand barefoot with both feet together and with eyes open. Next, the patient is asked to close his eyes, thus removing visual input. A significant increase in sway or loss of balance indicates a loss of proprioception in the lower extremities. If the patient does not maintain his balance with eyes open, although strength and cognition are intact, a cerebellar or cerebral lesion, or possibly a vestibular dysfunction, may be indicated.

Position Sense: Kinesthesia

Kinesthetic testing is performed in a similar manner to proprioception, however, the patient is asked to identify the direction the joint is moving as it is being moved. The patient is asked to respond with "moving up" or "moving down" as the digit is being moved. As with proprioception testing, the side of the digit being tested is grasped and moved slowly. If the patient does not respond until the digit stops moving, he is reminded to answer while the digit is moving, not when it stops. Testing kinesthesia in an entire extremity can be done by asking the patient to match the position of the opposite extremity while you are moving it. Once again, to accurately perform this test, normal motor function in the extremity the patient is moving must be present.

Pallesthesia (Vibration) Sense

In testing pallesthesia, the patient is asked to inform the examiner when the vibration is felt by stating "now" and when the vibration has stopped by stating "stopped." The patient is instructed not to respond to the sensation of feeling the fork but to the vibration of the fork. The feeling of the application of the fork versus the feeling of the fork vibrating on a bony prominence is demonstrated initially using a 128-Hz tuning fork held at the stem. The tuning fork is activated by striking the tines on the examiner's opposite hand or a padded plinth. The examiner intermittently may place a nonvibrating fork on the patient to ensure that the response is to the vibration, not to the pressure of the tuning fork. Vibration is tested over bony prominences and results are documented on a dermatome or nerve root chart. Common bony prominences tested include the digits (toes and fingers), malleoli, tibial crest, patellae, anterior superior iliac spine, vertebral spinous processes, radial and ulnar styloid processes, olecranon process, acromion process, and sternum.

Stereognosis: Object Recognition

Stereognosis is tested by having the patient identify small, familiar objects (eg, key, dice, coin, paper clip) that are placed in one hand.[37] In order for the patient to manipulate the object, motor function must be intact. An example of accuracy documented is "the patient is able to recognize eight of 10 objects placed in the palm of the right/left hand."

Graphesthesia

Graphesthesia is tested by tracing single digit numbers 3 to 4 centimeters high on the patient's palm and asking the patient to identify the numbers. An example of accuracy documentation is "the patient is able to recognize eight of 10 numbers drawn in the palm of the right/left hand."

Superficial Pain

Superficial pain perception is tested by asking the patient to respond with "now" or "yes" whenever he feels a pinprick. When introducing the sharp sensation, there should be ample force so that it is unpleasant but not enough to puncture the skin. Results should be documented on a dermatome or peripheral nerve chart. When the examination of superficial pain is completed, the safety pin should be disposed of in a sharps container.

Temperature Sensation

Temperature sensation assessment requires the patient to respond with "hot" or "cold" whenever he feels the stimulus. "Yes" and "no" is not an appropriate response, as this does not determine if the stimulus is hot or cold, and may indicate perception of the touch of the test tube on the area, as opposed to the temperature. To perform the test, two test tubes, one filled with hot water and the other filled with cold water, are used. A temperature difference of approximately 5° C is necessary to discriminate differences.

SPECIAL SENSE TESTING

Vision

Visual Acuity

A gross assessment of visual acuity, "a measure of the resolving power of the eye,"[43] can be made for both near and far vision. Far vision is tested with the patient sitting or standing at a specific distance (as indicated on the chart) from a standard eye chart. Corrective lenses, if needed, should be worn during the exam. The patient is asked to cover one eye and read the smallest line visible on the chart. Then the procedure is repeated with the other eye. The patient should be able to read the letters from the line marked "20 feet" with each eye. Visual acuity is expressed as the size of the smallest letters identified at 20 feet. For example, a letter that a person with perfect visual acuity can read at 60 feet, but is the smallest identified by the patient at 20 feet indicates a visual acuity or 20/60.

For near vision, the patient is asked to read newsprint (letters 1/16 inch). Normal vision allows newsprint to be read at a distance of 32 inches. Visual acuity is expressed as 0/32 if the patient can not read newsprint beyond 9 inches. Any abnormality in near or far vision that is not corrected by lenses should be further explored by an ophthalmologist.

Visual Field

The visual field of view, "the space within which an object can be seen while the eye remains fixed on one point,"[43] is examined with the patient sitting or standing with one eye covered. The patient is asked to focus on an object that is in the distance over the examiner's shoulder (eg, a picture on the wall). With the patient focusing, the examiner introduces a small white object (a die) from the periphery to the center of the visual field. This procedure is repeated while introducing the object from the superior, inferior, medial, and lateral direction in both eyes. The patient is asked to say "now" when the object is seen.

Visual Reflex

For direct light reflex testing, a light is shone into the patient's eye. This stimulus should cause the pupil to constrict. If the pupil does not constrict, this would indicate either a lesion in the afferent (CN II) reception of the light stimulus or a lesion in the efferent (CN III) motor response to the light stimulus. In the case where no direct light reflex is elicited, the consensual light reflex must be assessed.[32]

Consensual light reflex is tested by shining a light into the patient's eye and observing the contralateral eye for pupillary constriction. If the contralateral pupil constricts as a response to the light stimulus, this would indicate that the afferent (sensory) component of the reflex is intact. If no direct light reflex was elicited from the right eye, but a consensual light reflex was elicited from stimulating the right eye, this would indicate a lesion in the motor (CN III) innervation to the pupil.[32]

Interruption of the visual impulse anywhere along the pathway would result in stereotypic visual field loss and a functional limitation. For example, if light entering an eye is not detected because of a lesion in the eye itself or a complete lesion of the optic nerve, the patient would have a loss of peripheral vision in the affected eye and difficulty with depth perception. A lesion in the optic chiasm would cause "tunnel vision" in which peripheral vision would be lost in both eyes. A complete lesion in the optic tract would cause complete loss of the opposite visual field called ***homonymous hemianopsia***. In this case, a lesion of the right optic tract would cause a complete loss of the left visual field. A lesion affecting the left temporal part of the optic radiations would result in a right upper quadrant loss of the visual field; likewise, a lesion in the left parietal part of the optic radiations would result in a right lower quadrant loss of the visual field. The opposite would be true with right-sided lesions. Finally, a lesion in the occipital lobe may result in contralateral homonymous hemianopsia with sparing of central vision.

Visual Object Recognition

The patient is requested to name objects as they are presented. Common objects such as a toothbrush, comb, and paperclip should be used. The patient should be able to say the word as opposed to acting out the function of the object is used for. For example, when a comb is presented, the patient should say "comb" and not just act out combing the hair. The number of objects correctly named by the patient should be documented.

Vestibulocochlear Nerve Testing

Cochlear Division

Quantitative testing of hearing usually is performed by an audiologist, however, gross hearing testing can be performed in the physical therapy clinic. Minor hearing deficits may be detected by gently rubbing the thumb and forefinger together about 2 inches from the ear.

Vestibular Division

By slowly turning the patient's head side to side or up and down, a reflexive eye movement should occur. The occulovestibular response will cause the eyes to reflexively move to the left when the head is passively moved to the right and the eyes to the right when the head is moved to the left. When moving the head up, the eyes will move down, and when the head is moved down, the eyes will move up. In some patients, moving the head may induce vestibular response such as vertigo, blurred vision, nausea, dizziness, postural instability, and gait ataxia (see Chapter 11).

PEDIATRIC VARIATIONS/STANDARDIZED TESTS

The above sensory tests at the impairment level may not be appropriate when evaluating children. As previously described, the sensory systems mature at different times, therefore, children may not have the cognitive ability nor the physical ability to respond appropriately to the modalities introduced. Therefore, a gross observational examination may be performed to determine the function of the sensory systems in children. Somatosensory testing may be performed by introducing different tactile stimuli, including light touch and tickle to the extremities and trunk and observing for the response. A response, such as a smile, or moving the extremity away from the stimulus would indicate that the stimulus was perceived. Testing the auditory system may include using a bell, clapping, or a voice introduced at different levels of loudness and different locations. An appropriate response to the stimulus may be opening the eyes, looking toward the stimulus, or turning the head toward or away from the stimulus.

Examination of the visual system may be performed by presenting a bright object or a picture of a happy face to the child. This may result in tracking the object or accommodation (adjustment of the eyes to view a near object), which results in convergence of the eyes and pupillary constriction. The vestibular system can be examined by moving the child's head from side to side; placing the child in different positions, such as supine, prone, side lying, sitting, and standing; and noting the response to static position. Response to movement can be observed by placing the child on a ball, Sit and Spin, or suspended bolster or platform and noting the response. In addition to these gross observational methods, specific standardized tests, such as the Sensory Integration and Praxis Tests, Infant/Toddler Sensory Profile, Sensory Integration Inventory, or DeGangi Berk Test of Sensory Integration, can be administered.

Sensory Integration and Praxis Tests (SIPT)[44]

The SIPT is appropriate for children ages 4 to 8 years who do not have a diagnosis of neuromotor dysfunction. The therapist must be certified to administer the test, which takes approximately 2 to 2.5 hours to administer and 90 minutes to score. This may limit the participation of many children. Additionally, it is relatively expensive to administer. The test includes 17 subtests including:

1. Space visualization
2. Figure ground
3. Standing and walking balance
4. Design copying
5. Postural praxis
6. Bilateral motor coordination
7. Praxis on verbal command
8. Construction praxis
9. Postrotary nystagmus
10. Motor accuracy
11. Sequential praxis
12. Oral praxis
13. Manual form perception

14. Kinesthesia
15. Finger identification
16. Graphesthesia
17. Localization of tactile stimulus

Infant/Toddler Sensory Profile[45]

The Infant/Toddler Sensory Profile, a caregiver questionnaire, can be administered to children between birth to 36 months of age. The caregiver answers a series of questions in six categories including general, auditory, visual, tactile, vestibular, and oral sensory processing. The caregiver scores these questions by choosing one response for each question. The scoring is well defined in the questionnaire and includes the categories of "always," "frequently," "occasionally," "seldom," and "never." This questionnaire takes approximately 15 minutes to administer and 10 minutes to score. It is useful for gathering information about infant/toddler sensory processing.

Sensory Profile[46]

The sensory profile can be administered to children between 5 to 10 years of age. A questionnaire is given to the caregiver who answers with the same choices as the Sensory Profile in Infants and Toddlers. The test takes approximately 30 minutes to administer and 20 minutes to score. It is designed to capture information about the child's sensory processing, modulation, and behavioral and emotional responses. It links sensory processing to daily life and provides information for theory-based decision making.

Sensory Integration Inventory

The Sensory Integration Inventory is used to screen patients with developmental delays and disabilities for sensory integration dysfunction. It is an assessment of tactile, vestibular, proprioceptive, and general reactions. Scoring can be by observation or by caregiver report. Items are marked Yes if "typical behavior" and No if "not seen." It takes approximately 30 minutes to administer and can be used with adults and children.

The DeGangi Berk Test of Sensory Integration[47]

The DeGangi Berk Test of Sensory Integration is a direct assessment tool used to provide an overall measure of sensory integration for preschool children ages 3 to 5 years. The test is standardized and takes approximately 30 minutes to administer with an additional 15 minutes to score. Thirty-six items are tested in categories including postural control, bilateral motor integration, and reflex integration. Scoring is delineated in a protocol booklet with each item individually scored and summed to obtain a total score. The total score then is compared against a normed score.

Quantitative Testing

Examining sensory nerve function can be evaluated quantitatively by nerve conduction velocity testing and somatosensory evoked potential testing.[11,12] NCV testing is used to evaluate the function of peripheral nerves. Recording electrodes are placed at a specific distance along the surface of the skin overlying the course of the peripheral nerve. The skin at the most distal segment is stimulated and electrical activity is recorded along the length of the peripheral nerve by the recording electrodes. Conduction velocity of the impulse is determined by dividing the distance from the point of application of the stimulus to the recording electrode site (meters) by the time needed for the impulse to traverse the distance (seconds). In addition to velocity, amplitude also is recorded. Amplitude provides information about the number of axons conducting the impulse. Clinically, in diseases which cause demyelination of peripheral nerves, the NCV would be significantly slower than normal. Additionally, the exact location of a lesion can be identified by comparing the NCV between recording electrodes.

Somatosensory evoked potential recordings (SEPs) are similar to NCV as they examine the function of the peripheral nerve with the additional benefit of testing central nerve transmission. The skin over the peripheral nerve is stimulated with recording electrodes located on the skin of the upper cervical spinal cord and/or from the scalp over the primary somatosensory cortex. Once again, conduction velocity can be determined with additional information provided about the integrity of the dorsal roots, dorsal column, and brainstem. VEPs can be tested by introducing visual stimuli, such as a flashing light with variable patterns, and measuring the time for the impulse to travel to electrodes over the primary visual cortex. AEPs can be used to evaluate the cochlear division of CN III.[48] Electrodes record and time the activity in the primary auditory cortex after an auditory stimulus is presented.

Evaluation/Functional Level

The clinical tests as described previously are performed for a reason. Through testing, we can determine impairments, but the effect these impairments have on function is the true concern. Clinically, if peripheral afferent information is absent, the patient may exhibit lack of awareness of the limb. Lack of awareness of a limb leads to disuse in functional activities, thus producing a functional limitation. Functional limitation is defined as an inability to perform a physical action, task, or activity in an efficient, typically expected, or competent manner.[36] As stated, functional limitations are a result of impairment(s) and may affect performance in the execution of particular actions, tasks, and activities (eg, rolling, getting out of bed, lifting, carrying).[36] Specific sensory limitations causing motor dysfunction include perceptual difficulties, spatial orientation difficulties, slow responses or response times, and apraxia.

Perceptual difficulties include a disregard of body parts or space (neglect) or a loss of object recognition to any sensory modality. Neglect is a tendency to behave as if one side of the body and/or side of space does not exist.[30] Neglect can be tactile, visual, or auditory. Sensory neglect may be due to a lesion anywhere in the sensory pathway from the peripheral nerve to the cerebral cortex. A person with a complete laceration of a peripheral nerve would receive no somatosensation in the area perceived by that nerve; therefore, no response will result unless a second sensory system is involved in perception of the stimulus. Visual input often will provide the patient with the necessary sensory information. In a similar example, a person with a lesion in the dorsal column may have difficulty with proprioceptive input when performing functional activities. Difficulty perceiving proprioceptive input from the lower extremities may result in ataxia. To compensate for this, the patient may walk vigorously, slapping the feet flat on the floor with every step or tapping a cane vigorously on the ground to provide auditory input to the CNS, allowing some perception of the location of the limbs. In a similar compensation, people with dorsal column lesions may rely on their visual system for input; walking with their eyes watching their feet and the ground so they can see the location of their feet in relation to the ground.

A profound loss of awareness of one side of the body most commonly results from a CVA or tumor in the right parietal lobe. This produces mild to severe inattention to the left side of the body to somatosensory, auditory, and visual stimuli. In severe cases, patients will attend to only one side of the body and when oriented to the contralateral side, they will deny that the opposite side even belongs to them. If the patient does not acknowledge the existence of an entire side of the body, overall function for all activities will be severely impaired. The patient will not be able to roll to either side of the bed, steer a wheelchair, or transfer safely. Milder forms of inattention may not produce such profound functional limitations, however, functional limitations will exist. Spatial orientation can be examined by asking the patient to draw a picture of a symmetrical object such as a clock or a flower. The drawing may be of only one half of the object, or the picture will be distorted to one side of the paper. An additional assessment can be done by providing the patient with a piece of typed paper with the alphabet repeatedly printed on the page (Figure 9-3). The patient then is asked to identify, by circling or pointing to, all of the letter A's. The examiner then can count the number of A's missed and note the location of the majority of missed letters.

Intervention Strategies

In general, whenever it is possible, an attempt should be made to improve the function of a sensory system in which deficits are detected. For example, visual disregard can be addressed by activities to encourage the patient to look to the neglected side of space. Problems with visual acuity may be addressed by wearing glasses and a hearing impairment by wearing a hearing aid. Patients with deficits in somatosensation can participate in activities with eyes closed or with different tactile surfaces to draw their attention to somatosensation. In many cases, however, it is not possible to improve the functioning of a specific sensory system. In these cases, patients will need to be taught compensatory strategies, for example, using visual monitoring to compensate for impaired somatosensory or vestibular functioning.

Somatosensory

A loss of proprioception or kinesthesia will influence motor control. Individuals who cannot perceive where their limbs are in space or the direction of limb movement will produce inaccurate movements. They may be perceived as clumsy when performing activities. Interventions to improve proprioception include applying pressure by wrapping the patient in a blanket or special vest (Figure 9-4) to add somatosensation of pressure or warmth. New devices such as a weighted halo can assist with proprioception of head position (Figure 9-5). Often, individuals with a loss of position sense in the extremities will compensate with visual input. For example, they will carefully watch their feet as they move from location to location.

Visual

Color can excite or calm a person. Cool colors or a monotone room encourage relaxation and may allow a person with increased tone to perform a motor pattern they were not previously able to perform. Conversely, bright colors or repetitive even patterns may increase attention and alertness. Visual tracking can be emphasized by asking a patient to track an object as it is moved. More advanced tracking can be achieved by moving the object simultaneously with the patient who is moving on a movable surface.

Figure 9-3. The alphabet repeatedly printed on the page.

ABCDEFGHIJKLMNOPQRSTUVWXYZABCDEFGHIJKLMNOPQR
STUVWXYZABCDEFGHIJKLMNOPQRSTUVWXYZABCDEFGHIJK
LMNOPQRSTUVWXYZABCDEFGHIJKLMNOPQRSTUVWXYZAB
CDEFGHIJKLMNOPQRSTUVWXYZABCDEFGHIJKLMNOPQRST
UVWXYZABCDEFGHIJKLMNOPQRSTUVWXYZABCDEFGHIJKL
MNOPQRSTUVWXYZABCDEFGHIJKLMNOPQRSTUVWXYZABC

Figure 9-4. Neoprene vest used to improve proprioception.

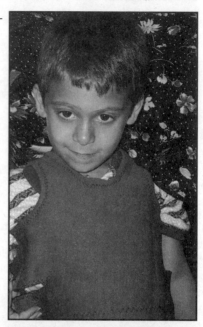

Figure 9-5. Weighted halo for improved proprioception to neck musculature; mobile platform to challenge vestibular function.

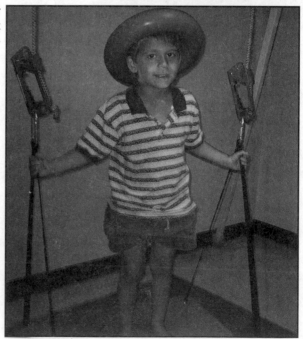

Auditory

Physical therapists do not think they use auditory stimuli to influence their patients, however, they probably do so without recognizing it. A voice can be soft or harsh, loud or a whisper. A loud or intermittent tone of voice may increase muscle tension, while a soothing, monotone voice may calm the patient, thereby improving motor control. Noise in the treatment room may have similar effects. Beepers, telephones, or overhead speakers may be overwhelming to a patient.

Vestibular

To stimulate the vestibular system, a change of static position or movement is introduced.[49,50] Muscle tension may change depending on the patient's position. A patient in supine may exhibit increased extensor tone, where more flexion may be exhibited in prone. This change in posture is due to the influence of the vestibular system on motoneuron excitability via the vestibulospinal tracts (see Chapters 3 and 12). In addition to position, the vestibular system influences the CNS in response to movement. The rate of vestibular stimulation will determine the effect. For example, a constant slow rocking tends to dampen the motor system; a fast spin or linear movement will heighten alertness and motor responses. Slow rhythmic rocking is most successful in reducing muscle tone when performed on a diagonal and can be done using a large ball, on a platform, on a suspended bolster (Figure 9-6), or on a swing. This stimulates all three semicircular canals producing the greatest effect. Just as slow rocking can decrease muscle tone, fast rocking in an anterior-posterior or angular direction can be used to increase muscle tone. This may be achieved with the patient sitting or in prone on a scooter board (Figures 9-7 and 9-8) or on a platform (see Figure 9-5). Arousal level can be influenced by massive vestibular input from spinning quickly, for example, on a Sit and Spin (Figures 9-9 and 9-10). Treatment for benign paroxysmal positional nystagmus (BPPN) and activities to promote specific balance strategies are covered in Chapter 11.

CASE STUDY # 1
Jane Smith

- *Age: 74 years*
- *Medical Diagnosis: Right hemiplegia, secondary to left CVA*
- *Status: 6 month post onset*
- *Practice Pattern 5D: Impaired Motor Function and Sensory Integrity Associated with Nonprogressive Disorders of the Central Nervous System—Acquired in Adolescence or Adulthood*

Figure 9-6. Suspended bolster used to provide proprioceptive and vestibular input.

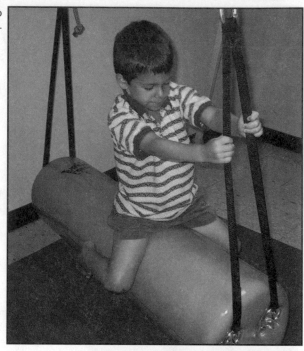

Figure 9-7. Scooterboard used to provide vestibular and proprioceptive input as well as used to challenge motor planning and execution.

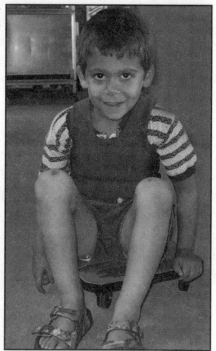

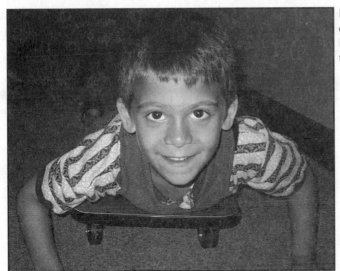

Figure 9-8. Prone on the scooter board to provide vestibular input and proprioceptive input to the abdomen and hands.

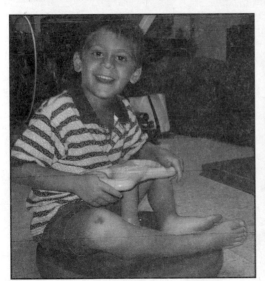

Figure 9-9. Sit and Spin.

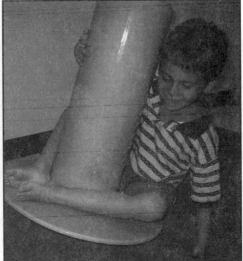

Figure 9-10. The patient is encouraged to volitionally execute the normally automatic forward trunk movements in anticipation of a rise.

EXAMINATION AND EVALUATION

Functional Limitations

Mrs. Smith requires assistance for all self-care activities, transfers, and standing activities. She can sit independently, although asymmetrically, in a wheelchair, but is unable to steer the wheelchair without bumping into objects. She is unaware of her limitations and is impulsive, attempting to stand or steer her wheelchair without assistance. Due to her sensory loss in the right upper extremity, she often bruises her arm by traumatizing the extremity when attempting to move.

Impairments

Mrs. Smith exhibits sensory impairments that include a right visual field cut, disregard for the right visual hemifield, sensory disregard and neglect for the right side of the body, asymmetric weight bearing while sitting and in supported standing, and with gaze and head/trunk rotation to the left.

PROGNOSIS/PLAN OF CARE

Goals

Treatment goals are for Mrs. Smith to:
1. Improve weight bearing symmetry while sitting, standing, and walking
2. Improve attention to the right hemifield
3. Demonstrate decreased neglect of the right side of the body
4. Improve bed mobility and transfers

Functional Outcomes

Following 3 months of therapy, Mrs. Smith will:
1. Achieve postural symmetry and maintain the head in neutral alignment while sitting, standing, and walking
2. Reach across midline to pick up objects placed to the affected side of the body, six of 10 times
3. Put on a house coat independently, four of six times
4. Perform bed mobility independently and transfer to her wheelchair with supervision five of six times

INTERVENTION

Neglect of the right side of the body and inattention to the right hemifield are playing a large role in Mrs. Smith's inability to accurately perform functional activities. For this reason, activities that bring attention to the right side are encouraged. Such activities include:
1. Sitting and supported standing while directing attention to a mirror placed in front of Mrs. Smith. In this manner she can be verbally cued to weight bear on the right lower extremity. Once sitting and standing symmetry is achieved, Mrs. Smith should work on deviating from center by leaning side to side or forward and back then returning to the sitting or standing symmetry.
2. Placing objects on a table on the involved side and encouraging her to identify all of the objects, directing her to the ones she missed. She can pick up each object, assisting the right upper extremity with the left, and place the object in a bucket set slightly to the right side of the table.

3. Asking her to identify pictures on the wall and drawing attention to the pictures in the right hemifield with the use of a flashlight by pulsing the light on the object, or asking her to track the light with her eyes as you bring it from the left hemifield to the right.

4. Incorporating movement of the right upper extremity into functional tasks. For example, asking her to apply lotion to her hands. This will orient her to both upper extremities, as well as provide some sensory input of light touch and temperature (the lotion may be warm or cold) to both upper extremities.

To reduce the risk of trauma to the right upper extremity due to loss of somatosensation, it would be prudent to provide Mrs. Smith with a trough for the right arm for use in the wheelchair. While in the chair, or during assisted walking, Mrs. Smith should work on steering around an obstacle course, using her legs and her left upper extremity to steer. Initially it may be difficult to identify objects in the right hemifield, so you may begin by asking her to follow a line of black tape that is placed around the room and having her follow the tape going clockwise and counterclockwise.

Functional skills such as rolling and transfers can be facilitated by the use of sensory stimulation. In supine, Mrs. Smith should work on clasping her hands together and, with visual tracking of the hands, rock from side to side to gain momentum. Once on her side (affected or unaffected), Mrs. Smith should be encouraged to use both upper extremities to push into sitting. Once in sitting, pressure to the outstretched right upper extremity with the fingers in extension will encourage joint compression and stimulate deep pressure receptors within the shoulder, elbow, and wrist.

CASE STUDY #2
Daniel Johnson

- *Age: 59 years*
- *Medical Diagnosis: Parkinson's disease*
- *Status: 4 years post initial diagnosis*
- *Practice Pattern 5E: Impaired Motor Function and Sensory Integrity Associated with Progressive Disorders of the Central Nervous System*

EXAMINATION AND EVALUATION

Functional Limitations

Mr. Johnson is experiencing increased difficulty with recreational activities including swimming and walking. He requires assistance when rising from a low chair. His walking is deteriorating with a festinating appearance (shortened stride length, progressive increase in speed), a loss of balance with turning, and difficulty regaining his balance when standing.

Impairments

Mr. Johnson exhibits mild to moderate rigidity of the upper extremities and mild rigidity of the lower extremities; decreased excursion of all extremities during movement, decreased flexibility of the trunk and pelvis; bradykinesia (slowness of movement); akinesia (difficulty initiating movement); dyskinesia (poor synergistic organization of movement); and poor postural control in sitting and standing.

PROGNOSIS/PLAN OF CARE

Goals

Treatment goals are for Mr. Johnson to:
1. Improve initiation of movement
2. Improve sit to stand transfers
3. Increase stride length during walking

Functional Outcomes

Following 3 months of therapy, Mr. Johnson will:
1. Initiate movement within 1 second for four of six upper extremity activities
2. Move from sit to stand independently 100% of the time
3. Walk 100 feet with a normal stride length

INTERVENTION

Mr. Johnson's bradykinesia and rigidity are impacting his functional activities. To begin treatment, general relaxation must be encouraged. This can be done in supine with gentle rocking and rotation exercises. Begin with side-to-side rocking of the head, gradually involving the entire body. Then maintain the rocking with gradual dissociation of the pelvis and trunk by rocking the pelvis in one direction and the shoulders (or head) to the other. Once Mr. Johnson is relaxed, functional training can begin. All functional exercises should encourage trunk rotation. Upper and lower extremity diagonal proprioceptive neuromuscular facilitation (PNF) patterns should be encouraged. Quick stretch of the extremity during the PNF patterning may carry over to aid in initiation of movement.

Sit to stand initiation should begin with a seat that is slightly higher than normal to practice and to ensure that the technique is mastered. As this action becomes easier, the chair height should be lowered. Begin standing by initially rocking the pelvis and trunk forward and backward (Figure 9-11), gradually increasing the excursion of the upper body beyond the feet. Once this excursion is mastered, move from sit to stand in a fluid forward movement. Tactile cues on the anterior hip will encourage hip extension during sit to stand.

Mr. Johnson would benefit from visual cues for gait enhancement. Black lines drawn approximately 20 inches apart on the floor (Figure 9-12) or marked with black electri-

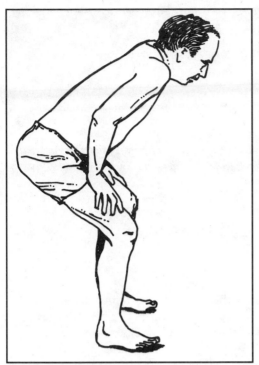

Figure 9-11. Patient is encouraged to volitionally execute the normally automatic forward trunk movements in anticipation of a rise.

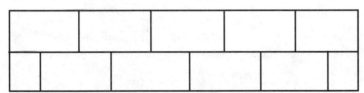

Figure 9-12. Visual cues for gait enhancement.

cal tape would help in cuing for longer step length. This task should be initiated in the parallel bars with Mr. Johnson being asked to step over the lines. The parallel bars could be used to assist with turning. Once he is able to step over the lines, similar lines can be drawn on the walking surface of the clinic. Another visual method used to improve gait is the use of an inverted cane. Mr. Johnson is asked to hold a cane by the tip, allowing the handle to dangle forward of the feet. This visual cue, first described by Dunne,[51] encourages longer step length and assists with step initiation. During turning, Mr. Johnson should be encouraged to take longer steps, slowly maintaining a wide base of support. In addition to visual cues, rhythmic auditory stimulation may be used to improve velocity, cadence, and stride length.[52,53] A metronome can be set to provide auditory cues at 100 to 120 beats per minute, or marching music can be played in combination with gait training.

CASE STUDY # 3
Shirley Teal

- *Age: 21 years*
- *Medical Diagnosis: Traumatic brain injury*
- *Status: 4 months post injury*
- *Practice Pattern 5D: Impaired Motor Function and Sensory Integrity Associated with Nonprogressive Disorders of the Central Nervous System—Acquired in Adolescence or Adulthood*

EXAMINATION AND EVALUATION

Functional Limitations

Ms. Teal limits the movement of her head on her body in an attempt to reduce dizziness and vertigo. She also is apprehensive to change position of her body, for example move from supine to sit, as this also produces vertigo and dizziness. She is unable to stand and walk independently.

Impairments

Ms. Teal exhibits astereognosia, vertigo and dizziness with change of position, BPPN, poor proprioception and kinesthesia, overall decreased strength, and impulsive, unsafe behavior.

PROGNOSIS/PLAN OF CARE

Goals

Treatment goals are for Ms. Teal to:
1. Demonstrate decreased movement-provoked symptoms of vertigo
2. Improve gaze stabilization
3. Improve overall strength

Functional Outcomes

Following 2 months of therapy, Ms. Teal will:
1. Move her head (full range) from side to side without producing vertigo nine of 10 times
2. Visually track an object for 1 minute
3. Walk 30 feet with one cane and minimal assistance

INTERVENTION

Movement therapy can be encouraged, but decreasing the vertigo resulting from movement must be immediately addressed. If vertigo persists with movement, Ms. Teal will not be cooperative and may appear combative during therapy. To address the vertigo, mechanical repositioning maneuvers should be administered initially (see Chapter 11). If this approach is not successful, habituation might be attempted.[54] This may be best received by doing this at the end of your therapy session. The head movement should be repeated in sitting, standing, and walking with close supervision of a therapist as a sudden onset of vertigo may result in loss of balance.

Gaze stabilization exercises such as those listed here should be performed in multiple positions. Examples are as follows:

1. Stand behind Ms. Teal as she faces a blank wall. Project a beam of light onto the wall with a flashlight or laser pointer. Have her focus her vision on the projected circle of light and slowly move the projection horizontally, vertically, clockwise, and counterclockwise. When Ms. Teal is able to follow the projection, gradually increase the speed of movement and the magnitude of excursion.

2. Follow the same procedure as above, but allow Ms. Teal to move her head to follow the projection of light. If she is apprehensive, increase the excursion, which would encourage her to move her head. This should be repeated with increasing speed of movement.

3. With Ms. Teal on a moving surface (eg, wheelchair, swing, therapeutic ball), ask her to focus her vision on a specific, stable object. Slowly move her horizontally and vertically while she maintains her focus. When she is able to maintain her focus, gradually increase the speed of movement.

4. With Ms. Teal on a moving surface ask, her to focus and follow a projected beam of light as it moves horizontally, vertically, clockwise, and counterclockwise. Alter the excursion and speed of movement of the projected beam of light, as well as the support surface.

Proprioception can be improved by asking her to visualize the movement that she is performing. Repetitive activities are helpful. Placing pegs in boards requires fine coordination and visual input. Functional activities such as sorting silverware into the appropriate bin will encourage the use of visual input; additionally, proprioception will be challenged with utensils of different weights. If tolerated, fluidotherapy may stimulate cutaneous receptors in the hand, which can play a role in proprioception. With her hands in the fluidotherapy, she can do an activity such as squeezing a ball or wrapping a ball with a shoestring. This will encourage movement of the fingers, enhancing proprioception with tactile stimulation.

Strengthening exercises can be facilitated by tapping the muscles prior to asking her to move them, for example, prior to extension of the right knee, vigorously tap the quadriceps to provide some sensory input and a slight stretch to the muscle, encouraging contraction. This also can be performed standing in the parallel bars to encourage knee extension for weight bearing.

CASE STUDY #4
Shawna Wells

- *Age: 4 years*
- *Medical Diagnosis: Cerebral palsy, spastic quadriparesis, mild mental retardation*
- *Status: Onset at birth*
- *Practice Pattern 5C: Impaired Motor Function and Sensory Integrity Associated with Nonprogressive Disorders of the Central Nervous System—Congenital Origin or Acquired in Infancy or Childhood*

EXAMINATION AND EVALUATION

Functional Limitations

Shawna is hesitant to play on movable toys, such as tricycles, scooters, and therapy balls. She refuses to use her walker on surfaces other than tile floors. She frequently loses her balance in both sitting and standing.

Impairments

Shawna demonstrates tactile hypersensitivity, postural instability, and a fear of movement, as well as difficulty processing sensory information during movement-based activities.

PROGNOSIS/PLAN OF CARE

Goals

Treatment goals are for Shawna to:
1. Improve balance and protective reactions during play activities
2. Participate in age-appropriate movement activities with improved motor coordination
3. Improve balance when walking with posterior walker on all surfaces

Functional Outcomes

Following 3 months of therapy, Shawna will:
1. Demonstrate appropriate protective reactions in the anterior/posterior and medial/lateral direction eight of 10 times during sitting or standing
2. Ride a tricycle independently for 100 feet within 10 minutes
3. Be able to walk with her walker from a carpeted area to a tiled area and back without hesitation eight of 10 times

INTERVENTION

Shawna's poor protective reactions may be contributing to her dislike of movement-based activities. Protective reactions and righting reactions can be elicited by rocking on a therapy ball or supported on a bolster (see Figure 9-10). Once protective reactions are consistently elicited, controlled falling should be a focus from the sitting and standing positions. Initially, this can be practiced on mats, then carpeting, and finally to hard surfaces.

Standing should be encouraged in her walker both with and without shoes on various surfaces including carpet, foam, and an exercise mat. She should wear her shoes and also stand or walk in her walker outside on grass and gravel.

Fear of movement may be overcome by beginning with activities she enjoys. She enjoys group activities including swimming and dance. These activities should be encouraged in the community. Therapy may focus on riding toys such as a tricycle or scooter. These activities should begin with Shawna well supported and progressed with less support provided. An example of this would be using a tricycle with a back support progressing to a tricycle without a back support, or a large scooter with a large base of support progressing to a smaller scooter with a narrower base of support.

CASE STUDY # 5
Robert Anderson

- *Age: 38 years*
- *Medical Diagnosis: Incomplete T9-10 spinal cord injury with left radial nerve damage*
- *Status: 6 months post injury*
- *Practice Pattern 5H: Impaired Motor Function, Peripheral Nerve Integrity, and Sensory Integrity Associated with Nonprogressive Disorders of the Spinal Cord*

EXAMINATION AND EVALUATION

Functional Limitations

Due to loss of sensation below the T9 level, Mr. Anderson has an increased tendency for skin breakdown, and, due to his radial nerve injury, he often drops items being held in his left hand.

Impairments

Mr. Anderson has a loss of sensation below the T9 level and decreased sensation in left radial nerve distribution.

PROGNOSIS/PLAN OF CARE

Goals

Treatment goals are for Mr. Anderson to:
1. Demonstrate understanding of areas of his body where sensation is absent
2. Improve ability to use visual information for mobility (ie, wheelchair or crutches)
3. Use visual information to monitor left hand function

Functional Outcomes

Following 3 months of therapy, Mr. Anderson will:
1. Maintain good skin integrity with no skin breakdown for the past 4 weeks
2. Walk and maneuver his wheelchair at the mall without bumping into objects or persons
3. Manipulate small objects using the left hand during ADLs and work-related tasks

INTERVENTION

Mr. Anderson is cooperative and motivated with no cognitive deficits. The loss of sensation below the T9 level makes Mr. Anderson a prime candidate for skin breakdown. He must first be educated on the risks of maintaining one position for an extended period of time. A wheelchair seat cushion designed to decrease pressure while sitting is indicated, however, he must still shift position frequently during the day. Sitting balance activities while on a mat and in the wheelchair are encouraged to increase his excursion for unweighting. A timer that is set to beep every 20 minutes can cue Mr. Anderson to shift position to prevent skin breakdown. A cushion should be used while he is driving and a mattress with viscoelastic properties is recommended for sleeping. Instruction to visually examine his lower extremities every morning and night is appropriate.

Mr. Anderson also should be encouraged to stand periodically throughout the day. A standing work station may be set up at his work to allow prolonged standing time to both unweight his buttocks as well as to discourage osteoporotic changes in the lower extremities.

Tactile stimulation of the left hand is encouraged with cloths of different textures, including cotton, wool, and corduroy. Additionally, tapping, quick icing, and electrical stimulation may provide sensory stimulation to encourage muscular contraction and reeducation. Mr. Anderson should be reminded to use visual input as an assist as he manipulates objects with his left hand and as he maneuvers himself through various environments.

REFERENCES

1. Ghez C, Krakauer J. The organization of movement. In: Kandell ER, Schwartz JH, Jessell TM, eds. *Principles of Neural Science*. 4th ed. New York, NY: McGraw-Hill; 2000:653-673.

2. Craik RL. Sensorimotor changes and adaptation in the older adult. In: Guccione AA, ed. *Geriatric Physical Therapy*. St Louis, Mo: Mosby; 1993:72-97.

3. Shumway-Cook A, Woollacott M. *Motor Control Theory and Practical Applications*. Philadelphia, Pa: Lippincott Williams & Wilkins; 1995:3-83.

4. Amaral DG. The anatomical organization of the central nervous system. In: Kandell ER, Schwartz JH, Jessell TM, eds. *Principles of Neural Science*. 4th ed. New York, NY: McGraw-Hill; 2000:317-336.

5. Juliano SL, McLaughlin DF. Somatic senses 2: discriminative touch In: Cohen H. *Neuroscience for Rehabilitation*. 2nd ed. Philadelphia, Pa: Lippincott Williams & Wilkins; 1999:93-110.

6. Bartzokis G, Beckson M, Lu PH, Nuechterlein KH, Edwards N, Mintz J. Age-related changes in frontal and temporal lobe volumes in men. *Arch Gen Psychiatry*. 2001;58:461-465.

7. Magnotta VA, Andreasen NC, Schultz SK, et al. Quantitative in vivo measurement of gyrification in the human brain: changes associated with aging. **Cereb Cortex.** 1999;9:151-160.

8. Lan LM, Yamashita Y, Tang Y, et al. Normal fetal brain development: MR imaging with a half-Fourier rapid acquisition with relaxation enhancement sequence. *Radiology*. 2000;215:205-210.

9. FitzGerald MJT. *Neuroanatomy Basic and Clinical*. 3rd ed. Philadelphia, Pa: WB Saunders; 1996:1-7.

10. Geidd JN, Blumenthal J, Jeffries NO, et al. Brain development during childhood and adolescence: a longitudinal MRI study. *Nat Neurosci*. 1999;2:861-863.

11. Kraemer M, Abrahamsson M, Sjostrom A. The neonatal development of the light flash visual evoked potential. *Doc Ophthalmol*. 1999;99:21-39.

12. Fagan ER, Taylor MS, Logan WJ. Somatosensory evoked potentials: part I: a review of neural generations and special considerations in pediatrics. *Pediatr Neurol*. 1987;3:189-196.

13. Pasman JW, Rotteveel JJ, Maassen B, Visco YM. The maturation of auditory cortical evoked responses between (preterm) birth and 14 years of age. *Eur J Paediatr Neurol*. 1999;3:79-82.

14. Mueller EA, Moore MM, Kerr DC, et al. Brain volume preserved in healthy elderly through the eleventh decade. *Neurol*. 1998;51:1555-1562.

15. Sandor T, Stafford AM, Kemper T. Symmetrical and asymmetrical changes in brain tissue with age as measured on CT scan. *Neurobiol Aging*. 1990;11:21-27.

16. Xu J, Kobayashi S, Yamaguchi S, et al. Gender effects on age-related changes in brain structure. *Am J Neuroradiol*. 2000;21:112-118.

17. Coffey CE, Lucke JF, Saton SA, et al. Sex differences in brain aging: a quantitative magnetic resonance imaging study. *Arch Neurol*. 1998;55:169-179.

18. Samorajski T. How the human brain responds to aging. *J Am Geriatr Soc*. 1976;24:4-11.

19. Steiner I, Gomori JM, Melamed E. Features of brain atrophy in Parkinson's disease. A CT scan study. *Neuroradiol*. 1985;27:158-160.

20. Howieson J, Kaye JA, Holm L, Howieson D. Interuncal distance: marker of aging an Alzheimer disease. *Am J Neuroradiol*. 1993;14:647-650.

21. McDonald WM, Krishnan KR, Doraiswamy PM, et al. Magnetic resonance findings in patients with early-onset Alzheimer's disease. *Biol Psychiatry*. 1991;29:799-810.

22. Paus T, Collins DL, Evans AC, Leonard G, Pike B, Zijdenbos A. Maturation of white matter in the human brain: a review of magnetic resonance studies. *Brain Res Bull*. 2001;54:255-266.

23. Gardner EP, Martin JH, Jessell TM. The bodily senses. In: Kandell ER, Schwartz JH, Jessell TM, eds. *Principles of Neural Science*. 4th ed. New York, NY: McGraw-Hill; 2000:430-450.

24. Jacobs SE, Lowe DL. Somatic senses 1: the anterolateral system. In: Cohen H, ed. *Neuroscience for Rehabilitation*. 2nd ed. Philadelphia, Pa: Lippincott Williams & Wilkins; 1999:77-92.

25. Jones L. Somatic senses 3: proprioception. In: Cohen H, ed. *Neuroscience for Rehabilitation*. 2nd ed. Philadelphia, Pa: Lippincott Williams & Wilkins; 1999:111-130.

26. Schmitz TJ. Sensory assessment. In: O'Sullivan SB, Schmitz TJ, eds. *Physical Rehabilitation Assessment and Treatment*. 4th ed. Philadelphia, Pa: FA Davis Co; 2001:133-156.

27. Lundy-Ekman L. *Neuroscience Fundamentals for Rehabilitation*. Philadelphia, Pa: WB Saunders Co; 1998:86-105.

28. Basbaum AI, Jessell TM. The perception of pain. In: Kandell ER, Schwartz JH, Jessell TM, eds. *Principles of Neural Science*. 4th ed. New York, NY: McGraw-Hill; 2000:472-491.

29. FitzGerald MJT. *Neuroanatomy Basic and Clinical*. 3rd ed. Philadelphia, Pa: WB Saunders Co; 1996:105-116.

30. Thomas CL, ed. *Taber's Cyclopedic Medical Dictionary*. 18th ed. Philadelphia, Pa: FA Davis Co; 1997:1646.

31. Pearson K, Gordon J. Spinal reflexes. In: Kandell ER, Schwartz JH, Jessell TM, eds. *Principles of Neural Science*. 4th ed. New York, NY: McGraw-Hill; 2000:713-736.

32. Wurtz RH, Kandel ER. Central visual pathways. In: Kandell ER, Schwartz JH, Jessell TM, eds. *Principles of Neural Science*. 4th ed. New York, NY: McGraw-Hill; 2000:523-547.

33. Wurtz RH, Kandel ER. Perception of motion, depth, and form. In: Kandell ER, Schwartz JH, Jessell TM, eds. *Principles of Neural Science*. 4th ed. New York, NY: McGraw-Hill; 2000:548-571.

34. Lundy-Ekman. *Neuroscience Fundamentals for Rehabilitation*. Philadelphia, Pa: WB Saunders Co; 1998:300-313.

35. Ayres AJ. *Sensory Integration and Learning Disorders*. Los Angeles, Calif: Western Psychological Services; 1972.

36. American Physical Therapy Association. Guide to physical therapist practice. 2nd ed. *Phys Ther.* 2001;81:S1-S738.

37. Berryman-Reese N. *Muscle and Sensory Testing*. Philadelphia, Pa: WB Saunders Co; 1999:421-496.

38. Patout CA, Birke JA, Horswell R, Williams D, Cerise FP. Effectiveness of a comprehensive diabetes lower-extremity amputation prevention program in a predominantly low-income African-American population. *Diabetes Care*. 2000;23:1339-1342.

39. Levin S, Pearsall G, Ruderman R. VonFrey's method of measuring pressure sensibility in the hand; an engineering analysis of the Weinstein-Semmes pressure aesthesiometer. *J Hand Surg*. 1978;3:211-216.

40. Nolan MF. Two-point discrimination assessment in the upper limb in young adult men and women. *Phys Ther*. 1982;62:965-969.

41. Nolan MF. Limits of two-point discrimination ability in the lower limb in young adult men and women. *Phys Ther*. 1983;63:1424-1428.

42. Nolan MF. Quantitative measure of cutaneous sensation: two-point discrimination values for the face and trunk. *Phys Ther*. 1985;65:181-185.

43. Thomas CL, ed. *Taber's Cyclopedic Medical Dictionary*. 18th ed. Philadelphia, Pa: FA Davis Co; 1997:2091.

44. Ayres A. *Sensory Integration and Praxis Tests*. Los Angeles, Calif: Western Psychological Services; 1989.

45. Dunn W, Daniels D. *Infant/Toddler Sensory Profile*. New York, NY: The Psychological Corp; 2000.

46. Dunn W. *Sensory Profile*. New York, NY: The Psychological Corp; 1999.

47. Berk RA, DeGangi GA. *DeGangi-Berk Test of Sensory Integration*. Los Angeles, Calif: Western Psychological Services; 1983.

48. Nelson C. Electrodiagnosis in neurological dysfunction In: Umphred D, ed. *Neurological Rehabilitation*. 3rd ed. St. Louis, Mo: Mosby; 1995:838-851.

49. Wilson Howle JM. Cerebral palsy. In: Campbell SK, ed. *Decision Making in Pediatric Neurologic Physical Therapy*. Philadelphia, Pa: Churchill Livingstone; 1999:23-83.

50. Rine RM. Vestibular dysfunction in children. *Advance for Physical Therapists & PT Assistants*. 2000;11:8.

51. Dunne JW, Hankey GJ, Edis RH. Parkinsonism: upturned walking stick as an aid to locomotion. *Arch Phys Med Rehabil*. 1987;68:380-381.

52. McIntosh GC, Brown SH, Rice RR, Thaut MH. Rhythmic auditory-motor facilitation of gait patterns in patients with Parkinson's disease. *J Neurol Neurosurg Psychiatry*. 1997;62:22-26.

53. Thaut MH, McIntosh GC, Rice RR, Miller RA, Rathbun J, Brault JM. Rhythmic auditory stimulation in gait training for Parkinson's disease patients. *Mov Disord*. 1996; 11:193-200.

54. Shumway-Cook A. Vestibular rehabilitation of the patient with traumatic brain injury. In: Herdman S, ed. *Vestibular Rehabilitation*. 2nd ed. Philadelphia, Pa: FA Davis Co; 2000:476-493.

SUGGESTED READING

FitzGerald MJT. *Neuroanatomy Basic and Clinical*. 3rd ed. Philadelphia, Pa: WB Saunders Co; 1996.

Jones L. Somatic senses 3: proprioception. In: Cohen H, ed. *Neuroscience for Rehabilitation*. 2nd ed. Philadelphia, Pa: Lippincott Williams & Wilkins; 1999.

Kandell ER, Schwartz JH, Jessell TM. *Principles of Neural Science*. 4th ed. New York, NY: McGraw-Hill; 2000.

O'Sullivan SB, Schmitz TJ, eds. *Physical Rehabilitation Assessment and Treatment*. 4th ed. Philadelphia, Pa: FA Davis Co; 2001.

Shumway-Cook A, Woollacott M. *Motor Control Theory and Practical Applications*. 2nd ed. Philadelphia, Pa: Lippincott Williams & Wilkins; 2001.

Issues of Cognition for Motor Control

Kathye E. Light, PhD, PT

INTRODUCTION

Physical therapists work with patients to assist the learning or relearning of movement control. We provide physical training for conditioning and work with patients on functional re-entry into the community. Many physical therapists do not see their role as that of a cognitive trainer. Cognitive training is thought to be the role of the psychologist. Learning or relearning movement control is not about cognitive processing. Movement does not require much cognitive processing, or does it?

The control of movement seldom is viewed as a cognitive process. Indeed, many of the traditional physical therapy neurophysiologic treatment techniques emphasize automatic movement ability and discourage the use of patient attentional processes. As therapists, we often attempt to mold the movements we perceive as best by facilitation techniques, and believe that if this facilitated movement is repeated often enough, the patient will automatically begin to move in the correct way.

Although facilitation is a common therapy technique for motor training, does facilitation actually enhance motor learning? By definition, motor learning is "a set of internal processes associated with practice or experience leading to relatively permanent changes in the capability for motor skill."[1] Consider yourself attempting to learn a new movement. If someone facilitates and manually guides you through the whole movement, are you then capable of performing that movement without help? When are guidance and facilitation useful and when do they hinder motor control? These are important questions for physical therapists.

In this chapter, the importance of cognitive or information processing ability for motor control will be discussed. Just as we must process information to interact appropriately with our environment, so must our patients with neurologic deficits. Just as we must hold movement plans in memory and use stages of memory and learning to function within the environment, so must our patients. Movement control involves highly integrated and interactive processing of central and peripheral neuromuscular mechanisms. Movement is meaningful only when executed appropriately with purpose, intention, and planning. Before a controlled intentional movement occurs, the brain receives, identifies, and recognizes sensory signals from the environment. Appropriate actions are chosen, and before the movement is executed, complicated neuromuscular integration, sequencing, timing, and coordination of motor output are required. This process of movement control is termed information processing and is necessary for producing environmentally useful movements. Information processing is interactive with the stages of memory for functionally directed movement control.

The purpose of this chapter is not to encourage physical therapists to become cognitive trainers or neuropsychologists, but to emphasize the role of cognitive processing in the training of movement control.

INFORMATION PROCESSING

The process of receiving, identifying, and recognizing environmental stimuli followed by selection and execution of planned actions has been defined by several different information processing models.[1-4] The most basic model, described by Schmidt, consists of three stages: 1. stimulus identification, 2. response selection, and 3. response programming.[1] This simple model is illustrated in Figure 10-1. Each of the stages of information processing requires time. Therefore, the total time necessary between receiving a cued environmental stimulus and beginning a movement output is an indicator of the individual's ability to process information and plan a movement.

Programming

Stages Defined

Stimulus identification, the first stage of the simple information processing model, entails the detection and neural encoding of sensory cues and identification and interpretation of the stimulus pattern. Basic factors known to affect processing speed within the stimulus identification stage are stimulus clarity, stimulus intensity, and pattern complexity.[1] The most easily processed sensory signal is a clear, intense cue with a simple pattern.

Response selection, the second stage of information processing, also is known as *response determination*.[2] In this stage, the decision is made about which response to execute. Two common factors that affect the processing time in the response selection stage are the number of stimulus-response (S-R) choices available to be made and the compatibility between the stimulus and the response. S-R compatibility can be viewed as the natural fit or match of a sensory signal to the desired motor output.[5] A simple example

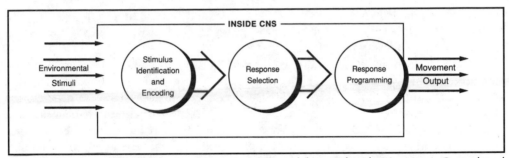

Figure 10-1. Stages of information processing (adapted from Schmidt RA. *Motor Control and Learning: A Behavioral Emphasis.* 3rd ed. Champaign, Ill: Human Kinetics; 1999).

of S-R compatibility is the ease of matching the visual appearance of an object to the motor output of touching the object. Visual cues indicating reaching toward an object are more compatible than sound cues indicating the same action. Many of us have experienced this reality when attempting to reach for the morning alarm clock without success, until we actually opened our eyes to visually locate the target. The simplest and fastest processing will occur through response selection when there are no choices involved (ie, a simple reaction time situation exists) and when the stimulus and response fit well together.

Some types of S-R compatibility appear to be natural sensorimotor connections. Other S-R compatibility is established and strengthened by learned association. After learning is intact for a particular S-R matching, interference in information processing occurs if the response is inconsistent with the learned association.[6] An example would be stepping on a surface that appears solid but is not.

The last stage of information processing, response programming, is the stage in which the movement is planned, structured, and centrally activated. This occurs after a movement output stimulus has been coded and identified, and the response selected.[1] Factors that affect response programming time are complexity of the movement, duration of the movement, and compatibility between the responses that are being performed simultaneously, in a sequence, or as choice alternatives.[3,4,7] This type of compatibility is known as response-response (R-R) compatibility.

R-R compatibility is a bit more difficult to understand than S-R compatibility. One of the most familiar examples of poor R-R compatibility is the difficulty we experience when attempting to pat our heads and rub our stomachs simultaneously. Much greater R-R compatibility exists between the two simultaneous responses of patting the head and patting the stomach or rubbing both the head and stomach.

Information processing stages are tested experimentally by chronometric techniques which involve reaction time instrumentation.[8] Because certain environmental factors affect particular stages of information processing, without affecting the processing time of other stages, experimental manipulation of those specific factors allows the central processing of particular stages to be determined.

Serial versus Parallel Processing

How can we function efficiently within our world if all movements are dependent on information processing? How can we account for our relative ease of functional movement if all environmental stimuli are processed one at a time and in series through the stages of information processing? Certainly not all of our movements are information processing dependent. We have simple, long loop, and cortical loop reflexes; triggered reactions; and subcortical motor programs which are feed-forward and executed without the need for sensory feedback.

Various types of movement outputs differ in the amount and degree of information processing required at each stage. Some types of movements are so complicated that each stage of information processing is challenged, and only one stage can proceed at a time. Other movements may be carried out simultaneously through mechanisms of central nervous system (CNS) parallel processing. Although there are individuals who suggest that all movements are single channel processed,[9] the theoretical notion of parallel processing is generally accepted.[10,11] Parallel processing implies that environmental stimuli can be processed simultaneously or in parallel, and that at least several stages of information processing may proceed simultaneously. Parallel processing of information is hypothesized to be a higher order function than serial processing. As tasks become well learned and practiced, the possibility exists that the motor learner shifts from serial processing to parallel processing of information.

MEMORY SYSTEMS

The process of memory development is one of the most debated and controversial topics in the study of information processing.[12] Information processing requires memory structures. The process of memory is a neurophysiologic phenomenon involving neural activity that is not totally understood, and a review of literature on the very complicated topic of memory is beyond the scope of this chapter. The development of memory traces for newly learned information appears to be dependent on plastic circuitry which allows the passage of neural activity between the hippocampal formation and neocortical association areas.[13,14] If this circuitry is disrupted, the result is a loss of retrieval of recently formed memory traces and an inability to form new traces.

Working memory, however, cannot be localized to a single location within the CNS. Researchers suggest that different neural structures are required for recall memory versus recognition.[15] In addition, memory subsystems for spatial movement tasks are not the same as those required for changing the timing and sequencing of a movement configuration.[16] Although an exact understanding of the neurophysiology of memory has not been achieved, a simplified conceptualization of memory processes is depicted in Figure 10-2.

The cognitive processes involved in the control of movement are not just those of information processing that allow an individual to react appropriately to environmental stimuli. Memory structures also are necessary to allow signals to be recognized and movement plans developed and recalled within the CNS. Many simultaneous events occur within the environment at each moment, and, although we are aware of these stimuli as they enter short-term sensory storage, we do not respond to all stimuli. Short-term sensory storage is a memory system that allows large amounts of sensory information to be stored for periods of less than 1 second.[17,18]

Pertinent sensory stimuli are processed into short-term memory from short-term sensory storage via the mechanism of selective attention. Short-term memory is a memory system with storage time up to approximately 1 minute and serves as a type of work area for movement plan processing.[19] Short-term memory is the working space for processing the input and output that direct goal-oriented movement and is considered to func-

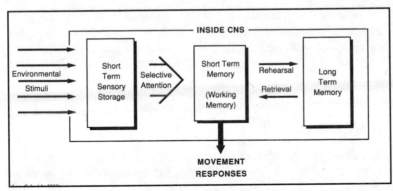

Figure 10-2. Memory compartments for movement control (adapted from Schmidt RA. *Motor Control and Learning: A Behavioral Emphasis*. 3rd ed. Champaign, Ill: Human Kinetics; 1999).

tion similar to the buffer in a personal computer. Both the computer memory and human short-term memory must be booted up before functioning and require input to process the output.

Long-term memory is a relatively permanent storage area for almost limitless amounts of information. Information can move into long-term memory by means of rehearsal or concentrated effort. Motor programs are stored in long-term memory, but must be brought into the short-term memory workspace before movement output is possible.[1] Information processing interacts with memory storage mechanisms to control functional movements within a constantly changing environment. Alteration of any mechanism involved in information processing or memory storage will alter environmentally appropriate, functional movement. Mechanisms that affect sensory storage, selective attention, attention switching, ability to rehearse, ability to concentrate and focus, and overall states of anxiety, arousal, or activation will influence learning and controlling movement.

The learning of cognitive information requires the process of declarative memory, and the learning of repetitious movement requires procedural memory. Exactly how these two systems work together in the learning of psychomotor functional activity is unclear, but the strong influences of practice and appropriate feedback are well established.[20-22] The amount of practice has the strongest influence on motor learning and memory.[1,20] The type of augmented feedback (ie, extrinsic information provided to the learner about the movement performance or outcome) also is very significant to the learning and memory process of movement control.[21-24]

Basic research themes on the method of providing feedback to motor learners suggest that continuous feedback is detrimental to motor learning and schedules of variable-faded feedback are preferred.[21,22] Janelle and colleagues[24] found that self-controlled solicitation of feedback was more beneficial to motor learning than feedback provided at the will of the instructor. Another important theme to future physical therapy practice is the successful use of augmented feedback presented during virtual learning environments.[23] The research on augmented feedback is important and relevant to the practice of physical therapy, but we must acknowledge that research on special clinical populations is scarce. When these special populations are explored, the results for the best type of extrinsic feedback may be different than that for nonclinical groups. Recent research on feedback provided to motor learners with Parkinson's disease resulted in considerable differences in the motor learning of those with Parkinson's disease as compared to nondisabled control subjects.[25] Although the control group demonstrated the usual benefit of variable feedback over continuous feedback for their motor learning, the opposite was discovered for the subjects with Parkinson's disease. Those individuals with Parkinson's disease appeared to benefit more from the continuous feedback schedule. Much more work with special clinical populations is needed in all areas of information processing.

BUILDING MOTOR PROGRAMS

Certainly not all of our everyday movements require attentional effort, decision making, rehearsal, intense concentration, attention switching, or other information processing and memory components mentioned previously. Most of us are capable of drinking a cup of coffee, writing our thoughts on paper, reaching quickly toward objects, and kicking a soccer ball without laboring cognitively over the movement itself. A number of motor control theorists hypothesize that the reason we can perform many movements quickly and without attentional demands is that we have developed motor programs for those tasks.[26]

Motor programming applies particularly to fast movements that are executed in a feed-forward manner and occur too quickly for the CNS to process and use sensory feedback. Closed loop movements, or those movements that occur slowly and allow feedback control, are never completely controlled by a motor program. Most slow movements are controlled by some degree of feedback during the course of movement; however, with learning, many movements that are initially controlled with feedback become faster and more automatic via motor programming.

The control of movement is extremely complicated. Consider the interaction among all the neural structures for inputting, processing, and outputting the appropriate neural signals. Consider as well the complicated process of moving the body's linked system, with its numerous range of motion possibilities built on an unstable base of support (ie, two rather small feet). Now, in addition to the actual control of the individual's central and peripheral mechanisms, consider how the environment changes from moment to moment. Not only must the individual process internal control signals and move the unstable linked system about, but the individual also must be able to interpret the external signals of the environment and keep the internal control mechanisms updated with all pertinent external information. This classic motor control problem, known as the *degrees of freedom* problem, is discussed in Chapter 2 and was first described by a Soviet scientist, Nicolai Aleksandrovitch Bernstein, in 1947. However, his work was not translated into English until 1967.[27]

The process by which degrees of freedom of the individual's central and peripheral structure are controlled, while interacting within the environment, is one of the most interesting issues facing contemporary motor control scientists. Schmidt promoted the schema theory of generalized motor programs to explain the way we develop efficiency of movement control.[28,29] According to Schmidt, a motor program is an abstract memory structure that is prepared in advance of a movement and, when initiated, results in the execution of efficient coordinated movement that does not require feedback or attentional demands.[1] Schmidt hypothesized that we gain movement efficiency by developing generalized motor programs that can be applied to whole classes of movements, regardless of the body part performing the movement. A generalized motor program is thought to consist of certain variant and invariant components. The variant components are those parameters of control that apply to a specific movement at a specific moment and which are not fixed in the motor program. Rather, the variant components are provided at the time of the required movement and consist of parameters such as the exact muscles required to perform the movement, the overall duration of the movement, and the overall force required to produce the movement. The components considered to be fixed or invariant in the motor program are order or sequence of events, phasing or temporal structure, and relative forces required to execute the actions of the program.[1]

Another group of motor control scientists disagree that the CNS must store programs for classes of movements. These researchers promote a dynamic systems approach to the control of movement.[30] Kelso and co-workers,[31,32] advocates of Bernstein's theory, emphasized that the body periphery (ie, the biomechanical linkages of muscles and joints) plays a significant role in movement, and that the CNS learns to take advantage of the laws of physics to control movement. According to dynamic systems theorists, skill in a motor task occurs through the development of a coordinative structure which writes equations of constraint between the CNS and the biomechanical linkages of the body periphery to control the degrees of freedom. More recently, Kelso and colleagues[30-32] have moved away from a purely biomechanical emphasis but continue to explain movement pattern coordination according to dynamic theory.

Regardless of how movement efficiency is developed between the CNS and periphery, motor skill in both closed and open loop tasks is established by the process of motor learning. Motor learning, or the relatively permanent change in the capacity to perform a motor task, is accomplished through basic stages often labeled as the *cognitive stage*, *associative stage*, and *autonomous stage*.

The cognitive stage learner struggles with understanding the motor task. At this stage, the patient needs to hear and repeat verbalized instructions, decide the goal of the task, establish what makes a good performance, and understand the sequencing of the parts. In the early stages of cognitive motor learning, the preparation to begin the task and initiation of the first few movement attempts require total attention of the patient. Concern for timing and accuracy is not possible in the cognitive stage, and the teaching therapist must be aware of potential overload. During the cognitive learning stage, motor skill develops primarily as a result of verbal-cognitive changes; therefore, the role of information processing at this stage of learning is extremely important.

While the patient is in the cognitive stage of learning, the most important component of therapy is to assist in the development of a reference of correctness. The patient must be clear on the goal of the movement that not only implies the outcome of the movement, but also involves the critical features of the movement performance. If, as the therapist, your goal includes symmetrical weight shift, a smooth movement trajectory, and a forward scapula, the patient must understand all of these components before a proper reference of correctness can be developed. Once the reference of correctness is achieved, the patient will be able to detect errors in the movement and make alterations through an internal locus of control.

A patient will be in the cognitive stage of learning during the first few weeks of rehabilitation following a neurologic insult; therefore, the issues of memory, information processing, and goal development are critical to early rehabilitation. During this time, the therapist's appreciation of cognitive components is important because movement ability and motor skill development progresses the most while the patient is in the cognitive learning stage.

Once the movement task is well understood, the goals and sub-goals are well established, and the patient has a reference of correctness for the motor skill, a natural progression toward the associative stage of learning occurs. During the associative stage of learning, the patient refines the motor skill. Much less verbalization about the task by the therapist or patient is needed. The patient must be allowed to experiment with movement control during the associative stage in order to determine the subtleties of an efficient movement plan. The amount and speed of motor skill improvement during the associative stage are less than during the cognitive stage of motor learning. Rather, the associative stage will be marked by gradual refinements in the timing, coordination, and movement efficiency of the motor patterns.

The last stage of motor learning, the autonomous stage, comes about slowly after a great deal of practice and experience with the motor task. When the patient reaches the autonomous stage, performance of the motor task will appear to be automatic. Little attention will be paid to the primary motor task, but rather a type of periodic checking in on the performance seems to be the method of control. When the patient reaches the autonomous stage, the motor skill can be accomplished under any type of environmental setting. The patient will not be affected by distractions and will be able to attend to and perform secondary tasks simultaneously with the primary motor skill.

MOTIVATION, PRACTICE, AND ADHERENCE

Most of us believe inherently that motivation is necessary to learn via any mechanism. Certainly, if learning is to be enjoyable, motivation is necessary. The reinforcement nature of motivation is, however, secondary in importance to motor learning.[1] Motivation is of primary importance to motor learning for its influence on practice.

As emphasized earlier, practice is the most powerful and influential factor in enhancing motor learning.[1,20,33] Variable and random practice appear to improve the learning outcomes, but the amount of practice is clearly the most significant practice issue.[1,20,33-35] When learners are motivated, self-selected practice is performed more readily, more often, and with greater attention. These secondary effects of motivation are directly related to the amount and quality of practice. Massed, effortful practice is clearly linked to positive motor learning and motor recovery outcomes.[20,36-38]

What can assist a person's motivational level to practice motor tasks? Certainly, physical therapists are aware of the lack of adherence or compliance many patients have with their home exercise programs. Strangely, the research literature on compliance and adherence to exercise is recent and sparse. The literature available is largely on non-clinical populations. Tools that appear to help individuals be motivated and to adhere to a planned practice schedule include: cooperative goal development between the trainer and trainee with both long-term specific and short-term specific goals; specific feedback on goal progress and fulfillment; exercise or practice diaries; activity log sheets; phone calls to allow questions, answers, and coaching; written contracts of agreement between trainer and trainee; and providing the opportunity for trainees to express how the changes in capabilities have affected their lives.

NEUROLOGIC DEFICITS

Clinical literature has documented that brain damage to different parts of the CNS results in a variety of movement control problems related to information processing. The obvious problems of stimulus identification occur when cortical primary or association areas of sensory processing are damaged. Deficits in visual attention and loss of appropriate visual scanning result from lesions of the parieto-occipital cortex.[33] Left hemisphere cerebrovascular accidents (CVAs) have been demonstrated to cause greater response programming deficits than right CVAs.[34] Controversy exists over the role of the basal ganglia in information processing, but it appears that basal ganglia structures have little to do with memory scanning, orientation, or attention to a stimulus.[35] The basal ganglia structures appear to be involved in movement initiation and execution,[36] but these deficits appear to be unrelated to perceptual impairment.[37] There is disagreement about the role of the basal ganglia in movement preparation.[35,36]

Because various types of movements may involve different memory subsystems,[16] specific types of lesions result in different control problems. Working memory structures for timing and force control appear to be damaged by lesions to the cerebellum or basal ganglia.[38,39] Working memory for spatial processing and targeting is affected by posterior cortical damage.[40] Memory for mimicking or copying sequences of movements or gestures results from cortical damage, particularly to the frontal lobes.[41] The research literature is clear that memory for movement control is not limited to the three boxes illustrated in Figure 10-2. Every type of self-initiated or environmentally directed movement made by an individual must, however, use the memory systems conceptualized in Figure 10-2. Evaluating the patient with pathology involving the CNS for the stages of memory, processes of selective attention and attention switching, and ability to rehearse or concentrate for adequate time periods will offer valuable direction to the physical therapist.

NEUROPLASTICITY OF LEARNING AND RECOVERY

Damage to the CNS may result in behavioral and sensory motor deficits. Are these deficits permanent, or is the CNS capable of alteration that will resolve these deficits? In the past, we considered the CNS to be arranged in an hierarchical fashion, and that damage to the higher centers of the CNS was permanent. Positive changes in patients following rehabilitation were considered to occur via mechanisms of central compensation, or the patient learning and using different strategies. Current research suggests that the CNS is quite capable of alteration following pathology. This alteration and subsequent reorganization are dependent on the types of activities that the patient engages in during the neurorecovery process[42,43] (see Chapter 4).

Use-dependent and learning neuroplasticity are areas of active research among motor control and neuroscience researchers. There are studies being undertaken to explore how the CNS responds to damage and the processes underlying recovery and use-dependent plasticity.[44] Physical therapists are most interested in two research agendas that have implications for clinical practice. These are constraint-induced movement therapy for individuals following a CVA[45,46] and intensive treadmill training for individuals who have sustained CNS damage to the spinal cord and/or brain.[47]

Compensation versus Training

Not all neurologic deficits are resolvable. The practical problem faced each day by the physical therapist is how to spend valuable treatment time in the most efficient manner. The physical therapist has control over three different aspects of neurologic rehabilitation. We control the teaching of movement, including physical guidance, encouragement, and verbal instruction. We also control the practice schedule, deciding how much and how hard a patient should work at a task. Finally, we have control over the physical or exercise training of strength, endurance, flexibility, and coordination.

Our overall physical therapy goal is to assist functional independence at the highest level of each patient's potential. Because the environmental demands of total independence in our ever-changing world are endless, we all must set limits and develop a degree of structure to the environmental challenges we undertake. As physical therapists, we help to establish those limits for our patients. We assist the patient in improving movement and functional abilities, and then we help the patient and caregivers to structure the world within the capabilities of the patient.

After evaluating the patient's overall functional abilities, we establish intervention programs to achieve specific functional outcomes. Most of these outcomes will necessitate that the patient be able to perform certain movement patterns with appropriate timing, sequencing, and control. Many goals of physical therapy will necessitate the patient having improved strength, flexibility, and endurance. As therapists, we must not forget that the principles of exercise physiology apply to the training of strength, flexibility, and endurance of all patients, not just patients with cardiac or orthopedic problems. In addition to exercise training, the training of functional movement patterns will be accomplished best by applying the principles of motor learning. The types of training appropriate depend on the patient's information processing ability and the stage of motor learning for the particular functional task being taught.

Generally, movement training proceeds from simple to complex. We find what the patient can do, and then we add complexity. For example, by requiring more steps, a different context, or greater accuracy of the movement, we increase the difficulty of the task requirements. The concept of simple to complex is useful in training movements controlled by information processing. Following analysis of the patient's information processing ability, the stimulus identification requirements can be made more complex after starting with clear, intense, and simple patterned stimuli. Two examples of simple stimulus identification requirements are the use of one-word instructional commands given in a quiet setting and the placement of one object on a table for the patient to reach out and touch. Gradually, the stimuli should be made less intense and require greater pattern complexity, such as commands given in sentences in the middle of a busy rehabilitation gymnasium.

Response selection complexity also can be increased. The simplest situation is no choice being required and the motor response being easily matched to a stimulus, such as a verbal command to reach toward a visualized object. A more complex situation is one where the patient must make decisions about which activities to do and must respond to stimuli that do not fit so easily with the motor output.

Response programming is the most common stage of information processing manipulated by the physical therapist as the patient progresses. Movement complexity can initially be kept simple with one-step unilateral limb responses. Progression to movements requiring multilimb compatibility coordination with movements sequenced in fast pro-

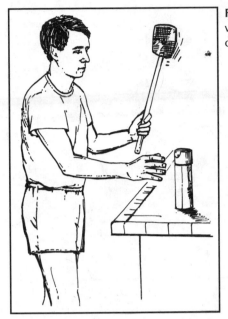

Figure 10-3. Simultaneous reaching for the fly spray while swatting the fly are movements with poor R-R compatibility.

gression then can occur. Movement duration of task demands can be gradually increased. R-R compatibility can be progressed from doing only one movement at a time to movements performed synchronously with two or more limbs. Further progression involves movements that do not have R-R compatibility performed simultaneously or in rapid succession, such as slow reaching with one limb while the opposite limb performs a ballistic hitting response (Figure 10-3).

The progression of the intervention program should be dependent on the patient's level of motor learning for the specific task. Training protocols and methods should vary appropriately as motor learning progresses. The principles of practice and feedback presented by Schmidt[1] and Winstein[48] are helpful in determining what types of practice and feedback are most appropriate during the three stages of learning.

CASE STUDIES

Evaluation

Information processing and memory systems testing were performed with the five patients. The case studies present the findings of the examination and evaluation, as well as general intervention approaches to address each individual's functional limitations.

Clinical evaluation of patients' information processing abilities would be detected best with chronometric testing equipment.[8] Because this type of equipment is not readily available in the clinic, a simple reaction time evaluation system has been developed, consisting of a telegraph key connected to a millisecond timer.

Before attempting to determine reaction time under various conditions, stimulus identification ability was tested by requesting the patient to point with the most easily controlled upper extremity toward a visual light stimulus, an auditory bell stimulus, and

Figure 10-4. Auditory and visual discrimination testing.

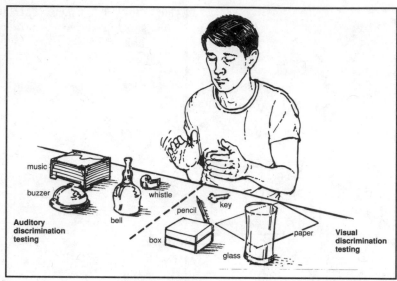

a somatosensory vibration stimulus placed within appropriate sensory fields. This testing was increased in complexity by presenting combinations of two or more stimuli sequentially or simultaneously and testing the patient's ability to detect all of the stimuli presented. This testing also allowed examination of short-term sensory store.

Once basic stimulus detection was tested, stimulus identification ability of the least impaired sensory fields was examined. The ability to differentiate stimuli was tested by presenting multiple stimuli and asking the patient to point toward the named stimulus. Visual discrimination was tested with five common objects: pencil, glass, key, piece of paper, and small box. Auditory discrimination was tested by presenting five sounds: music, ringing bell, buzzer, whistle, and clapping (Figure 10-4). Somatosensory discrimination was tested with a stereognosis test using objects from the visual discrimination test. Somatosensory discrimination was tested by simultaneous stimulus presentation of vibration, pinprick, or light touch and requesting the patient to point toward the named stimulus.

Response selection was tested first by observing simple reaction times for releasing a start switch. Using the more controlled hand, the patient was required to reach quickly to turn off a switch at the sound of a bell. Another test was performed by the therapist first giving the command "Get ready" and then allowing variable warning periods between 1 and 3 seconds before saying "Go." Reaction time was measured as the time in milliseconds after the sound of the bell or the "Go" command until the patient released the start key. This simple reaction time was compared to the reaction time for releasing the start switch when a choice was required. The choice was between reaching for the bell switch when it rang versus reaching for a buzzer switch when it sounded. Additional sounds were added to increase the number of choices required. Response selection ability was judged by the change in reaction time for releasing the start position key for the bell stimulus under simple and progressively more difficult choice situations. This test also helped determine the patient's short-term memory for movement to accomplish the goal. Selective attention requirements were increased by adding environmental distractors of visual, auditory, and somatosensory stimuli. The patient's performance was compared under the nondistracting and visual, auditory, and somatosensory distracting conditions.

Response programming ability was determined by the simple reaction time for releasing a switch under three progressively difficult tasks for movement execution. The tasks were releasing the start key; releasing the start key and reaching 12 inches; and releasing the start key and reaching first sideways to the right 12 inches, then sideways to the left 12 inches, and returning to the start position.

CASE STUDY #1
Jane Smith

- *Age: 74 years*
- *Medical Diagnosis: Right hemiplegia, secondary to left CVA*
- *Status: 6 months post onset*
- *Practice Pattern 5D: Impaired Motor Function and Sensory Integrity Associated with Nonprogressive Disorders of the Central Nervous System—Acquired in Adolescence or Adulthood*

EXAMINATION AND EVALUATION

Functional Limitations

Mrs. Smith demonstrates general disregard of the right side of her body and right visual space. She is at risk for injury to her right extremities because she is not always aware of the position of either the upper or lower extremity and often is unaware of objects in the right side of space. She has difficulty using her right hand for bilateral fine motor activities, and her upper extremity movements are slow and often inaccurate when she attempts to perform self-care tasks.

Impairments

Examination reveals extreme deficits in stimulus identification ability for the right visual field, somatosensory fields of the right upper extremity, and right lower leg and foot. Auditory fields appear to have no deficits. Once basic stimulus detection was tested, stimulus identification ability of the least impaired sensory fields was examined. The ability to differentiate visual stimuli appeared intact when visual objects were placed in the left visual field. Auditory discrimination appears intact overall. Somatosensory discrimination for tests of stereognosis was intact with the left hand, but Mrs. Smith could not differentiate between the key and the pencil or between the small box and glass with the right hand. Somatosensory discrimination, tested by simultaneous paired presentations of vibration, pinprick, or light touch, revealed marked deficits on the right side of the body.

Mrs. Smith has extreme deficits in response selection as indicated by her 500% faster performance under the simple reaction time condition versus two choice conditions. The deficits became much more apparent as more choices were added.

Response programming for movements performed with either the right or left upper extremity also is impaired, although deficits are greater for graded complexity with the right upper extremity. The response programming problem does not appear to be as great as the problem with response selection. Mrs. Smith did not perform movements crisply and smoothly with either arm until numerous practice trials with verbal feedback corrections were given. She then could perform the left arm movements with good coordination. This indicates, however, that Mrs. Smith may not have an appropriate internal reference of correctness for the required movements with the left arm that she can hold as a standard for the right arm.

Four distinct areas of impairment were identified. These impairments were difficulty with stimulus identification, response selection, and response programming, as well as having a poor reference of correctness.

PROGNOSIS/PLAN OF CARE

Goals

Treatment goals are for Mrs. Smith to:
1. Improve ability to identify tactile and somatosensory stimuli, especially in the right hand
2. Improve visual attention to the right side of space
3. Improve speed of response selection
4. Increase accuracy in response programming
5. Demonstrate improved reference of correctness

Functional Outcomes

Following 3 months of therapy, Mrs. Smith will:
1. Visually track individuals as they move from left to right in her field of vision
2. Demonstrate improved response selection by turning during sitting to right or left on verbal command, with 90% accuracy, and looking to ceiling or floor on verbal command with 50% accuracy while standing in the walker
3. Correctly sort forks and spoons using the right hand while removing utensils from her dishwasher
4. Lift a partially filled glass to her mouth without spillage with the left hand three times, then with the right hand three times
5. Demonstrate improved awareness of the right upper extremity by not bumping the arm into environmental objects

INTERVENTION

Examples of treatment for improving awareness of the right side of space include practicing visual tracking of objects (such as swinging objects suspended from the ceiling) from left to right and right to left. Visual scanning practice of the environment in all visual fields will be included. Somatosensory difficulties will be addressed by practicing identification of common objects (eg, a key, pencil, or small box) with the right hand after first identifying them with the left and receiving touch and proprioceptive input to the left and then to the right side.

To improve response selection, a slow progression in the process of decision making will be attempted. Initially, Mrs. Smith does not have to make choices, but carries out simple one-step commands. Then simple two-choice responses are required, such as when the therapist names the object in the therapist's right hand, Mrs. Smith looks toward the therapist's right hand. However, if the therapist names the object in her left hand, Mrs. Smith should look to the left hand. Another example of two-choice responding would be if, while practicing sitting balance, the therapist tells Mrs. Smith to move as quickly as possible toward a forward lean when the therapist says "forward" and to lean back as quickly as possible after hearing the "back" command. This task could be progressed in decision making by adding left and right commands. This type of response selection activity should be included throughout the therapy session.

The treatment plan for increasing accuracy in response programming includes having the therapist progress the task complexity and movement duration of the tasks used for functional training. This progression includes unilateral single-step movements with the less involved left hand and progressing the left hand activities by adding movement steps in the activity sequence. The left hand and foot then could be worked together in a coordinated activity, such as putting on a slipper. After practicing with the left extremities, the same tasks are practiced with the right extremities. Then all four extremities are coordinated in a multilimb task with progressive steps, such as putting on and taking off shoes with Velcro closures.

To achieve an improved reference of correctness, Mrs. Smith practices functional tasks with the left extremities to improve the sense of movement requirements before practicing the identical movements with the right extremities. Movements that require bilateral activity or balance control are aided by visual feedback with a mirror, verbal feedback from the therapist, or other appropriate sensory feedback.

CASE STUDY #2
Daniel Johnson

- *Age: 59 years*
- *Medical Diagnosis: Parkinson's disease*
- *Status: 4 years post initial diagnosis*
- *Practice Pattern 5E: Impaired Motor Function and Sensory Integrity Associated with Progressive Disorders of the Central Nervous System*

EXAMINATION AND EVALUATION

Functional Limitations

Mr. Johnson is demonstrating increasing problems with remembering and executing multistep motor activities, such as getting up from a chair, retrieving the channel changer for the television set, and sitting back down in the chair. His movements are slow, and it is taking him an increasingly longer time to complete self-care and functional household tasks.

Impairments

The primary information processing problems observed during the evaluation of Mr. Johnson were related to task execution. He appears to perceive sensory stimuli adequately and has no notable problems with attention or response selection. As tasks were graduated in movement complexity by increasing the number of steps in the movement, or by asking him to perform two types of movements simultaneously, Mr. Johnson essentially stopped all execution attempts.

Careful examination of Mr. Johnson's responses revealed the following three major problems related to information processing: response programming deficits, short-term memory difficulty, and difficulty with open loop tasks.

PROGNOSIS/PLAN OF CARE

Goals

Treatment goals are for Mr. Johnson to:
1. Demonstrate improved response programming
2. Increase short-term memory for motor tasks
3. Improve performance of open loop tasks

Functional Outcomes

Following 3 months of therapy, Mr. Johnson will:
1. Walk 30 feet in 15 seconds
2. Hold a piece of paper with his left hand while cutting out a pattern with scissors with his right hand
3. Accurately recall and verbally explain initial treatment activity at the end of a treatment session, four of five sessions
4. Remember and demonstrate the correct sequence of a three part motor task from one session to another
5. Sequentially place 15 household objects into three drawers placed in front of him within 20 seconds, and displace 10 spoons from a tray in 10 seconds

INTERVENTION

The length of time requested for Mr. Johnson to perform repetitive tasks such as stationary cycling, ambulation, folding papers, and pulling nonresistive reciprocal pulleys gradually will be progressed to improve his response programming. Task requirements will be graduated first by increasing the repetition time of the same task, and then by increasing the number of steps in a required movement sequence. Task complexity will be increased further by requiring him to shift between types of movements, such as switching between ballistic reaching, tying a shoestring, wrapping an object, carrying an object, bending to retrieve an object from the floor, and kicking a ball. Finally, task difficulty will be enhanced by decreasing R-R compatibility. R-R compatibility will be high initially, such as requesting Mr. Johnson to clap both hands simultaneously. Then, similar types of movements of one hand and one foot will be requested, followed by requests for simultaneous dissimilar movements of the hands, such as tapping with one hand while the other hand reaches for an object or opens a drawer. R-R compatibility challenges will be progressed by providing coordination tasks with functional relevance that require more than one extremity (eg, holding the telephone receiver to the ear while dialing a number with the other hand).

For improving short-term memory, Mr. Johnson will be requested to perform a movement activity during the first few minutes of therapy, perform another task requirement, and then will be asked to recall and demonstrate the first activity. After the demonstration, other activities will proceed. At the end of the therapy session, he will be asked to again demonstrate the first activity. During each session, a new memory activity will be requested.

Open loop or feed-forward tasks are difficult for Mr. Johnson. He will be asked to perform short, quick responses such as pressing a lever to ring a bell, knocking with his fist on a door, or pulling a light switch cord to a lamp. Tasks will be progressed in open loop complexity by requiring fast two-step and then three- to four-step movements. All fast movements will be performed as quickly and briskly as possible, without feedback until the task is completed.

CASE STUDY # 3
Shirley Teal

- *Age: 21 years*
- *Medical Diagnosis: Traumatic brain injury*
- *Status: 4 months post injury*
- *Practice Pattern 5D: Impaired Motor Function and Sensory Integrity Associated with Nonprogressive Disorders of the Central Nervous System—Acquired in Adolescence or Adulthood*

Examination and Evaluation

Functional Limitations

Ms. Teal has difficulty sustaining her attention to complete motor activities. She also demonstrates poor bilateral coordination of the upper extremities in tasks such as washing and drying her hands and dressing and undressing. She is unable to consistently follow two- or three-part directions during her therapy sessions.

Impairments

During the evaluation, Ms. Teal lost interest and focus on each task presented. She failed to notice new items and tasks as attention switching requirements were challenged. Although aware of pinprick, vibration, and light touch overall, she could not discriminate common objects consistently in tests of stereognosis of either hand.

Ms. Teal followed simple instructions well but appeared to be dramatically affected when movement requests were altered in duration, complexity, or R-R compatibility. This finding suggested the need for additional evaluation of response programming. When simple and choice reactions times were compared, she had notable slowing in reaction times as the number of choices increased. At times, when choices were presented, Ms. Teal failed to react and would appear to lose attention for the task. She appeared to forget what she was doing and would begin another task.

The overall testing of information procession ability for Ms. Teal suggested the following three major problem areas: stimulus identification problems for stereognosis discrimination bilaterally, response selection and motor planning difficulties, and difficulty with maintenance of concentration and inability to switch attention between tasks or objects within the environment.

Prognosis/Plan of Care

Goals

Treatment goals are for Ms. Teal to:
1. Improve stimulus identification ability in both hands
2. Improve response selectivity and motor planning
3. Increase ability to concentrate
4. Improve attention switching ability

Functional Outcomes

Following two months of therapy, Ms. Teal will:
1. Match three-dimensional circle and square forms using tactile and proprioceptive cues (without vision) with 75% accuracy with either hand
2. Place a hat on her head with left or right or both hands on verbal command with 50% accuracy
3. Propel her wheelchair forward and backward by using both lower extremities
4. Draw a line with the left hand through a simple maze with five or fewer errors
5. Mimic 10 upper extremity activities without being distracted from the task
6. Attend visually to new objects when presented, 50% of the time

INTERVENTION

All treatment will be done initially in sitting. Activities will be progressed gradually to other positions, such as standing.

To improve stimulus identification ability, Ms. Teal will practice observing three-dimensional shapes and objects, close her eyes, palpate an object with eyes closed, and locate a matching object. Common objects, such as a washcloth, hairbrush, glass, pencil, and doorknob, will be used for discrimination. With eyes closed, Ms. Teal will be asked to palpate a common object and then demonstrate its usage.

Choices for response selection will be increased gradually. Initially, Ms. Teal will receive a simple one-step command for execution of a simple movement. An example is the placement of a soccer ball on the floor and asking her to kick the ball. This will be progressed to a two-choice command by using the terminology left or right to indicate which foot to use to kick the ball. Gradually, this simple activity will be progressed to a four-choice situation by using the commands: left foot/right foot to kick the ball or left hand/right hand to bat a suspended balloon.

These activities also will improve concentration and attention switching ability. Therapy directed toward the problems of concentration maintenance and inability to appropriately switch attention will be progressed slowly to ensure patient success. For example, Ms. Teal will be asked initially to focus on the therapist. She then will be asked to mimic the therapist's left hand movements immediately after the therapist performs each movement. The therapist will begin by simply raising her left hand, then returning the hand to her left knee. Ms. Teal then imitates the movement. This task will be repeated for five to six trials with variable time intervals between each movement. Then attention switching will be progressed slowly by asking Ms. Teal to focus on both the therapist's left hand and left foot. She will be required to mimic the therapist's movements of the left hand or left foot for simple lifting movements. Concentration requirements will be progressed by slowly increasing the length of time spent in the activity and by increasing the attention switching requirements. Attention switching will be progressed by having Ms. Teal mimic more and more types of movements, until she has to mimic quickly and immediately any movement that the therapist performs. In order to progress Ms. Teal's ability to concentrate appropriately for functional environmental demands, the length of time spent on tasks should vary intermittently.

CASE STUDY #4
Shawna Wells

- *Age: 4 years*
- *Medical Diagnosis: Cerebral palsy, spastic quadriparesis, mild mental retardation*
- *Status: Onset at birth*
- *Practice Pattern 5C: Impaired Motor Function and Sensory Integrity Associated with Nonprogressive Disorders of the Central Nervous System—Congenital Origin or Acquired in Infancy or Childhood*

EXAMINATION AND EVALUATION

Functional Limitations

Shawna demonstrates general impulsivity when performing fine motor activities that are performed at home or at school. She has difficulty with selective attention and, often, when she does concentrate on an activity, she tends to perseverate and has difficulty shifting her attention to a new task. She often avoids activities involving object manipulation (eg, coloring, cutting, or hair brushing).

Impairments

As with most young children, evaluation of Shawna's information processing ability was a challenge. Shawna demonstrated good identification ability for all auditory stimuli. She could visually locate and point to all objects during testing. The tested objects were presented in all visual fields. Shawna did not cooperate well with the examination of somatosensory location testing of vibration, pinprick, and light touch, but appeared to feel each sensation. She could discriminate the pencil, paper, and key, but could not differentiate between the glass and box during testing of stereognosis. When holding objects, Shawna complained of palm itchiness, became inattentive, and wanted to move from the test position.

When testing response selection, Shawna could perform relatively well under the simple reaction time condition. However, she often produced errors by reacting to the warning signal rather than to the stimulus signal. When two choices were presented, Shawna could not switch between the stimuli. She often persisted with the same response to both stimuli. Her responses were variable, with long delays before reacting. Under the choice condition, Shawna appeared to forget what she was supposed to do, and frequently would perform a movement unrelated to the task requirements. After a short time under the choice testing condition, Shawna became fussy and would not continue.

Shawna did not appear to be unduly slow in her reaction times when movement requirements became more complex (within her limited skilled movement repertoire). Response programming ability was, therefore, determined to be adequate for her level of functioning.

Two problems in information processing were determined. These included her difficulties in somatosensory stimulus detection and avoidance, as well as her difficulty in selectively attending to tasks.

PROGNOSIS/PLAN OF CARE

Goals

Treatment goals for Shawna are to:
1. Demonstrate improved discrimination of somatosensory stimuli
2. Decrease avoidance responses to tactile stimuli
3. Demonstrate improved selective attention to academic and self-care tasks

Functional Outcomes

Following 3 months of therapy, Shawna will:

1. Manipulate classroom materials to complete academic tasks such as coloring, cutting, and pasting
2. Use a hairbrush and a toothbrush appropriately with verbal cues only
3. Attend to a table activity for 5 minutes without being distracted by two other children working at the same table
4. Shift her attention from one fine motor task to another with verbal cues only

INTERVENTION

To improve Shawna's willingness to experience somatosensory stimuli, sensory experiences will progress from general whole body contact to specific hand manipulation tasks. For example, Shawna could be wrapped in a cotton blanket then asked to remove the blanket. Then she could wrap her own arms with a towel and unwrap the towel with guidance and assistance. She could scrub her forearms and hands with a dry washcloth before engaging in activities to manipulate large solid objects, then progressing to hold large soft objects, smaller hard objects, and, finally, small soft objects. Shawna then could participate in fine motor activities currently required in her classroom. Shawna's selective attention may be improved by having her focus initially on a specific single task in a quiet, isolated physical environment. Progressively, tasks will be increased in the number of attention requiring components, and the treatment environment will become more typical (eg, increasing amount of visual and auditory stimuli in environment, increasing number of other children in close proximity). A structured classroom and home program for carry over of strategies to improve attention will be essential, and the therapist will need to develop these strategies in conjunction with Shawna's classroom teacher and family.

CASE STUDY # 5
Robert Anderson

- *Age: 38 years*
- *Medical Diagnosis: Incomplete T9-10 spinal cord injury with left radial nerve damage*
- *Status: 6 months post injury*
- *Practice Pattern 5H: Impaired Motor Function, Peripheral Nerve Integrity, and Sensory Integrity Associated with Nonprogressive Disorders of the Spinal Cord*

EXAMINATION AND EVALUATION

Functional Limitations

Initially following his motorcycle accident, Mr. Anderson demonstrated problems with short-term memory due to his concussion. Subsequent testing revealed that these problems had resolved and his cognitive function appears to be normal.

Impairments

No impairments noted in cognitive information processing areas. Therefore, no intervention in this area is necessary.

REFERENCES

1. Schmidt RA. *Motor Control and Learning: A Behavioral Emphasis*. 3rd ed. Champaign, Ill: Human Kinetics; 1999.

2. Theios J. The components of response latency in simple human information processing tasks. In: Rabbitt PMA, Domic S, eds. *Attention and Performance, Vol 5*. New York, NY: Academic Press; 1975:418-439.

3. Light KE. Information processing for motor performance in aging adults. *Phys Ther.* 1990; 70:820-826.

4. Light KE. Effects of adult aging on the movement complexity factor of response programming. *Journal of Gerontology: Psychological Sciences*. 1990;45:107-109.

5. Hommel B, Prinz W, eds. *Theoretical Issues in Stimulus-Response Compatibility*. Amsterdam, Holland: Elsevier; 1997.

6. Proctor RW, VanZandt T. *Human Factors in Simple and Complex Systems*. Boston, Mass: Allyn and Bacon; 1994.

7. Light KE, Spirduso WW. Age-related response preparation differences for response-response compatibility. *Journal of Aging and Physical Activity*. 1996;4:179-193.

8. Posner MI. *Chronometric Explorations of the Mind*. Hillsdale, NJ: Erlbaum; 1978.

9. Welford AT. The psychological refractory period and the timing of highspeed performance—a review of theory. *Brit J Psych*. 1952;43:2-19.

10. Keele SW. *Attention and Human Performance* (Chapter 4). Pacific Palisades, Calif: Goodyear; 1973.

11. Keele SW. Motor control. In Kaufman L, Thomas J, eds. *Handbook of Perception and Performance*. New York, NY: John Wiley; 1986.

12. Anderson JR. **Learning and Memory: An Integrated Approach.** New York, NY: John Wiley; 1995.

13. Halgren E. Human hippocampal and amygdala recording and stimulation: evidence for a neural model of recent memory. In: Squire L, Butters N, eds. *The Neuropsychology of Memory*. New York, NY: Guilford; 1984:165-181.

14. Squire LR, Cohen N, Nadel L. The medial temporal lobe in memory consolidation: a new hypothesis. In: Weingartner H, Pardner E, eds. *Memory Consolidation*. Hillsdale, NJ: Erlbaum; 1984:185–210.

15. Hirst W, Johnson MK, Kim JK, et al. Recognition and recall in amnesics. *J Exp Psych*. 1986; 12:445-451.

16. Smyth MM, Pendleton LR. Working memory for movements. *Quart J Exp Psych*. 1989; 41 A(2):235–250.

17. Sperling G. The information available in brief visual presentations. *Psychological Monographs*. 1960;74(11): whole no. 498.

18. Bliss JC, Crane HD, Mansfield K, et al. Information available in brief tactile presentations. *Perceptions and Psychophysics*. 1966;1:273–283.

19. Atkinson RC, Shiffrin RM. The control of short term memory. *Sci Amer*. 1971; 225:82 – 90.

20. Light KE, Reilly MA, Behrman AL, et al. Greater benefits of practice on reaction time in older versus younger subjects. *Journal of Aging and Physical Activity.* 1996;4:27-41.

21. Proteau L, Blandin Y, Alain C, at al. The effects of the amount and variability of practice on the learning of a multi-segmented motor task. *Acta Psychologica.* 1994;85:61-74.

22. Schmidt RA, Wulf G. Continuous concurrent feedback degrades skill learning: implications for training and simulation. *Human Factors.* 1997;39:509-525.

23. Todorov E, Shadmehr R, Bizzi E. Augmented feedback presented in a virtual environment accelerates learning of a difficult motor task. *Journal of Motor Behavior.* 1997;29:147-158.

24. Janelle CM, Barba DA, Frehlich SG, et al. Maximizing performance feedback effectiveness through videotape replay and a self-controlled learning environment. *Research Quarterly for Exercise and Sport.* 1997;68:269-279.

25. Guadagnoli MA, Leis B, Van Gemmert AAW, et al. The relationship between knowledge of results and motor learning in Parkinson's patients. Manuscript in review, 2001.

26. Pratt J, Abrams RA. Practice and component submovements: the roles of programming and feedback in rapid aimed limb movements. *Journal of Motor Behavior.* 1996;28:149-156.

27. Bernstein NA. *The Coordination and Regulation of Movements.* Oxford, England: Pergamon Press; 1967.

28. Schmidt RA. A schema theory of discrete motor learning. *Psych Rev.* 1975;82:225–260.

29. Schmidt RA: The schema concept. In: Kelso JAS, ed. *Human Motor Behavior: An Introduction.* Hillsdale, NJ: Erlbaum; 1982:219–235.

30. Jeka JJ, Kelso JAS. The dynamic pattern approach to coordinated behavior: a tutorial review. In: Wallace SA, ed. *Perspectives on the Coordination of Movement.* Amsterdam, North Holland: Elsevier Science Publishers B V;1989:3-45.

31. Kelso JAS. *Human Motor Behavior, An Introduction.* Hillsdale, NJ: Erlbaum; 1982: 239–287.

32. Kelso JAS, Schoner G. Self-organization of coordinative movement patterns. *Human Movement Science.* 1988:7;27–46.

33. Lynch JL, McLaren JW. Deficits of visual attention and saccadic eye movements after lesions of parieto-occiptal cortex in monkeys. *J Neurophys.* 1989;61(1):74–89.

34. Haaland KY, Harrington DL, Yeo R. The effects of task complexity on motor performance in left and right CVA patients. *Neuropsychologia.* 1987;25:783–794.

35. Rafal RD, Posner MI, Walker JA, et al. Cognition and the basal ganglia. *Brain.* 1984;107: 1083–1094.

36. Marsden CD. The mysterious motor function of the basal ganglia. The Robert Wartenberg Lecture. *Neurology.* 1982;32:514–539.

37. Stelmach GE, Phillips JG, Chau AW. Visuo-spatial processing in Parkinsonians. *Neuropsychologia.* 1989;27:485–493.

38. Keele SW, Ivry RI. Timing and force control: a modular analysis. *International Research Conference on Motor Control.* Moscow: March 1987.

39. Margolin DI, Wing A. Agraphia and micrographia: clinical manifestations of motor programming and performance disorders. *Acta Psych.* 1983;54:263-283.

40. DeRenzi E, Faglioni P, Previdi P. Spatial memory and hemispheric locus of lesion. *Cortex.* 1977;13:424–433.

41. Basso A, Luzzatti C, Spinnler H. Is ideomotor apraxia the outcome of damage to well defined regions of the left hemisphere? *Journal of Neurology, Neurosurgery and Psychiatry.* 1980;43:118–126.

42. Nudo RJ, Plautz EJ, Milliken GW. Adaptive plasticity in primate motor cortex as a consequence of behavioral experience and neuronal injury. *Seminars in Neuroscience.* 1997;9:13-23.

Balance Deficits: Examination, Evaluation, and Intervention

Mary Ann Seeger, PT, MS

INTRODUCTION

Researchers, including clinicians, from a variety of disciplines have contributed to the knowledge base on postural control. New divergent perspectives and methodologies have been built on previous theories, and the neural mechanisms underlying postural control have continued to be explored.[1-11] Our understanding of neuromuscular behavior,[12-23] approaches to recovery of impaired balance,[24-28] and methods of evaluating balance[4,10,29-41] continues to evolve. Physical therapists have been involved extensively in this information gathering. In spite of this explosion of new information, physical therapists' evaluation and intervention protocols have been slow to adapt. Horak stated "scientists view balance as an emergent property of a complex, multicomponent sensorimotor system, whereas clinicians often think of it as a single set of automatic reactions. The implications for how to assess and treat balance disorders based on these different assumptions about neural control of balance are immense."[42] The future holds great promise, for even more precise information on balance and technology has brought research closer to the clinician. Additionally, as research broadens to a more holistic approach of studying movement during natural activities versus laboratory simulations, the physical therapist is able to understand important clinical applications. The purpose of this chapter is to discuss current information on postural control and to update evaluation and intervention approaches to balance disorders in the patient with pathology involving the nervous system. The term *balance* will be used interchangeably with *stability* and *postural control*.

Balance is the ability to maintain the position of the body relative to stability limits.[43] It involves controlling the body's position in space for the purposes of *stability* and *orientation*. Orientation is the ability to maintain an appropriate relationship between the body segments and between the body and environment for a task.[44] For most tasks we maintain a vertical orientation using multiple sensory references (eg, gravity, support surface, and relationship of the body to objects in the environment). Stability and orientation are two distinct goals of the postural control system. Some tasks, needing a particular orientation, are accomplished at the expense of stability. Examples are looking at a high corner shelf while standing on a ladder and extending sideways and riding a bicycle around a tight corner thereby leaning into the curve. In both instances the person would have orientation against gravity but would be vulnerable to instability. Another example would be diving sideways toward the ground to catch a ball. Therefore, most tasks have postural control as a requirement, but the demands of stability and orientation change with each task.[10,44]

Models

In rehabilitation science, there are a variety of conceptual models that can describe the neural control of posture and movement. Two will be discussed in this chapter: the traditional reflex/hierarchical model and the more contemporary systems model. A reflex/hierarchical model suggests that balance results from hierarchically organized reflex responses within the individual.[12,14,15] Alternatively, the systems model suggests that balance involves an interaction between the individual and his environment.[2] Recently, Shumway-Cook and Woollacott have added "task" to the interaction, completing an important loop which needs to be considered therapeutically.[8,10] Each model has implications for evaluating and treating balance disorders in the patient with neurologic involvement, and clinical assumptions are made based on the theoretical model of postural control, thereby influencing intervention strategies.

Reflex/Hierarchical Model

According to the reflex/hierarchical model, balance is the ability to correctly deploy a set of interacting, hierarchically organized reflexes and reactions which support the body against gravity.[14-16] The reflex/hierarchical model of motor control is based on Sherrington's model of reflex chaining, which demonstrated that a single stimulus can result in varying responses.[1]

In this model, it is proposed that sequential maturation of ascending levels of the central nervous system (CNS) hierarchy results in the emergence of higher levels of behavior, which in turn modify immature behaviors organized at lower levels. Therefore, during development, the young child is first dominated by primitive reflexes which are controlled hierarchically at low levels within the CNS. With maturation of higher brainstem and mid-brain levels within the CNS, righting reactions emerge which modify or inhibit primitive reflexes. Finally, with maturation of the cortex, considered the "highest" level of the CNS, the emergence of equilibrium reactions occurs.

Equilibrium reactions were defined by Weisz as automatic reactions by the body in response to labyrinthine inputs.[12] Equilibrium reactions, or tilting reactions, have been described as emerging first in prone, then in supine, in sitting, in quadruped, and finally in standing. It is assumed that mature or partially mature equilibrium reactions must emerge at each stage of development (eg, in sitting prior to quadruped, in quadruped prior to stance) before the maturing child can achieve the next developmental milestone.[30]

According to the reflex/hierarchical model, instability demonstrated by a patient is the result of release of spinal and brainstem reflexes which are no longer modified or inhibited by higher CNS structures.[34] Lesions in the cerebral cortex of an adult patient result in the reappearance of primitive reflexes which dominate motor function and prevent the expression of normal equilibrium.

Based on the reflex/hierarchical model of motor control and development, a number of reflex profiles have been developed and integrated into clinical assessments.[33,45,46] Examination of reflexes and equilibrium reactions has traditionally been considered an essential part of the clinical evaluation of patients with neurologic impairments, since persistence and dominance of primitive reflexes are considered to be major deterrents to independent stability and mobility. Treatment based on this model has stressed facilitation of more "normal" righting and equilibrium reactions and inhibition of competing primitive reflexes.[15]

Systems Model

The study of postural control using a systems model has emerged in the last decade with the advent of advanced technology.[7,10,11,44] This model is based on work by Bernstein, but recently has been expanded to include an operational model for motor control focusing on goal-directed neural organization of multiple, interacting systems.[10,11,44,47] (Figures 11-1 and 11-2).

Perception (integration of sensory information assessing the position and motion of the body in space), *action* (ability to generate forces for controlling the body position), and *cognition* (attention, motivation, intent, or goal) are all required for the stability and orientation of postural control. In a systems model, therefore, we think of postural control as a complex interaction of musculoskeletal, neuromuscular, and cognitive components (Figure 11-3).[10] Sensory and motor strategies for postural control based on a systems model are described in the following sections. Because multiple interacting systems contribute to postural control, it can be difficult to discern the relative contributions of individual impairments to balance disorders. For example, there may be anatomical differences in the musculoskeletal system and underlying pathology, and factors such as age, prior medical history, prior movement experiences, and current therapeutic interventions including medications all play a role in postural control.

STRATEGIES FOR POSTURAL CONTROL

Sensory Strategies

Studies have examined the behavior, motor output, and biomechanics of normal subjects when sensory inputs for postural control were varied.[25,48,49] Each sense provides specific information regarding gravity, the environment, and relationships about motion, as well as position or a frame of reference for postural control. In environments where a sense is not accurately reporting self-motion, an alternative sense may be selected for

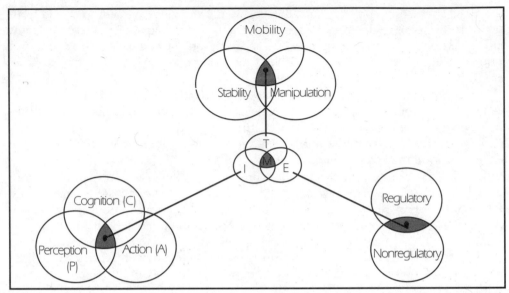

Figure 11-1. Motor control emerges through the interaction among the individual (I), the task (T), and the environment (E) (reprinted with permission from Shumway-Cook A, Woollacott MH. *Motor Control: Theory and Practical Application.* 2nd ed. Philadelphia, Pa: Lippincott Williams & Wilkins; 2001).

Figure 11-2. Systems model for the emergence of motor strategies (reprinted with permission from the American Physical Therapy Association from Horak FB, Henry SM, Shumway-Cook A. Postural perturbations: new insights for treatment of balance disorders. *Physical Therapy.* 1986;66:10).

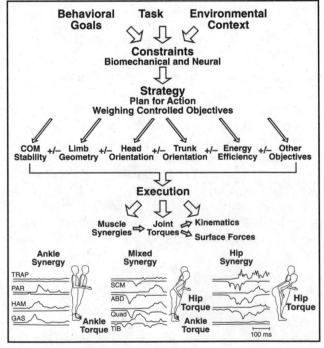

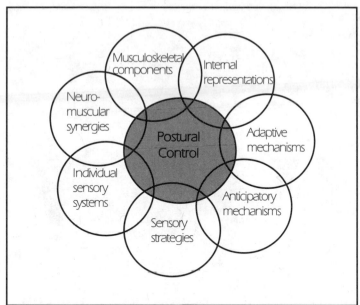

Figure 11-3. Systems contributing to postural control (reprinted with permission from Shumway-Cook A, Woollacott MH. *Motor Control: Theory and Practical Application.* 2nd ed. Philadelphia, Pa: Lippincott Williams & Wilkins; 2001).

orientation. Because of the redundancy of sensory information available for orientation, normal individuals are able to maintain stability in a variety of environments where one or more senses are unavailable for balance.

Research suggests that the CNS organizes and adapts sensory information for postural control. A hierarchical weighting of sensory input based on accuracy is done regarding the body's position and movements in space. If sensory information is not complete, for example, when one is in a darkened room, the weight of visual information is reduced and the weight of other more accurate or complete sensory information is increased. The weighting of sensory input may depend on the person's age, the environment, and the task. Somatosensory information for postural control apparently is weighed more heavily than vision and vestibular inputs.[10,48,50,51] This may explain the clinical observation that when elderly people have sensory neuropathy in their feet, a slight decrease in either of the other two senses (vision or vestibular) causes them to become posturally unstable. Research suggests, however, that while nondisabled adults tend to rely most on somatosensory inputs, children tend to rely more on visual information.[10]

The nervous system must adapt its use of sensory information under changing tasks and conditions. One approach to investigating this adaptation is the use of a moving platform with a moving visual surround.[48] Body sway is measured while the person stands quietly under six conditions that alter the availability and accuracy of visual and somatosensory inputs for postural orientation (Figure 11-4). A clinical simulation for posturography is seen in Figure 11-5 and will be discussed in Examination of Sensory Strategies.

Motor Strategies

Balance requires the generation, scaling, and coordination of forces effective in controlling the center of mass (COM) relative to desired limits of stability. Postural move-

Figure 11-4. Six conditions of the sensory organization test (reprinted with permission from the American Physical Therapy Association from Duncan P, ed. *Balance: Proceedings of the APTA Forum*. Alexandria, Va: APTA; 1990:8).

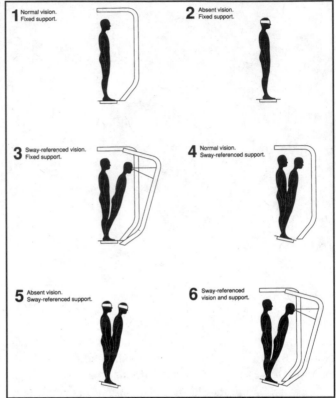

Figure 11-5. Six positions and devices used for manipulating the senses of the clinical test for sensory interaction for balance (reprinted with permission from the American Physical Therapy Association from Shumway-Cook A, Horak F. Assessing the influence of sensory interaction on balance. *Phys Ther.* 1986;66:10; 1548-1554).

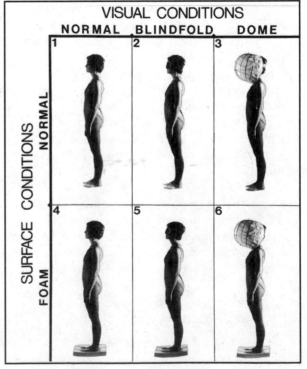

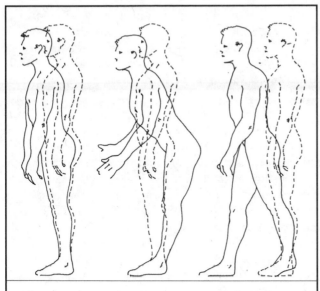

Figure 11-6. Three postural motor strategies used by normal adults for control of upright sway (reprinted with permission from Thieme Medical Publishers from Shumway-Cook A, Horak F. Vestibular rehabilitation: an exercise approach to managing symptoms of vestibular dysfunction. *Seminars in Hearing.* 1989;10:2).

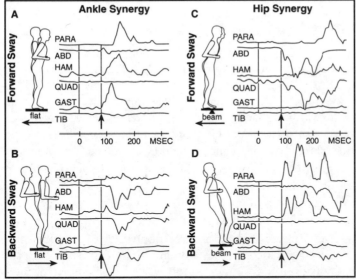

Figure 11-7. Sequencing of EMG activity and joint motions during response to forward and backward perturbations (reprinted with permission from the American Physiological Society from Horak FB, Nashner L. Central programming of postural movements: adaptation to altered surface configurations. *J Neurophysiol.* 1986;55).

ment strategies are viewed as using both feedback and feed-forward or anticipatory activation to achieve or restore balance in a variety of circumstances. Studies documenting this feed-forward control of posture and synergistic style are important to understanding normal timing of muscle activation for balance.[3,52-54]

Using a moving platform to study postural motor reactions, Nashner and others [17,24,25,55] have described movement patterns or strategies used for recovery of perturbed stance. These include an ankle strategy of recovery, a hip strategy, and a stepping strategy. These movements are illustrated in Figure 11-6. Patterns of muscle activity or synergies used for postural recovery also have been described with electromyography (EMG). (Figure 11-7). The *ankle movement strategy* restores the COM to stability around the ankle joint using identified muscle activity while on flat surfaces, and when small excursions of recovery are required. Motion (ie, translation) of the platform in a backward direction, for example, causes the individual to sway forward, thus producing ankle dorsiflexion and hip extension. Use of the ankle strategy requires adequate range of motion and strength in the ankles. Muscle activity to recover balance begins at 90 msecs in the gastrocnemius, followed by activation of the hamstrings (116 msecs), then paraspinal muscles (117 msecs).

In contrast, the hip strategy is activated when needing a large and/or fast recovery from COM displacement. Examples are walking on a compliant surface or where the surface is small, such as quick recovery while walking tandem on a beam or when slipping on ice. The hip and head move in opposite directions and the muscle activation is from proximal to distal.[25] When a postural perturbation is of sufficient magnitude to displace the COM outside the base of support of the feet, or a hip or ankle strategy is insufficient to recover balance, a step or reach is normally taken.[56] Maki and McIlroy[52] demonstrated that a stepping strategy is used in many conditions even when the COM is within the base of support. Examples are trips, active reaching too far, and misjudging the distance needed for a step. A suspensory strategy also has been described.[41] It is used when lowering the center of gravity is needed, as in a squatting motion, thereby lowering the COM in activities such as skateboarding or skiing.

EXAMINATION OF POSTURAL CONTROL

In traditional approaches to evaluating balance, clinical examination of postural and equilibrium responses is done by tipping or tilting the individual. Postural responses can be tested in a developmental progression from supine to standing with the individual maintaining balance in response to movement of a movable support base or by displacing the individual sideways, forwards, or backwards. Appropriateness of responses to tilt or perturbation and the movement patterns used by the patient are noted.[33,34]

Using a systems approach, three areas of balance should be evaluated. These are:

1. Sensory, motor, and cognitive impairments or constraints to normal postural control

2. Sensory and motor strategies used to recover from imbalance and sensory strategies available to detect imbalance in various environments and tasks

3. Functional skills assessed through self-report questionnaires and performance tests. After data are gathered and identified regarding impairments, strategies, and functional skills, an evaluation of the information should be completed, goals identified, and an intervention plan established with a specific time frame. An example of a Balance Examination and Evaluation is outlined in Table 11-1.

Identifying Constraints to Normal Postural Control

Examination of Neurosensory Impairments

Abnormal postural control can result from damage within an individual sensory system (eg, visual, vestibular, or somatosensory) or from deficits in central sensory organization processes as described in the Sensory Strategies section.[50,57-60] The visual system detects information regarding motion of self in regard to the stationary environment, to objects, and to moving objects or people. For example, the visual system determines the

TABLE 11-1

Balance Assessment Format

Balance Examination & Evaluation

History/Diagnosis:_____

Chief Complaint:_____

Pain:_____ Dizziness:_____ Falling:_____ Weakness:_____ Dysfunction:_____

Other:_____

Circumstances/conditions/environment Problems:_____

Medications:_____ Fall: Frequency/1st/Last:_____

Vestibular/CNS Tests:_____

Activity Difficulty: Driving ___ Recreation ___ Fitness ___ Personal Care ___ Shopping ___

Subsystem Impairments/Constraints: Pain:_____ ROM:_____

Strength:_____ Tone:_____ Leg length:_____

Proprioception/Touch/Pressure in Feet:_____

Coordination: RAM-UE:_____ LE:_____ Finger to Nose:_____

Oculomotor Control:

Gaze Control: Nystagmus:_____ Acuity:_____ Exo/esophoria:_____ R/L:_____

Smooth Pursuits: Smooth:_____ Ragged:_____ Teaming:_____

Saccades: Past Point:_____ Slow:_____ Search:_____ Teaming:_____

Visual-Vestibular Interaction (Dyscoordination, jumpy, nausea, imbalance, duration, speed):

	Head Movement—Still Target (in phase)	Head and Eye Movement Moving Target (suppression of VOR)
Sitting		
Standing (Feet Touching) 1/2 Tandem/		
Feet Separated		
Comments		

V VOR/2:_____

Cervical Screen (body/neck rotation on head):_____

Jacobson Dizziness Handicap Inventory:_____ /100

Static Postural Control:

Posture	Trunk	Neck	Shoulder	Hips	Knees	Ankles	COG	Equality
Sitting								
Standing								

continued

Static Postural *Motor* Strategies:
(complaints, % mechanical LOS excursion, dyscoordination)

Sitting	Anterior		Posterior		Lateral	
	EO	EC	EO	EC	EO	EC
Self Initiated Shifts						
Reactive Strategies						
Anticipated/Predicted						

Standing	Anterior		Posterior		Lateral	
	EO	EC	EO	EC	EO	EC
Self Initiated Shifts						
Reactive Strategies						
Anticipated/Predicted						

Static Balance Skills: Time (trial, ability to assume positions, fear, need of support, etc)

	Eyes Open	Eyes Closed
On Toes		
On Heels		
Stand on Left Leg		
Stand on Right Leg		
Tandem Stand		

Clinical Test of *Sensory* Interaction for Balance (CTSIB):
(complaints, fall, strategy, direction, fear)

	Time	Quality	Tandem
EO firm surface			
EC firm surface			
Dome firm surface			
EO foam surface			
EC foam surface			
Dome foam surface			

Dynamic Postural Control (Walking):
Assistive devices:_____ Orthotics:_____
Functional status including environments/tasks:_____
Assumed walking speed:_____ Ability to slow/speed up:_____
Walk-Stop ability:_____ Pivot turns:_____
Walk with head turns, head and eye turns (complaints, dyscoordination, vision, nausea, dizzy, stagger, etc.): _____
Walking pattern: (time on each foot, base of support, heel strike, step length, antalgic, stagger, en bloc, etc.[with and without walking device]):_____
Dynamic gait index:_____ Timed up and go test:_____
Berg balance static balance score:_____/56 Tinetti POMA (Gait and/or balance):_____

continued

Vertiginous Positioning: (position testing, complaints, intensity 1-10, nystagmus)

	Right	Left
Baseline		
Head movement		
Rolling		
Bend toward knee		
Sit to stand		
Hallpike		

Assessment/Problems:
Impairments/Constraints (circle): Dizzy, gaze stabilization, proprioception, vision, V VOR, motor behaviors, strength, pain, coordination, headaches, weight, ROM, posture, flexibility, other:_____.
Strategies:
Sensory:_____ Motor:_____
Balance Skills:
Performance Tests:_____

Dynamic Postural Control (Gait):

Functional Limitations:

Goals/Functional Outcomes:

Intervention:

speed of oncoming people who are walking to determine the individual's self route of walking. If the visual system does not distinguish between self-motion and surrounding motion, there may be misinterpretation with resultant inaccurate motor output.

Somatosensory (ie, proprioception, kinesthesia) input provides information regarding the body with reference to the supporting surface. Slopes and uneven ground are best detected by somatosensors. Ankle strategies can be stimulated by proprioceptive input. If an individual does not use an ankle strategy effectively, diminished or absent proprioception may be the reason.[10,50,61]

Vestibular information signals the head's position and movement. The semicircular canals detect angular acceleration of the head, and the otoliths signal linear position and acceleration. Gravity is a stimulus and therefore the otoliths detect position in relation to the vertical. The vestibular system alone cannot detect complete information regarding the head in relation to the COM, such as distinguishing between head movement during bending at the waist which is similar to head movement when moving the head down only. Proprioceptive, visual, and vestibular information are assessed together to determine the position of the head on the body versus the head moving in space. Complaints of dizziness are common in individuals with vestibular impairments that also may include vertigo, imbalance, and visual complications.[23,58-61]

The visual, vestibular, and somatosensory systems are critical for providing the sensory information necessary for balance. The examination of hemianopsias, field cuts, visual acuity, double vision, gaze control, pursuits, and saccades are all important to include, even in cursory tests.[62-64] Identification of any vestibular impairment's contribution to imbalance is important.[10,65,66] For example, gaze stabilization during head movement is a function of the vestibular system. Vertigo or frank spinning may be due to a vestibular impairment that impacts balance, posture, movement, fear of movement, and function.[65] Administering clinical tests of eye/head movement in conjunction with static balance or dynamic balance (walking) is critical. Patients with a vestibular component to their imbalance may function well in static tests and even when walking in a straight line. However, when asked to turn around or turn their heads while looking at a stationary target or a moving object, their balance may be compromised. Observations of dyscoordination, complaints of nausea, "jumpy" vision, imbalance, or decreased speed of movement are all variables that can be identified on the baseline evaluation and then used for subsequent measures of progress. A Borg Scale, used to subjectively identify severity of pain, is typically used. Cervical screening tests, such as having the patient move the body with the head versus moving the head on the body, can isolate neck proprioceptive from vestibular contributions in individuals with complaints of dizziness.[66-68] Vertiginous positioning testing should be done if the patient's history is indicative of movement-provoked dizziness.[69] It is important to identify if dizziness is provoked with particular head movements or head movement in general, remembering there are many reasons for dizziness, such as cardiovascular disorders or side effects of medication. Current reviews of dizziness have been published by Cavanaugh,[70] Shepard and Solomon,[71] and Parikh and Bid.[72] Head movement-provoked dizziness is the key to identifying the vestibular system as a contributor to deficits in postural control.[65,70,73] The Dix-Hallpike Tests for benign paroxysmal positional nystagmus or vertigo, BPPN(V), are provided in Figure 11-8. Signs of involvement in the ipsilateral posterior canal are: rotary nystagmus with fast phase to the downward ear; a spinning sensation after a few seconds delay; and, lastly, an extinction of this nystagmus and sensation. A blow to the head, infection, aging, and iatrogenic reasons are all possible etiologies of BPPN (V). Recently, effective treatment resolutions have been identified for BPPN (V). It is essential that therapists screen for this potentially debilitating problem.[74]

Somatosensory deficits can impair reception of correct feedback from the support surface (eg, ground). Testing pressure and vibration sense can be effective in making judgments regarding the status of somatosensory feedback potentially lacking in the elderly patient or as a complication of diabetes, leading to ineffective or limited ankle strategies. Weakness can be a associated with poor sensation, since strengthening ankle musculature in people with very poor sensation in their feet can improve balance when ankle strategies are necessary.

Examination of Neuromotor and Skeletal Impairments

Musculoskeletal restrictions can limit movement strategies used in balance. For example, insufficient range of motion (ROM) in the ankles can compromise a needed ankle

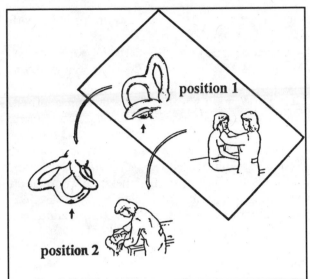

Figure 11-8. Hallpike Test for anterior or posterior canal BPPV showing the debris moving to its dependent position in the posterior canal. The head is turned 45 degrees and then taken to 20 degrees effectively off the horizontal to observe for nystagmus and spinning sensations (reprinted with permission from Herdman SJ. *Vestibular Rehabilitation.* 2nd ed. Philadelphia, Pa: FA Davis; 2000).

strategy and those movements that are necessary at the hip and knee. Any limitation in joint ROM, whether head, trunk, or upper or lower extremities, can have a negative impact on postural control.

Since stability requires the ability to generate forces necessary for moving the COM, upper motoneuron lesions producing limitations in strength may produce concomitant limitations in stability. Studies involving strength impairments in CNS lesions recently have been completed.[75,76] The correlation between impairments in strength and in stability in individuals with CNS lesions suggests a rationale for including strength training in treatment interventions. Instability due to abnormalities of coordination within postural muscle synergies also has been reported in patients with a wide range of conditions. Examples include significantly delayed onset of postural responses and abnormal sequencing of muscles in patients with diagnoses of traumatic brain injury (TBI),[69] cerebrovascular accident (CVA),[77] cerebellar disorders,[78] or Parkinson's disease.[79,80] In addition, involuntary movements and tremors can affect the ability of patients to control movements of the center of mass, thus impeding maintenance and recovery of stability.

Tests for ROM, strength, coordination, pain, and muscle tone can be done in a traditional fashion.[10,34,81] It is important to note areas of abnormalities to determine possible constraint contributions to reactive and predictive motor strategies. Inspection of the feet and assessment of ankle ROM is necessary for knowledge of the patient's biomechanical excursions of ankle motion for ankle strategies and potential interferences to weight bearing. General static posture can be examined with traditional tests for mechanical alignment and possible perceptual contributions to balance (see Chapter 8).

Examination of Cognitive and Perceptual Impairments

Impairments in sensory function can affect perceptual interpretations (eg, spatial relations), praxis, body scheme, and body identification. Poor cognitive functioning in areas such as attention, memory, organization, sequencing, and orientation may impact efficient and effective interaction with the environment. These cognitive factors are all challenging and compete with balance. They have been identified as increasing the risk of falling and impeding progress in the elderly,[10,82-89] as well as in patients with Parkinson's disease,[90,91] multiple sclerosis,[92,93] and Alzheimer's disease.[94,95]

Cognitive and perceptual tests have been designed for the elderly, for patients post-CVA, and for patients with TBIs.[62,64,96-101] Psychologists, speech pathologists, and occupational therapists have been actively involved in designing tests and treating such problems. More recently, cognition and information processing have been recognized, studied, and evaluated as potential influences on balance.[102-104] Testing sway during quiet stance while demanding cognitive information, or testing accuracy and speed of cognitive information while doing a balance skill, can provide information regarding processes for motor skill versus processes for cognition. Obtaining baseline information of strictly cognitive processing should be done prior to testing the same information while doing a balance skill. Impairments such as apraxia, spatial deficits, poor discrimination, impaired memory, impaired figure/ground, diminished visual information processing, decreased motility, and neglect all have clinical implications.[10,64]

Identifying Motor and Sensory Strategies

Examination of Motor Strategies (see Table 11-1)

Examination of coordinated ankle, hip, and stepping strategies in stance and movement activities may be done under various task conditions. First, patients are asked to voluntarily sway, then stop (performed in all directions), while the type of movement pattern used to maintain stability and the process of weight shifting are observed (ie, self-initiated voluntary or active weight shifts). The distance of excursion or percent of mechanical limits of stability (LOS), synergistic style of active movement, and complaints or fear of movement can be noted. Differences in strategy with eyes open or eyes closed can be noted. Next, reactive strategies can be documented during resistive pressure at the hips then, when released, noting reactive balance using ankle strategies. The same test can be done with resistance at the shoulders for hip strategies. While the patient is attempting to recover balance, the therapist should look for behaviors suggestive of motor incoordination, for example, excessive flexion of the knees, asymmetric movements of the body, or excessive flexion or rotation of the trunk.

Figure 11-9 compares movement associated with normal and abnormal sequencing of muscle activity in response to backward sway. Figure 11-9A shows that in response to backward sway, normal muscle activation begins in the tibialis anterior (numbered 1) and moves proximally to the quadriceps muscles (numbered 2), then the abdominal muscles (numbered 3). This pattern of muscle activity produces joint torques (shown as arrows) causing ankle-centered movement propelling the COM forward.

EMG studies of abnormal synergy patterns have been done demonstrating patterns of dyscontrol.[57,80,105] For example, movement in a patient with motor incoordination resulting from abnormal sequencing of muscle activation is seen in Figure 11-9B. Backward sway results in activation of the quadriceps muscles first (numbered 1), followed by the abdominal muscles (numbered 2), and finally, the tibialis anterior (numbered 3). This pattern of muscle activation results in hyperextension of the knee and forward flexion of the trunk, a pattern seen commonly in patients with hemiplegia.

Anticipated or predictive motor strategies are only grossly observed with clinical examination. A greater perturbation is required for the clinical observation of arm movement prior to the actual hip, ankle, or step strategy, indicating the individual's greater perceived need for safety. More refined and exact arm or head strategies in anticipation

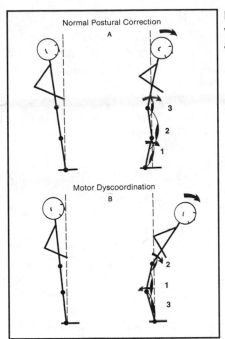

Figure 11-9. Comparison of body motions associated with normal versus abnormal sequencing of muscle activity in response to backward sway.

of displacement have been documented.[54] These motor strategies can be tested in sitting or standing, on different surfaces, with eyes open or closed, or with distracting sounds or cognitive demands. These variations of demands should be done in a progressive fashion. Safety during a balance evaluation can be difficult. The goal is to determine at what level of balance challenge the person becomes unstable, yet not allow him to fall. Touching the patient adds an additional sensory cue so no touching should occur. Close guarding without touch is possible. If the patient's COM moves outside his BOS and his motor strategy is not sufficient to recover balance, it will be necessary to intervene to prevent a fall.

Examination of Sensory Strategies

Shumway-Cook and Horak[106] designed a Clinical Test of Sensory Interaction for Balance (CTSIB) based on posturography concepts of Nashner.[48] Posturography was designed to distinguish vestibular disorders from other sensory integrative problems. El-Kashlan and Telian[107] established that the CTSIB with dynamic posturography is a screening tool for sensory problems. The CTSIB requires the patient to maintain standing balance for 30 seconds under six different sensory conditions that either eliminate visual input or produce inaccurate visual and surface orientation inputs. Patients are tested in two positions, Classic or Standard Romberg (feet together) and tandem (heel/toe position), in the sequence shown in Figure 11-5. It is important to gain consistency in the procedures, such as always having shoes off, or feet 4 inches apart, or placing the hands on the hips to observe upper extremity reactive or anticipatory balance responses. Using condition one as a baseline reference, the therapist observes the patient for changes in the amount and direction of sway, complaints, strategies used to keep balance, asymmetries, and time balanced. The test is repeated with the subsequent five conditions. A more sophisticated method for assessing sensory strategy interaction is posturography as described by Nashner.[108] A model for interpreting results of the CTSIB or posturography has been proposed.[10] Strategy dysfunction can be described as "visually dependent" with problems in Conditions 2, 3, and 6; "surface dependent" with problems in Conditions 4, 5, and 6; "vestibular loss" with poor performance in Conditions 5 and 6; and a "sensory selection dysfunction" with problems in Conditions 3, 4, 5, and 6, when people are unable to adapt to changing environments.

Identifying Functional Skills through Self-Report Questionnaires and Performance Tests

Examination of physical performance should be included in a postural control evaluation. Determining if there is a balance problem can be accomplished by using one or two of many performance tests that have been developed over the past 15 years. Self-report questionnaires provide a perception of skill ability, fear, or trust of capability. Appropriate functional performance tests coupled with self-report questionnaires may quantify and document the patient's status thereby helping to describe the person's functional abilities. The most common tests used are: timed Get Up and Go,[39] Berg Balance test,[40] Tinetti balance and Gait test,[38] physical performance test,[109] modified Gait-Abnormality Rating Scale (GARS-M),[110] modified seated step test,[111] 6-minute walk test,[112] Gait speed,[113] and modified outcome study SF–36.[114] Many of these tests were designed for elderly persons in relation to predicting falls and continuing wellness. Some were designed for a more global population of individuals with disabilities and others to document functional activities of daily living (ADLs) post-CVA. Balance skill tests such as standing on one leg, tandem stance, standing on toes, and standing on heels continue to be used for measuring balance.[115] However, it must be considered that these tests originally were normed on healthy young men and probably are not useful for elderly or disabled populations. Self-reporting measures have been developed and assist in describing function and often are used when nonprofessional staff are obtaining data.[116-120]

It is evident that selection of examination tools should be based on practicality of administering the test, the target population, and psychometric properties. We are continually learning the limits and appropriateness of such tests. Recently, comparisons among performance tests regarding sensitivity and specificity of tests, validity, reliability, appropriate settings to administer some tests, and establishing baseline performance of patients to more objectively document change in functional performance have been done.[121-127] Future studies should continue to identify new performance and functional balance tests for patients with various dysfunction and will contribute to evolving knowledge of our present tools.

INTERVENTION FOR BALANCE IMPAIRMENTS

General Considerations

A systems approach to treatment of balance deficits will be described. After an examination, an evaluation and interpretation of results must be done. Then functional limitations are identified and a problem list of impairments developed. At this point, goals and an intervention plan can be established.

Goals for treating patients with balance deficits should include: resolving, reducing, or preventing impairments; developing effective task-specific sensory and motor strategies for postural control; and retraining functional tasks with varying demands, under changing environmental contexts.[10] Examples of problems at the impairment level could be: asymmetry of static weight bearing (left greater than right); excessive sway around hips with feet 2 inches apart and eyes open; fused left ankle at 10 degrees of plantarflexion; nausea that exists following head movement; constant blurry vision in the left eye due to a cataract; no vibration sense on right foot bony prominence; and "jumpy" vision when fast turning to the left. Each problem should be described with specificity or in context, such as in what environment, after how much time, or lasting for how long.

When determining interventions, decisions whether to alleviate or compensate for the impairments need to be made.[10,41,128,129] For example, a physical therapist is not able to correct peripheral neuropathy or "fuzzy" vision due to macular degeneration in a patient. However, the patient should be instructed in the use of a cane to compensate for the neuropathy and "fuzzy" vision and strongly encouraged to see an ophthalmologist. Decisions regarding the possibility of immediate corrections of impairment versus treatment over time need to be decided by the therapist. An example of decision-making would be the treatment of a painful corn on the foot prior to teaching symmetry of weight bearing. Another example would be treating BPPN prior to addressing balance strategies. However, it is not uncommon to treat impairments in alignment, strength, ROM, visual-vestibular adaptation, or self-confidence in conjunction with strategy training. Allison and Fuller[41] provided examples of diagnoses as they relate to impairments from a systems model. Decisions whether to stimulate, facilitate, or force usage versus emphasizing substitution, compensation, and education were outlined.

Treatment should be progressive. To improve balance, there should be balance challenges. As the patient gains ability to do a task in a given environment, the challenge of the task or environment should be increased. Designing safe progressive balance exercises in a home program can be difficult. Safe exercise positions can be created, however, by having the patient perform activities next to walls, in corners, by counters or chairs in front of the patient, or by walking in halls. Careful thought about the demands on one system or multiple systems and the adding of slight balance challenges over time should be done. Strengthening exercises also have been used successfully with patients with neurologic deficits.[130] In addition, motor learning principles related to practice schedules and feedback should be considered when designing a home program.

Vestibular Impairments

Treatment of vestibular impairments has advanced over the past decade. Head injury, stroke, cerebellar insults, aging, and peripheral labyrinthine dysfunction are all etiologies of vestibular impairments with resulting balance limitations. It is imperative to screen for such impairments with subjective self-report of dizziness and/or imbalance with head movement. Enhancing the gain of the vestibulo-ocular reflex (VOR), or clinically the visual-vestibular ocular reflex (VVOR), is done by moving the head and attempting to focus on a stationary target. General eye/head coordination combinations are imposed progressively and are done to adapt the vestibular system or to make long-term changes in the neuronal response to sensory input.[65,73,131,132] Progressively increasing the challenge with increasing speed or duration, as well as changes in surface, environment, or cognitive demands should be planned to increase gaze stabilization during balance challenge when the head is moving.[129]

Treatment for BPPN (V) has been modified recently from habituating the symptoms by repeated movements in the provocative position, to a mechanical repositioning maneuver to move the displaced otoconia from the semicircular canal(s).[74,107,133,134] The posterior is the most commonly involved canal, however, recently, the horizontal and anterior canals also have been identified as being involved.[74,107,135]

Cognitive Impairments

Cognitive abilities and constraints are important to identify. Cognitive impairments can be a distraction and impede learning and limit balance progressions in treatment. The therapist should consider the patient's cognitive abilities to avoid overtaxing the CNS, resulting in poor performance in physical tasks such as balance. Balance challenge should progress by using more difficult cognitive challenges in combination with balance challenges as appropriate. Communicating and coordinating intervention strategies with speech pathologists, occupational therapists, and psychologists can enhance the overall outcome for the patient.

Motor Strategies

Treatment of poor, ineffective, or inappropriate motor strategies can be based on intervention for specific impairments hypothesized to cause abnormal patterns and/or by treating the abnormal movement strategies directly. Choosing the task to encourage the appropriate or needed strategy is important.[10] For example, with a patient with cerebellar impairments of past-pointing and an inability to control an ankle strategy while standing, the therapist may want to have the patient kneeling and to progressively decrease the patient's touch on the wall while exploring limits of stability around the knee against the mat. Babst boards, pivot turns, twisting around ankles, swaying to music, as well as standing and balancing on tilt boards are all examples of promoting ankle strategies. Hip strategy promotion can be done by progressing to tandem stand and walk, start/stop movements, feet static with low reaching tasks, and large and quick reaction balance tasks. Standing using visual biofeedback, instead of attention to proprioception or touch, when testing the limits of stability exploration and training needs to be incorporated. The amount of touch or physical feedback or assistance should be considered with balance strategy training. The therapist's touch provides actual proprioceptive feedback, thereby possibly giving false information to the patient as to the limits of stability and balance security. Home programs should be designed so physical assistance is given only when needed. The goal should be to do the task without touch, and only with close guard. Using goal-oriented tasks such as putting Post-It notes at designated levels for progressive excursion around the COM while standing, sitting, or kneeling can be effective in manipulating the environment and instructing the patient in designated balance challenges. Including variables of timing, expectation, scaling, and force in treatment is necessary. Incorporation of carrying various loads that may be unpredictable can contribute to predictive flexibility in strategy operations. Walking on different surfaces to encourage flexibility in strategies also is necessary. Walking on slopes, then demanding quick movements, encourages the demand of changing motor strategies from a stabilizing ankle strategy to a quick recovery of a hip strategy in order to get the COM over the base of support. Encouraging stepping strategies is important in many patients with CNS problems. For example, patients with cerebellar dysfunction, hemiplegia, or visual-perceptual disorders may not have effective stepping strategies. Using progressive stepping such as onto or from a piece of paper to plywood to a higher step coupled with step/stop exercises can be beneficial. Playing catch with a rolling or bounced ball that is outside of static limits of stability also can promote stepping. Actively stopping after an action to "break down" the action can encourage the patient to attend to using correct senses, components of graded movement, and correct strategies. Moving the feet for turning instead of twisting around the ankles should be practiced with a variety of goal-oriented tasks to promote stepping strategies. Home programs must be creative and challenging, however, safety always should be considered.

Sensory Strategies

Sensory strategy training is based on which senses are available and how the patient is selecting the sense for each environment. Again, the progression should be selection of available senses for motor strategy training, then introduction of second senses, and then movement to less accurate senses or more complicated motor activities or environments.

"Visual dependence" impairment is treated by encouraging attention to proprioception for correct orientation within various environments, then incorporating greater visually distracting environments. "Grounding" exercises can be progressed to combining eye/head movement thereby stimulating the vestibular system. Patients with vestibular impairments need encouragement to use compensating and more accurate senses of vision and proprioception appropriately with various tasks and environments so they do not develop maladaptive balance strategies. The remaining vestibular information can be enhanced by gradually reducing availability of visual and somatosensory inputs. "Surface over dependence" frequently seen in the elderly is treated by changing the surface gradients gradually and reducing visual cues. Voluntary ankle excursions with limits of stability exercises and providing knowledge of results using mirrors, a balance master, or body awareness and attention training can be practiced.

General Fitness

Long-term retention of impairments and ongoing strategy training should always be considered in the planning of intervention. Fitness training, tai chi classes, aerobic classes, swimming, home program exercise regimes, or other general movement programs should be incorporated into the treatment plan. Walking for conditioning and balance, considering the environment and need for supervision, also may be recommended.

SUMMARY

Specific evaluation methods, treatment goals, and intervention strategies reflect the physical therapist's underlying assumptions regarding both the neural basis for normal balance and underlying pathology contributing to instability in the patient. This chapter presented two models for the neural control of postural stability: the reflex/hierarchical model and the systems model. Examination and treatment interventions presented were based primarily on the systems model. Our knowledge of motor control has expanded over the past decade and we have gained greater breadth in examination tools and information for evaluating postural control (ie, balance) and understanding the neurophysiologic bases for intervention. Our therapeutic decisions are based on this continually developing knowledge.

CASE STUDY #1
Jane Smith

- *Age: 74 years*
- *Medical Diagnosis: Right hemiplegia, secondary to left CVA*
- *Status: 6 months post onset*
- *Practice Pattern 5D: Impaired Motor Function and Sensory Integrity Associated with Nonprogressive Disorders of the Central Nervous System—Acquired in Adolescence or Adulthood*

EXAMINATION AND EVALUATION

Functional Limitations

Mrs. Smith is unable to walk without a hemi-walker more than 30 feet or with one person for assistance. She is dependent on others to accomplish or assist her in most ADLs. She has difficulty with transfers, with standing, and needs assistance. She has poor awareness of her balance problems and, therefore, has poor appreciation regarding safety factors and is at risk for falls.

Impairments

Mrs. Smith has the following impairments: limited flexibility into ankle dorsiflexion, weakness in right extremities, poor sensory appreciation, right visual field deficit, problems with response selection and programming, and decreased motor function on the right side of her body, typically posturing in a total flexor synergy in the upper extremity.

PROGNOSIS/PLAN OF CARE

Goals

Treatment goals for Mrs. Smith are to:
1. Increase flexibility of right ankle
2. Increase strength of trunk and right lower extremity
3. Improve appreciation of symmetry in sitting and standing posture
4. Increase ability to bear weight on right lower extremity
5. Increase standing posture independence

6. Improve motor strategies for maintaining balance
7. Improve transfer ability
8. Improve appreciation of safety factors
9. Increase locomotion

Functional Outcomes

Following 3 months of intervention, Mrs. Smith will:

1. Demonstrate a 15 degree increase in ROM in right ankle dorsiflexion in assisted forward sway in standing
2. Achieve flexion of right hip and knee (without abduction) adequate for toe clearance with ankle foot orthosis (AFO) while walking in parallel bars
3. Achieve neutral alignment in sitting and standing in front of a mirror with eyes open (five of five attempts), then with eyes closed (two of five attempts)
4. Be able to bear weight equally on lower extremities while standing on bathroom scale or balance master three of five trials
5. Stand independently at the bathroom counter and remain standing for 30 seconds without assist
6. With hinged AFO locked at 5 degrees of dorsiflexion, demonstrate an adequate hip strategy during reaching 10 inches, four of five attempts
7. Transfer safely from her bed to a chair with supervision (with AFO) 100% of the time
8. Walk 100 feet. with her hemi-walker with minimal assistance two times per day

INTERVENTION

Because Mrs. Smith is seen by her physical therapist two times each month, her program will be designed as a home program to be done with supervision and assistance because of her cognitive and physical status. Her therapist will increase the balance challenge each visit compatible with her progress, caregiver ability, and goals. The program will be written for the caregiver and Polaroid pictures will be given to Mrs. Smith of each exercise and activity.

Increasing flexibility (Goal 1) of the ankle would best be done by standing with the ball of the right foot on a 1-inch thick book, keeping the heel on the floor. Manual stretching while supine would be an alternative, but would depend on the strength of her caregiver. For strengthening (Goal 2), active movements of knee extension and ankle dorsiflexion can be done sitting. Standing weight shifts, such as backward sway, promote dorsiflexion of the ankles and also can be used for strengthening. Sitting weight shifts (eg, backwards) promote knee flexion. Visual cues should be used. Standing and performing hip flexion with knee flexion should be included.

Verticality (Goals 3, and 4) exercises can be done sitting and standing with a mirror (eyes open and closed), with stripes on her shirt to align with stripes on the mirror, and use of physical margins to denote end goal of weight shift.

For greater weight bearing on the right leg (Goal 4) with use of the AFO, small excursions of ankle strategies in standing can be done. The stopped dorsiflexion at the ankle promotes knowledge of security that the ankle and knee will not collapse. This exercise should be done with verbal, visual, or physical feedback as to weight acceptance and knowledge of results (KR) that the goal was met. Steps with the right foot only 6 inches forward and stepping with the left foot can be done. This provides small but manageable challenges of weight acceptance. The right foot step length can be increased very slowly.

Standing independence (Goal 5) can be actively practiced by touching a counter while standing with progressive decrease of contact, and increased reaching and weight shifting in small excursions with her hand on the counter top to provide sensory input and stability.

Improvement of motor strategies (Goal 6) can be done sitting and standing. Sitting or standing and reaching with her left hand to various targets can encourage hip strategies. The distance to the targets should be progressively moved away from center in all directions exploring her limits of stability. Ankle strategies standing can be practiced with active weight shifts with feet slightly set apart with one foot slightly in front of the other, with shift/stop commands, reaching for high targets at various positions. Slight inclines can be used for verticality and ankle strategy exploration. Because of her moderate to severe impairments, the AFO should be used.

Transfers (Goals 7, and 8) can be done throughout the day during functional activities. Safety, proper foot placement, hand holds, weight shifts, and steps all should be done within the functional setting.

Walking (Goal 9) can be practiced within daily activities or as a form of exercise. Using principles of weight shifting, as described above, such as short 6 inch steps using the right leg and encouraging active hip flexion while discouraging external rotation with circumduction at the hip, could be done.

Motor learning principles should be used with program practice and scheduling. Goals of a specific walking destination with gradually increasing distances on level ground over the next 3 months should be stressed to provide maximum opportunity for success.

CASE STUDY #2
Daniel Johnson

- *Age: 59 years*
- *Medical Diagnosis: Parkinson's disease*
- *Status: 4 years post initial diagnosis*
- *Practice Pattern 5E: Impaired Motor Function and Sensory Integrity Associated with Progressive Disorders of the Central Nervous System*

EXAMINATION AND EVALUATION

Functional Limitations

Mr. Johnson is experiencing gradually diminishing mobility skills. These include problems in initiating transitions of movement and maintaining a normal stance and walking pattern. He does not rotate his trunk during active movement, resulting in en bloc movements. His slowed onset of postural adjustments in response to instability results in a tendency to fall forward.

Impairments

Mr. Johnson exhibits neurologic impairments impacting his function including dyskinesia, tremor, and bradykinesia. Musculoskeletal impairments are decreased flexibility and ROM particularly in the trunk and pelvis. Additionally, abnormal body alignment (posture) in sitting and standing is present. He stands with his head, trunk, and center of mass displaced forward. His balance is poor during walking. He exhibits signs of depression.

PROGNOSIS/PLAN OF CARE

Goals

Treatment goals for Mr. Johnson are to:
1. Increase ROM and flexibility in trunk and pelvis
2. Increase speed of response to perturbations to balance in upright positions
3. Improve speed and safety during transitions of movement
4. Improve posture and body alignment
5. Increase activity level

Functional Outcomes

Following 3 months of therapy, Mr. Johnson will:
1. Rotate his upper trunk in a sitting position to reach for an object placed out to the side and slightly behind him 100% of the time (increase actual LOS, to 70% of mechanical LOS)
2. Report increased ease of rolling for changing positions in bed
3. Initiate sit to stand maneuver from a chair within 5 seconds of a verbal signal
4. Walk an obstacle course of 25 feet with six objects to circumvent, within 5 minutes
5. Participate in a Parkinson's disease support group exercise program two times per week

INTERVENTION

Traditional physical therapy techniques for increasing flexibility of the trunk and particularly counter-rotation between the upper and lower trunk segments can be used. For example, while sitting, doing "windmill" exercises, touching opposite toes could be done. Verticality exercises using a mirror during transitions of movement such as coming to stand can be practiced. Leaning against a wall, standing, then moving away from the wall for his stooped posture could give tactile feedback. Raising his arms forward

Figure 11-10. Raising arms forward to encourage back extension, to improve vertical posture, and to facilitate an ankle strategy.

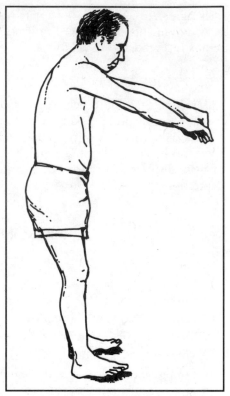

also could help strengthen his upper back muscles and contribute to his vertical posture (Figure 11-10). Coming to stand using various tactile targets can be used and balancing while sitting on a ball to get weight shift also would be helpful to promote the motor program of weight shifting. Rolling and coming to sit using functional tasks also can be done.

Limits of stability exercises should be incorporated, including standing on a slight incline (downward) to promote weight shifting backward. Ankle strategy exercises in all directions should be done to promote correction of imbalance starting with small excursions and progressing to greater distances of need for correction. A static force plate retraining system also may assist him for visual biofeedback of limits of stability training. A pegboard with various targets at various heights and widths can be used to encourage rotation and excursions of limits of stability. Timed exercises should be incorporated.

Walking with head turns and pivot turns around a figure 8 could be practiced to decrease his en bloc pattern of movement. Having visual targets and encouragement to move his head with his eyes should be done. Increasing his speed of movement to change his center of mass should be incorporated into the above exercises. Timed shifting could be done for goal training. Start/stop mixed with backward and sideways walking can be incorporated into his practice schedule. Stepping over small height objects can be done as a precursor to more functional tasks, such as walking up stairs. Changing walking surfaces should be done to promote flexibility in the use of sensory strategies.

Use of visual and/or auditory cues prior to a voluntary movement may assist Mr. Johnson with initiating movement and increasing speed of performance.

CASE STUDY # 3
Shirley Teal

- *Age: 21 years*
- *Medical Diagnosis: Traumatic brain injury*
- *Status: 4 months post injury*
- *Practice Pattern 5D: Impaired Motor Function and Sensory Integrity Associated with Nonprogressive Disorders of the Central Nervous System—Acquired in Adolescence or Adulthood*

EXAMINATION AND EVALUATION

Functional Limitations

Functionally, Ms. Teal is limited to minimal assist with transfers and standing and is unable to walk. Her mobility is limited to household wheelchair and limited community mobility.

Impairments

Neuromuscular impairments include positional vertigo with positive left Hallpike, visual dependence, increased muscle tone on the right, decreased ROM in right lower extremity joints, increased stiffness, and decreased strength of right extremities. Weight distribution in static and dynamic balance is poor with listing to the left and poor weight transfer to the right. Balance is poor. Problems with initiation and coordination of movement, concentration, attention, memory, and behavioral outbursts impact her goals and interventions.

PROGNOSIS/PLAN OF CARE

Goals

Treatment goals for Ms. Teal are to:
1. Demonstrate a resolved or greatly reduced left posterior canal BPPN
2. Increase ROM of right ankle dorsiflexion, hip and knee extension
3. Increase strength in right extremities
4. Increase symmetry during sitting and stance
5. Improve motor strategies during recovery from imbalance

6. Increase flexibility of sensory strategies
7. Ambulate with a wheeled walker
8. Perform independent transfers

Functional Outcomes

Following two months of intervention, Ms. Teal will:
1. Independently manage her dizziness
2. Perform five standing to semi-squat exercises while holding onto a support and retrieving an object from a bench
3. Achieve 75% of mechanical LOS to the right, forward, and backwards 75% of the time in sitting and standing
4. Stand independently with a cane for 1 minute, 100% of time
5. Walk and stand with a wheeled walker with close supervision on various surfaces and with recognition of change in surfaces to recover balance 75% of time
6. Complete all transfers with only verbal cues

INTERVENTIONS

Treatment of her left posterior canal BPPN (Goal 1) is accomplished by administering a left canalithic repositioning procedure (CRP) with the usual precautions. Considering her poor memory and compliance with precautions post-treatment, more than one procedure may be necessary. Other canals should be checked for positive reactions, if vertigo persists. Habituation of provoking positions should be done if resolution of BPPN cannot be resolved with CRPs. Treatment of BPPN should be done immediately considering the impact of vertigo on attention.

Treatment for right plantarflexion contracture (Goal 2) should be conservative considering the short time post onset. This would include stretching in standing, as tolerated. However, considering the severity of contracture, cognitive deficits, and potential gain, botulinum injections into plantarflexors, nerve blocks, or surgery (SPLAT or Z Plasty) should not be ruled out as future interventions.

Strengthening and motor strategy training (Goals 3, and 4) could be done with similar activities as in Case Study 1. Visual dependence training should begin after treatment of BPPV to allow the vestibular system to participate appropriately. Eyes closed training with safety of walls, counters, or bars should be done to force attention on proprioception for balance during limits of stability training. Progressing to standing on various surfaces to facilitate flexibility in sensory strategies should be done.

Standing balance and ambulation training (Goals 5 through 7) should be very structured considering impairments of ankle ROM so maladaptive motor behaviors will not be promoted unnecessarily. However, accommodating to the contracture with wedging could be done to establish symmetry of weight bearing. Practicing ankle and hip strategies and stepping strategies with a short 6 inch step on the right and increasing the excursions to a full step with weight acceptance on the right could be incorporated. Practice turning to the right, keeping the right foot slightly behind the left could be done. Stepping onto visual targets for stepping strategies and reaching high and low and left and right for hip and ankle strategies also can be included in treatment. A wheeled walker should be used to promote symmetry of the trunk, upper extremity control, and increased step lengths. Later a cane could be used. A quad cane on the left is not recommended since it would encourage asymmetry because of the ease of putting weight on it rather than the right side of the body.

Transfers in and out of her wheelchair (Goal 8) should be incorporated into her daily routine with caregivers being consistent about verbal and tactile cues. Careful documentation of her ability to assist and perform specific transfers will assist in progressing her from moderate to minimal assistance and, eventually, to total independence.

CASE STUDY #4
Shawna Wells

- *Age: 4 years*
- *Medical Diagnosis: Cerebral palsy, spastic quadriparesis, mild mental retardation*
- *Status: Onset at birth*
- *Practice Pattern 5C: Impaired Motor Function and Sensory Integrity Associated with Nonprogressive Disorders of the Central Nervous System—Congenital Origin or Acquired in Infancy or Childhood*

EXAMINATION AND EVALUATION

Functional Limitations

Shawna demonstrates delayed and slowed protective responses to changes in COM with reliance on stepping strategies. She requires minimal assistance walking with posterior control walker, however, she can only walk on smooth surfaces and moves too slowly to keep up with her nondisabled peers. Shawna has difficulty with learning and retaining new motor skills.

Impairments

Neuromuscular impairments include decreased coordination and reciprocation of the lower extremities and inability to sustain full knee extension and dorsiflexion during stance. Musculoskeletal impairments include decreased ROM in ankle dorsiflexion, as well as in knee extension and trunk flexibility. Shawna has difficulty with selective attention and memory, and her performance on IQ tests indicates mild mental retardation.

PROGNOSIS/PLAN OF CARE

Goals

Treatment goals are for Shawna to:
1. Increase flexibility of plantarflexors, hamstrings, and trunk
2. Increase lower extremity reciprocation

3. Improve motor strategy execution
4. Improve motor control of knee extension in stance
5. Improve sitting and standing balance
6. Improve sensory strategy organization

Functional Outcomes

Following 3 months of treatment, Shawna will:
1. Put on socks with minimal assist in floor sitting
2. Perform five "windmill" exercises (ie, right hand to left toe, left hand to right toe) in standing with assist during her adaptive physical education class
3. March in time to slow music for 30 seconds while holding her walker
4. Regain her balance in standing following slight displacements left or right without using a stepping strategy, three of five trials (while holding onto her walker)
5. Maintain knee extension on either leg while lifting the opposite leg up on a step five times in succession while walking up stairs holding the rail
6. Sway independently forward and backward in her walker using an ankle strategy, three or five trials
7. Walk safely down a hallway with her walker at school 100% of time when lights are dimmed

INTERVENTION

Active-assistive exercises to increase active ROM in gastrocnemius/soleus and hamstring muscle groups should be stressed. Daily functional activities should be devised to maintain ROM so that daily stretching does not have to be done. An example would be having Shawna sit in long sitting with sandbags over her knees in the classroom or at home for 10 minutes each day to maintain hamstring elongation. If her hamstrings become tighter, her program can be modified to increase the duration or frequency of stretch.

Activities in sitting and standing to increase Shawna's limits of stability should be included in her program. These activities would include passive, active, anticipated, and unanticipated displacements.

A variety of sensory inputs should be incorporated to increase awareness of her body parts and position in space as well as to challenge her balance. Examples would be walking barefoot, walking on different textures, and walking in rooms with variable lighting available using her walker. Activities that are of high interest and motivating to Shawna should be used. One example is the use of music, which she enjoys. Practicing active weight shifts to music (dancing) and reciprocation (marching) will be more successful if she is motivated and attending to the task.

CASE STUDY # 5
Robert Anderson

- *Age: 38 years*
- *Medical Diagnosis: Incomplete T9-10 spinal cord injury with left radial nerve damage*
- *Status: 6 months post injury*
- *Practice Pattern 5H: Impaired Motor Function, Peripheral Nerve Integrity, and Sensory Integrity Associated with Nonprogressive Disorders of the Spinal Cord*

EXAMINATION AND EVALUATION

Functional Limitations

Functional limitations include difficulty with transferring from sit to stand with knee ankle foot orthoses (KAFOs) to bed, floor, bath, car, and wheelchair. Mr. Anderson is unable to stand independently but must use forearm crutches and KAFOs. He is unable to walk in the community with KAFOs.

Impairments

Mr. Anderson has loss of sensation below T10 and is at risk for problems with skin integrity. He has increasing muscle spasms and stiffness in the lower extremities, weakness in radial nerve innervated muscles, loss of muscle power in the lower extremities, and poor endurance.

PROGNOSIS/PLAN OF CARE

Goals

Treatment goals for Mr. Anderson are to:
1. Demonstrate knowledge and awareness of skin integrity risks
2. Demonstrate knowledge and awareness of problems associated with decreased ROM
3. Demonstrate knowledge of secondary impairments
4. Perform all transfers independently
5. Don and stand with KAFOs independently
6. Walk with crutches and KAFOs for short distances during community outings

Functional Outcomes

Following 3 months of intervention, Mr. Anderson will:
1. Recite accurate information regarding risks associated with skin integrity and demonstrate ability to relieve pressure while sitting and lying and inspect skin 100% of time

2. Recite accurate information regarding risk of contractures and demonstrate ROM of all joints correctly

3. Recite information regarding secondary impairments such as decreased cardiovascular fitness and infections

4. Demonstrate independence in all transfers 100% of time

5. Demonstrate donning and coming to stand with KAFOs and forearm crutches from wheelchair, bed, and captain's chair independently, 90% of time

6. Demonstrate walking with crutches and KAFOs 300 feet., turning around both on level surfaces and slight inclines without loss of balance

INTERVENTION

Flexibility exercises, education, and training regarding ROM should be done each visit. Education regarding pressure relief techniques and risks of skin breakdown and importance of visual skin checks also should be done. Information regarding the risks of fractures, cardiovascular complications, and other secondary complications should be provided.

Activities to promote weight shifting and balance should be included in Mr. Anderson's physical therapy intervention. He will need to learn to rely more on visual and vestibular information for balance. His intact visual and vestibular systems will assist him in compensating for loss of somatosensory information below the level of his spinal cord lesion. He will be able to use this intact sensory information to accurately perceive his position in space, to maintain balance, and to initiate appropriate postural responses and strategies. He will need to rely on his upper extremities, however, to provide the stability and postural reactions necessary for efficient movement.

Training for transfers and functional independence such as putting his wheelchair in and out of car would be emphasized. Endurance training such as using a supported treadmill system and a weight training program also could be included in his intervention.

REFERENCES

1. Sherrington C. *The Integrative Action of the Nervous System.* 2nd ed. New Haven, Conn: Yale University; 1947.

2. Bernstein N. *The Coordination and Regulation of Movement.* London, England: Pergamon; 1967.

3. Cordo P, Nashner L. Properties of postural adjustments associated with rapid arm movements. *J Neurophysiol.* 1982;47:24-287.

4. Schmidt RA. *Motor Control and Learning.* 2nd ed. Champaign, Ill: Human Kinetics; 1988.

5. Gordon J. Assumptions underlying physical therapy intervention: theoretical and historical perspectives. In: Carr JH, Shepherd, RB, Gordon J, et al. eds. *Movement Sciences: Foundations for Physical Therapy in Rehabilitation.* Rockville, Md: Aspen; 1987:1-30.

6. Horak F, Shumway-Cook A. Clinical implications of posture control research. In: Duncan P, ed. *Balance, Proceedings of the APTA Forum.* Alexandria, Va: APTA; 1990.

7. Horak FB, Henry SM, Shumway-Cook A. Postural perturbations: new insights for treatment of balance disorders. *Phys Ther.* 1997;77:517-533.

8. Woollacott M, Shumway-Cook A. Changes in posture control across the life span: a systems approach. *Phys Ther.* 1990;70:799-807.

9. Perry SB. Clinical implications of a dynamical systems theory. *Neurology* Report. 1998;22:4-10.

10. Shumway-Cook A, Woollacott MH. *Motor Control: Theory and Practical Application.* 2nd ed. Philadelphia, Pa: Lippincott Williams & Wilkins; 2001.

11. Newton RA. Contemporary issues and theories of motor control: assessment of movement and posture. In: Umphred DA, ed. *Neurological Rehabilitation.* 4th ed. St Louis, Mo: Mosby; 2001.

12. Weisz S. Studies in equilibrium reaction. *J Nerv Ment Dis.* 1938;88:150-162.

13. McGraw M. *Neuromuscular Maturation of the Human Infant.* New York, NY: Hafner; 1945.

14. Martin JP. *The Basal Ganglia and Posture.* London, England: Pitman Med Publ; 1967.

15. Bobath B. *Abnormal Postural Reflex Activity Caused by Brain Lesions.* London, England: Heinemann Publ; 1975.

16. Wyke B. The neurological basis of movement—a developmental review. In: Holt K, ed. *Movement and Child Development.* Philadelphia, Pa: Lippincott; 1975:19-33.

17. Dichgans J, Diener HC. The contribution of vestibulo-spinal mechanisms to the maintenance of human upright posture. *Acta Otolargyngol (Stokh).* 1989;107:338-345.

18. Winter DA. *Biomechanics and Motor Control of Human Movement.* New York, NY: Wiley; 1990.

19. Patla AE. Visual control of human locomotion. In: Patla AE, ed. *Adaptability of Human Gait.* Amsterdam, Netherlands: Elsevier Science Publ BV; 1991: 55-97.

20. Gordon J, Ghez C. Muscle receptors and spinal reflexes: the stretch reflex. In Kandel E, Schwartz JH, Jessell TM, eds. *Principles of Neuroscience.* 3rd ed. New York, NY: Elsevier; 1991: 564-580.

21. Martin JH, Jessell TM. Anatomy of the somatic sensory system. In: Kandel E, Schwartz JH, Jessel TM, eds. *Principles of Neuroscience.* 3rd ed. New York, NY: Elsevier, 1991.

22. Goodale MA, Milner AD. Separate visual pathways for perception and action. *Trends in Neurosci.* 1992;15:20-25.

23. Horak FB, Shupert CL. Role of the vestibular system in postural control. In: Herdman SJ, ed. *Vestibular Rehabilitation (Contemporary Perspectives in Rehabilitation).* 2nd ed. Philadelphia, Pa: FA Davis; 2000.

24. Nashner LM, McCollum G. The organization of human postural movements: a formal basis basic and experimental synthesis. *Behav Brain Sci.* 1985;8:135-172.

25. Horak FB, Nashner L. Central programming of postural movements: adaptation to altered surface configurations. **J Neurophysiol.** 1986;55:1369-1381.

26. McIlroy WE, Maki BE. Adaptive changes to compensatory stepping responses. *Gait and Posture.* 1995;3:43-50.

27. Macpherson JM. The force constraint strategy for stance is independent of prior experience. *Exp Brain Res.* 1994;101:397-405.

28. Shupert CL, Horak FB, Black FO. Hip sway associated with vestibulopathy. *J Vestib Res.* 1994;4:231-244.

29. Brunnstrom S. Motor testing procedures in hemiplegia: based on sequential recovery stages. *Phys Ther.* 1966;46:357-375.

30. Milani Comparetti A, Gidoni E. Routine developmental examination in normal and retarded children. *Dev Med Child Neurol.* 1967;9:631-638.

31. Stockmyer S. An interpretation of the approach of Rood to the treatment of neuromuscular dysfunction. *Am J Phys Med.* 1967;46:950-955.

32. Bayley N. *Bayley Scales of Infant Development*. San Antonio, Tex: Psychological Corporation; 1969.

33. Fiorentino MR. *Reflex Testing Methods for Evaluating CNS Development*. Springfield, Ill: Charles Thomas; 1973.

34. Bobath B. *Adult Hemiplegia: Evaluation and Treatment*. London, England: Heinemann Publishing; 1974.

35. Folio RM, Fewell RR. *Peabody Developmental Motor Scales*. Allen, Tex: DLM Teaching Resources; 1983.

36. Carr JH, Shepherd RB, Nordholm L, et al. Investigation of a new motor assessment scale for stroke patients. *Phys Ther*. 1985;65:175-180.

37. Gentile A. Skill acquisition: action movements and neuromotor processes. In: Carr J, Shepherd R, eds. *Movement Science: Foundations for Physical Therapy in Rehabilitation*. 2nd ed. Rockville, Md: Aspen Systems; 2000:111-187.

38. Tinetti M. Performance oriented assessment of mobility problems in elderly patients. *J Am Geriatr Soc*. 1986;34:119-122.

39. Podsiadlo D, Richardson S. The Timed "Up and Go" test: a test of basic functional mobility for frail elderly persons. *J Am Geriatr Soc*. 1991;39:142-148.

40. Berg K, Wood-Dauphinee SL, Williams JT. Measuring balance in the elderly: validation of an instrument. *Can J Public Health*. 1992;83:9-11.

41. Allison L, Fuller K. Balance and vestibular disorders. In: Umphred DA, ed. *Neurological Rehabilitation*. 4th ed. St Louis, Mo: Mosby; 2001.

42. Horak FB. Balance strategies: 2000 and beyond. In: Reynold JP. *Balance Monograph*. Alexandria, Va: APTA;1997:13.

43. McCollum G, Leen T. Form and exploration of mechanical stability limits in erect stance. *J Motor Beh*. 1989;21:225-238.

44. Horak FB. Assumptions underlying motor control for neurologic rehabilitation. In: Lister MJ, ed. *Contemporary Management of Motor Control Problems: Proceedings of the II Step Conference*. Alexandria, Va: Foundation for Physical Therapy Inc; 1991.

45. Haley S. Sequential analyses of postural reactions in nonhandicapped infants. *Phys Ther*. 1986; 66:531-536.

46. Carr J, Shepherd R. *A Motor Relearning Programme for Stroke*. Rockville, Md: Aspen; 1983.

47. Umphred DA, Bly N, Lazaro RT, et al. Interventions for neurological disabilities. In: Umphred DA, ed. *Neurological Rehabilitation*. 4th ed. St Louis, Mo: Mosby; 2001.

48. Nashner LM. Adaptation of human movement to altered environments. *Trends Neurosci*. 1982;5:358-361.

49. Forssberg H, Hirschfeld H. Postural adjustments in sitting humans following external perturbations: muscle activity and kinematics. *Exp Brain Res*. 1994;97:515-527.

50. Horak FB, Shupert CL, Dietz V, et al. Vestibular and somatosensory contributions to responses to head and body displacement in stance. *Exp Brain Res*. 1994;100:93-106.

51. Peterka RJ, Black FO. Age-related changes in human posture control: sensory organization tests. *J Vestib Res*. 1990;1:73-85.

52. Maki BE, McIlroy WE. The role of limb movements in maintaining upright stance: the "change–in-support" strategy. *Phys Ther*. 1997;77:488-507.

53. Brown JE, Frank JS. Influence of event anticipation on postural actions accompanying voluntary movement. *Exp Br Res*. 1987;67:645-650.

54. McIlroy WE, Maki BE. Early activation of arm muscles follows external perturbations of upright stance. *Neurosci Lett*. 1995;184:177-180.

55. Nashner L. Adapting reflexes controlling the human posture. *Exp Brain Res*. 1976;26:59-72.

56. Nashner L, Woollacott M, Tuma G. Organization of rapid responses to postural and loco-motor-like perturbations of standing man. *Exp Brain Res.* 1979;36:463-476.

57. Di Fabio RP, Badke MB. Relationship of sensory organization to balance function in patients with hemiplegia. *Phys Ther.* 1990;70:543-548.

58. Herdman SJ. Advances in the treatment of vestibular disorders. *Phys Ther.* 1997;77:602-618.

59. Patla AE. Understanding roles of vision in the control of human locomotion. *Gait Posture.* 1997;5:54-69.

60. Pozzo T, Berthoz A, Lefort L, et al. Head stabilization during various locomotor tasks in humans: 2. Patients with bilateral peripheral vestibular deficits. *Exp Brain Res.* 1991; 85:208-217.

61. Kristinsdottir EK, Jarnlo G, Magnusson M. Aberrations in postural control, vibration sensation and some vestibular findings in healthy 64-92 year old subjects. *Scand J Rehab Med* 1997;29:257-265.

62. Scheiman M. *Understanding and Managing Vision Deficits: A Guide for Occupational Therapists.* Thorofare, NJ; SLACK Incorporated; 1997.

63. Coffey B, Seeger MA. *Visual-Vestibular Rehabilitation. Course Notes.* Victoria, British Columbia; 1998.

64. Chaikin LE. Disorders of vision and visual-perceptual hypofunction. In: Herdman SJ, ed. *Vestibular Rehabilitation.* 2nd ed. Philadelphia, Pa: FA Davis; 2000.

65. Herdman, SJ. Physical therapy assessment of vestibular hypofunction. In: Herdman SJ, ed. *Vestibular Rehabilitation.* 2nd ed. Philadelphia, Pa: FA Davis; 2000.

66. Gill-Body KM, Benianato M, Krebs DE. Relationship among balance impairments, functional performance, and disability in people with peripheral vestibular disorders. *Phys Ther.* 2000;80:748-758.

67. Bogduk N. Cervical causes of headache and dizziness. Chapter 22. In: Greive G, ed. *Modern Manual Therapy: The Vertebral Column.* 2nd ed. London, England: Churchill Livingstone; 1994:317-331.

68. Wrisley DM, Sparto PH, Whitney SL, et al. Cervicogenic dizziness: a review of diagnosis and treatment. *J Orthopaed Sports Phys Ther.* 2000;30:755-766.

69. Shumway-Cook A, Olmscheid R. A systems analysis of postural dyscontrol in traumatically brain-injured patients. *J Head Trauma Rehabil.* 1990;5:51-62.

70. Cavanaugh JT. Examining the patient with dizziness of unknown etiology. *Neurol.* 1999;247:100-113.

71. Shepard NT, Solomon D. Practical issues in the management of the dizzy and balance disorder patient. *The Otolaryngol Clinics North Am.* 2000;33:455-469.

72. Parikh SS, Bid CV. Vestibular rehabilitation. In: DeLisa JA, Gans BM, eds. *Rehabilitation Medicine: Principles and Practice.* 3rd ed. Philadelphia, Pa: Lippincott-Raven Publ; 1998.

73. Shumway-Cook A, Horak F. Vestibular rehabilitation: an exercise approach to managing symptoms of vestibular dysfunction. *Semin Hearing.* 1989;10:196-205.

74. Herdman SJ. Benign paroxysmal positional vertigo. In: Herdman SJ, ed. *Vestibular Rehabilitation.* 2nd ed. Philadelphia, Pa: FA Davis; 2000:451-475.

75. Andrews AW, Bohannon RW. Distribution of muscle strength impairments following stroke. *Clin Rehabil.* 2000;14:79-87.

76. Teixeira-Salmela LF, Olney SJ, Nadeau S, et al. Muscle strengthening and physical conditioning to reduce impairment and disability in chronic stroke survivors. *Arch Phys Med Rehabil.* 1999;80:1211-1218.

77. Badke MB, Di Fabio RP. Balance deficits in patients with hemiplegia: considerations for assessment and treatment. In: Duncan P, ed. *Balance: Proceedings of the APTA Forum.* Alexandria, Va: APTA; 1990.

78. Bastian AJ, Martin TA, Keating JG, et al. Cerebellar ataxia: abnormal control of interaction torques across multiple joints. *J Neurophysiol.* 1996;76:492-509.

79. Horak FB, Nashner LM, Nutt JG. Postural instability in Parkinson's disease: motor coordination and sensory organization. *Neurology Report.* 1988;12:54-55.

80. Horak FB, Nutt JG, Nashner LM. Postural inflexibility in parkinsonian subjects. *J Neurol Sci.* 1995;111:46-58.

81. Duncan P. Physical therapy assessment. In: Rosenthal M, Bond M, Griffith ER, et al, eds. *Rehabilitation of the Adult and Child with Traumatic Brain Injury.* 2nd ed. Philadelphia, Pa: FA Davis; 1990.

82. Brown LA, Shumway-Cook A, Woollacott MH. Attentional demands and postural recovery: the effects of aging. *J Gerontol.* 1999;54:165-171.

83. Chen H-C, Schultz AB, Ashton-Miller, et al. Stepping over obstacles: dividing attention impairs performance of old more than young adults. *J Gerontol Med Sci.* 1996;51:116-122.

84. Marsh AP, Geel SE. The effect of age on the attentional demands of postural control. *Gait Posture.* 2000:12:105-113.

85. Melzer I, Benjuya N, Kaplanski J. Age-related changes of postural control: effect of cognitive tasks. *Gerontol.* 2001;47:189-194.

86. Quintana LA. Evaluation of perception and cognition. In: Trombly CA, ed. *Occupational Therapy for Physical Dysfunction.* 4th ed. Baltimore, Md: Williams & Wilkins; 1995:201-223.

87. Wade MG, Jones G. The role of vision and spatial orientation in the maintenance of posture. *Phys Ther.* 1997;77:619-628.

88. Geurts ACH, Ribbers GM, Knoop JA, et al. Identification of static and dynamic postural instability following traumatic brain injury. *Arch Phys Med Rehabil.* 1996;77:639-644.

89. LaJoie Y, Teasdale N, Bard C, et al. Attentional demands for static and dynamic equilibrium. *Exp Brain Res.* 1993;97:139-144.

90. Morris M, Iansek R, Smithson F, et al. Postural instability in Parkinson's disease: a comparison with and without a concurrent task. *Gait Posture.* 2000;12:205-216.

91. Brown RG, Marsden CD. Dual task performance and processing resources in normal subjects and patients with Parkinson's disease. *Brain.* 1991;114:215-231.

92. Frzovic D, Morris ME, Vowels L. Clinical tests of standing balance: performance of persons with multiple sclerosis. *Arch Phys Med Rehabil.* 2000;81:215-221.

93. Krupp LB, Elkins LE. Fatigue and declines in cognitive functioning in multiple sclerosis. *Neurology.* 2000: 10;55:934-9.

94. Chong RK, Jones CL, Horak FB. Postural set for balance control is normal in Alzheimer's but not in Parkinson's disease. *J Gerontol A Biol Sci Med Sci.* 1999;54:M129-35.

95. Alexander N. Postural control in older adults. *JAGS.* 1994;42:93-108.

96. Lawler KA, Terregino CA. Guidelines for evaluating and education of adult patients with mild traumatic brain injuries in an acute care hospital setting. *J Head Trauma Rehabil.* 1996;11:18-28.

97. Gronwall DMA. Paced auditory serial addition test. *Percept Mot Skills.* 1997;44:367-373.

98. Stroop JR. Studies of interference in serial verbal reactions. *J Exp Psychol.* 1935;18:643-662.

99. Gentilini M, Paldo N, Schoenruber R. Assessment of attention in mild head injury. In: Levin HS, Eisenberg HM, Benton AL, eds. *Mild Head Injury.* New York, NY: Oxford University Press; 1989:163-175.

100. Schmitter-Edgecomb M. Effects of traumatic brain injury on cognitive performance: an attentional resource hypothesis in search of data. *J Head Trauma Rehabil.* 1996;11:17-30.

101. Sohlberg MM, Mateer CA. *Introduction to Cognitive Rehabilitation.* New York, NY: Gilford Press; 1989.

102. Geurts ACH, Knoop JA, van Limbeek J. Is postural control associated with mental functioning in the persistent post concussion syndrome? *Arch Phys Med Rehabil.* 1999;80:144-149.

103. Shumway-Cook A, Woollacott M. Attentional demands and postural control: the effect of sensory context. *J Gerontol A Biol Sci Med Sci.* 2000;55:10-16.

104. Light KE. Information processing for motor performance in aging adults. *Phys Ther.* 1990;70:820-826.

105. Inglis JT, Horak FB, Shupert CL, et al. The importance of somatosensory information in triggering and scaling automatic postural responses in humans. *Exp Brain Res.* 1994;101:159-164.

106. Shumway-Cook A, Horak F. Assessing the influence of sensory interaction on balance. *Phys Ther.* 1986;66:1548-1550.

107. El-Kashlan HK, Telian SA. Diagnosis and initiating treatment for peripheral system disorders; imbalance and normal hearing. *Otolaryngol Clin North Am.* 2000;33:563-577.

108. Nashner LM. Sensory, neuromuscular, and biomechanical contributions to human balance. In: Duncan P, ed. *Balance: Proceedings of the APTA Forum.* Alexandria, Va: APTA; 1990:5-12.

109. Reuben DB, Sir AL. An objective measure of physical function of elderly outpatients: the physical performance test. *J Am Geriatr Soc.* 1990;38:1105-1112.

110. VanSwearingen JM, Paschal KA, Bonino P, et al. The modified Gait Abnormality Rating Scale for recognizing the risk of recurrent falls in community-dwelling elderly adults. *Phys Ther.* 1996;76:994-1002.

111. Smith EL, Gilligan C. Physical activity prescription for the older adult. **The Physician and Sportsmedicine.** 1983;11:91-101.

112. Butland RJ, Pang J, Gross ER, et al. Two-, six-, and 12 minute walking tests in respiratory disease. *Br Med J (Clin Res Ed).* 1982;284:1607-1608.

113. Wolfson L, Judge J. Strength is a minor factor in balance, gait, and the occurrence of falls. *J Ger Series A.* 1995;50:64-67.

114. Ware JE, Sherbourne CD. The MOS 36-Item Short-Form Health Survey (SF-36), I: conceptual framework and item selection. *Med Care.* 1992;30:473-483.

115. Graybiel A, Fregly AR. A new quantitative ataxia test battery. *Acta Otolaryngol.* 1996;61:292-312.

116. Jette AM, Davis AR, Cleary PD, et al. The Functional Status Questionnaire: reliability and validity when used in primary care. *J Gen Intern Med.* 1986;1:143-149.

117. Tager IB, Swanson A, Satarino WA. Reliability of physical performance and self-reported functional measures in an older population. *J Gerontol.* 1998;53:295-300.

118. Washburn RA, Smith KW, Jette AM, et al. The Physical Activity Scale for the Elderly (PASE): development and evaluation. *J Clin Epidemiol.* 1993;46:153-162.

119. Tinetti ME, Richman D, Powell L. Falls efficacy as a measure of fear of falling. *J Gerontol.* 1990;45:239-243.

120. Jacobson GP, Newman CW. The development of the dizziness handicap inventory. *Arch Otolaryngol Head Neck Surg.* 1990;116;424-427.

121. VanSwearingen JM, Brach JS. Making geriatric assessment work: selecting useful measures. *Phys Ther.* 2001;81:1233-1252.

122. Shumway-Cook A, Brauer S, Woollacott M. Predicting the probability for falls in community-dwelling older adults using the Timed Up & Go Test. *Phys Ther.* 2000;80:896-903.

123. Harada N, Chiu V, Damron-Rodriguez J, et al. Screening for balance and mobility impairment in elderly individuals living in residential care facilities. *Phys Ther.* 1995;75:462-9.

124. Shields RK. Evaluation of health-related quality of life in individuals with vestibular disease using disease-specific and general outcome measures. *Phys Ther.* 1997;77:890-903.

125. Di Fabio RP, Seay R. Use of the "Fast Evaluation of Mobility, Balance, and Fear" in elderly community dwellers: validity and reliability. *Phys Ther.* 1997;77:904-917.

126. Creel GL, Light KE, Thigpen MT. Concurrent and construct validity of scores on the Timed Movement Battery. *Phys Ther.* 2001;81:789-798.

127. Rozzini R, Frisoni GB, Bianchetti A, et al. Physical performance test and activities of daily living scales in the assessment of health status in elderly people. *J Am Geriatr Soc.* 1993;41:1109-1113.

128. Duncan P, Badke MB. Determinants of abnormal motor control. In: Duncan P, Badke MB, eds. *Stroke Rehabilitation: The Recovery of Motor Control.* Chicago, Ill: Year Book Medical Publ; 1987:135–159.

129. Seeger MA. *PT 611: Balance Disorders. Graduate Program in Physical Therapy.* Memphis, Tenn: University of Memphis; 2001.

130. Bohannon RW, Walsh S. Nature, reliability, and predictive value of muscle performance measures in patients with hemiparesis following stroke. *Arch Phys Med Rehabil.* 1992; 73:721-725.

131. Gizzi M. The efficacy of vestibular rehabilitation for patients with head trauma. *J Head Trauma Rehabil.* 1995;10:60-77.

132. Norre ME. Rationale of rehabilitation treatment for vertigo. *Am J Otolaryngol.* 1987;8:31-35.

133. Brandt T, Steddin S, Daroff RB. Therapy for benign paroxysmal positioning vertigo, revisited. *Neurol.* 1994;44:796-800.

134. Epley JM. The canalithic repositioning procedure; for treatment of benign paroxysmal positional vertigo. *Otolaryngol Head Neck Surg.* 1992;107:399-404.

135. Appiani GC, Catania G, Gagliardi M. A liberatory maneuver for the treatment of horizontal canal paroxysmal positional vertigo. *Otol Neurotol.* 2001;22:66-69.

Spasticity and Motor Control

Carol A. Giuliani, PhD, PT

INTRODUCTION

We think of normal movement as the ability to perform a well-coordinated movement by controlling multiple extremity segments in space and arriving at a target with some degree of accuracy and control. Performing even the simplest movement often is a frustrating task for patients with neurologic disorders. To choose an intervention for these patients, the therapist must first identify the underlying movement problem(s). Disorders of spasticity and tone are often associated with movement problems in patients with upper motor neuron lesions; however, the role of spasticity in movement dysfunction is not well understood. As is reflected in this book, movement problems are complex, and therapists need to understand these complexities as current research and clinical evidence become available. This chapter will address the topics of spasticity and muscle tone, as they may be associated with movement abilities and with interventions in patients with pathology involving the nervous system.

THEORETICAL FRAMEWORK

For years therapists have been operating under the assumption that spasticity is the primary cause of abnormal motor control. The clinical assumptions we make are important because they bias our choices for examination, evaluation, and intervention. In the past 10 years, many therapists and other scientists have questioned our traditional assumptions and the causal relationship between spasticity and movement. Recently, research studies have begun to explore this relationship, and results suggest that spasticity alone cannot explain the movement problems exhibited by patients with neurologic disorders. Some of the difficulty in understanding the relationship between spasticity and motor control has been because of the multiple definitions of spasticity, the confusion between spasticity and muscle tone, the difficulty of adequate measurements, and a lack of research designed to test our clinical assumptions.

Katz and Rymer suggested that muscle tone related issues are central in origin and that spasticity is a peripherally mediated phenomenon.[1] These two mechanisms should not be confused as they relate to motor control. Our terminology increases confusion of the issue because therapists and other professionals often use the terms spasticity and tone to mean the same thing. I will try to clarify these terms because they become important to understanding the relationship between spasticity and motor control. Lance defined spasticity as a velocity-dependent hyperexcitability of the stretch reflex.[2] In contrast, Bobath described spasticity as a phenomenon that can be assessed by observing the patient's movements.[3,4] The Bobath definition of spasticity includes hypertonus caused by tonic reflexes, muscle co-contraction, and abnormal movement patterns.

Muscle tone typically is defined as the state of muscle contraction and examined physiologically by electromyography (EMG) and clinically by the resistance to passive stretch.[2] Hypertonus is a description of excessive muscle activity and hypotonus is inadequate or less than expected muscle activity. Clinicians also are aware that muscle tone changes readily with position, posture, activity (resting or during movement), excitement, illness, and other factors. The fluctuations in tone related to internal or external factors also contribute to difficulties measuring muscle tone. Because of the dynamic nature of tone, therapists often are unsure about when and under what conditions they should measure or describe tone. Therapists may describe tone when a patient is at rest, when standing, during movement, during different states of alertness, or during a specific task. The problem is that it would be difficult to measure tone as a resistance to movement in each of these conditions. Likewise the level of tone during one condition may not predict the same level of tone during another condition. Katz and Rymer suggested that muscle tone is a result of the central nervous system (CNS) output that occurs with spontaneous and voluntary movement, as opposed to spasticity that is a reflexive mechanism that increases muscle activity in response to a sensory stimulus (ie, muscle stretch).[1] Spasticity and tone therefore do not describe the same phenomenon.

What Is the Relationship Between Spasticity and Voluntary Movement?

Results from studies that examined or discussed the relationship between spasticity and movement ability provide conflicting evidence. Much of this conflict can be explained by differing definitions of spasticity. If spasticity is defined as the presence of abnormal movement patterns, then spasticity may be strongly related to movement function. On the other hand, if spasticity is defined as a hyperactive velocity dependent response to muscle stretch, then it may have a weak association with movement function. In addition to the problem of different definitions, methods of measurement may affect study outcomes.[5-10] Although the Modified Ashworth Scale (MAS)[11] is the most commonly used clinical measure of spasticity, two recent studies questioned the use of this measure.[12,13] Pandyan et al[13] suggested that the Ashworth scale can be used to measure resistance to passive movement, but not spasticity, because resistance to movement may be the result of several factors, only one of which is spasticity. Recently, Shaw et al[6] examined the relationship among several clinical measures of tone and spasticity (ie, the Modified Ashworth Scale–MAS[11], handheld dynamometry[7], the H-reflex, and the pendulum test[9]). Shaw defined spasticity as only one dimension of hypertonicity. In his study, tone is the umbrella term and spasticity (hyperreflexia) is one component. Although all the measures in this study showed differences between the hemiplegic and the less affected extremity in patients following a cerebrovascular accident (CVA), the measures were not necessarily related to each other. Furthermore, clinical measures of spasticity and tone were not related to laboratory measures. These findings support the notion that any one measure that assesses some aspect of tone or spasticity is not necessarily related to other aspects. It appears that tone is multidimensional and the dimensions are related differentially. The results of this study also suggest that we do not understand just what it is that we are measuring and how these dimensions of spasticity and tone are related to movement ability.

To help understand the role of spasticity related to movement ability, consider the consequences of a brain lesion. As discussed in other chapters of this book, these patients may have many impairments, such as cognitive deficits, cardiovascular endurance problems, sensory loss, paresis, abnormal tone, spasticity, and other sensorimotor changes depending on the site and extent of the lesion. All or any of these impairments, not just tone or spasticity, can alter movement performance and functional ability. Lesion effects and patient examination may be organized using the Nagi model of disablement.[14] In this model, there is a pathology that, for this discussion, is a CNS lesion. The pathology results in associated impairments such as those listed above, and then these impairments may contribute to losses in function, and eventually to disability. Subsequently, reduced function may create secondary and tertiary impairments. The literature suggests that there is little evidence of a direct or causal relationship between spasticity and movement when spasticity is defined according to Lance et al.[2,15-24] For example, if we tested the severity of spasticity in a child with cerebral palsy, it may not tell us anything about the movement ability of that child.[22] Consistent with earlier literature, a recent study examined factors associated with loss of dexterity after a CVA during a spatial temporal arm-tracking task.[25] In this study, dexterity was defined as difficulties with muscle coordination. Difficulty with dexterity appeared to be more related to problems controlling agonist muscle activation than to spasticity or muscle co-contraction. It appears that difficulties with control of muscle tone at rest or during movement may be associated with movement problems.

Results of studies that examined medical treatments intended to reduce spasticity and improve function also raised questions regarding the relationship between spasticity and movement. Posterior dorsal rhizotomy is a surgical procedure used with children who have cerebral palsy to reduce spasticity by severing dorsal rootlets entering the spinal cord.[26] This procedure decreases afferent stimuli to both spinal segmental and supraspinal centers from all sensory afferents, not just afferents from the muscle spindle. Essentially the result is a decreased neural drive to motor neuronal pools, interneurons, and other areas of the CNS. The initial rationale for rhizotomy was that by reducing spasticity, function would improve, or that reduction in spasticity would give therapists a window of opportunity to improve function. Our work and that of others show that initially after the dorsal rhizotomy spasticity is either reduced or eliminated and passive range of motion (ROM) usually increases in selective joints.[19, 26-28] However, there is not necessarily an immediate improvement in movement patterns or voluntary movement ability. Abnormal movement patterns, such as toe walking, may remain after the rhizotomy. Many children do experience improvements in movement patterns, but usually after periods of intense physical therapy, and even then abnormal movement patterns may persist. The persistent abnormal patterns represent the central motor control problems of regulating the timing and magnitude of muscle activity that are unaffected by reduced neural drive. Understandably, the children still have cerebral palsy. They continue to have the accompanying motor control and musculoskeletal problems that sometimes require therapy or corrective orthopedic surgery in order to improve movement or personal care.

Several current pharmacological treatments such as botulinum toxin (Botox,Allergan Inc, Irvine, Calif)[29-33] and baclofen[34-37] are intended to reduce spasticity and improve function. The research evidence indicates that improvement in function after pharmacological treatment also is associated with intense periods of physical therapy after and sometimes before the treatment. Botox is injected into target muscles and works to reduce muscle activity by blocking acetylcholine release at the neuromuscular junction. Spasticity and tone are reduced because of the localized reduction in muscle activity without affecting the CNS control parameters of movement. The timing of the effects varies with dosage but generally the effect peaks about 3 to 4 weeks after injection and may last for several months.[30-32,38] This reduction in muscle activation provides a window of opportunity for an intense period of physical therapy to improve motor control factors, such as strength and force control of both the agonist and antagonist muscles. A recent study by Hesse and colleagues[39] suggested that using electrical stimulation for the affected muscles also may enhance the effectiveness of post Botox rehabilitation for the upper extremity.

Baclofen, a gamma-amino butyric acid agonist, acts at the spinal cord level to impede the release of excitatory neurotransmitters believed to mediate spasticity.[40] Continuous intrathecal Baclofen infusion has been used to treat spasticity in children with cerebral palsy and adults with diagnoses of CVA, traumatic brain injury (TBI), and multiple sclerosis.[36,37,40,41] When administered intrathecally, Baclofen can be given in adequate dosage to reduce spasticity without the stuporous side effects associated with oral administration. Baclofen appears to be effective in reducing spasticity and improving function in selected cases. It appears most effective in individuals with severe spasticity to improve hygiene and reduce caregiver assistance. Again, as is true with other medical treatments, most benefits of improved function are associated with a concomitant period of intense therapy.

The evidence suggests that the mere presence or absence of spasticity may not be a good indicator of functional ability. For example, if we observed knee spasticity in a patient while supine, we would not be able to predict if the spasticity was going to interfere with the patient's gait pattern. To determine if spasticity is interfering with movement, the therapist needs to observe muscle activity during a specific task. The relationship between hyperactive reflexes and central control of movement is unclear. The evidence suggests it is not causally related. Spasticity and tone may be two different processes that, in fact, share components of similar neural circuits.

Is Effortful Exercise Detrimental in Patients with Spasticity?

Fowler et al[42] tested the clinical assumption that effortful strengthening exercises were detrimental to children with spastic cerebral palsy. Knee extensor muscle spasticity was tested in children with spastic cerebral palsy and nondisabled children before and after one session of intense knee extensor strengthening exercise. Spasticity was measured with a pendulum test[9] (see Chapter 8).

Following exercise, there were no changes in spasticity as measured by swing excursion, number of oscillations, and duration of oscillations. Similarly, Brown and Kautz[43] tested the same clinical assumption in adult subjects with hemiparesis following a CVA. In this study, force output and EMG were examined during pedaling at 12 random work speeds. During pedaling, subjects increased the net mechanical work appropriately for each workload. There was no increase in inappropriate (antagonist) lower extremity muscle activity. Dawes et al[44] also used high intensity cycling in a patient with brain injury and reported increased elbow extension without any detrimental effects on function. Weiss et al[45] conducted a 12-week progressive resistive lower extremity exercise program with seven patients who were more than 1 year post-CVA. Increased strength was associated with improvement in rising from a chair, balance, and motor performance. Damiano et al[46,47] used a resistive exercise program to strengthen leg muscles in patients with spastic cerebral palsy. Strength in these muscles increased without a concomitant increase in spasticity. Smith et al[48] also reported increases in hamstring muscle strength and decreased spasticity in patients who were post-CVA. These recent studies and others provide evidence that patients with neurologic involvement can perform effortful exercise with spastic muscles and increase muscle strength without the negative effects of increased spasticity or decreased function. There may be some instances where resistive or effortful exercise could have detrimental effects on tone or functional performance. If the therapist observes this negative effect, as with any intervention, a reevaluation of the patient and the intervention would be indicated. The current evidence suggests that the *clinical assumption* of the negative effects of effortful exercise appears to be unfounded.

COMPONENTS OF MOTOR CONTROL

Factors Affecting Movement Patterns

As described in previous chapters, a major aspect of motor control involves initiating and controlling voluntarily generated patterns of movements. Functional movements are composed of a series of events involving several joints and using many muscles that are activated at the appropriate time and which produce the correct amount of force so that smooth, coordinated movement occurs. Isolated strength of an individual muscle or muscle group may have little to do with using that muscle or muscles in concert with others to perform a specific task. Sequencing and timing of muscle agonists, antagonists, and synergists are important. Not surprisingly, static tests of muscle strength do not always predict movement performance. Likewise, performance on one type of task does not necessarily predict performance on another type of task because the task requirements are different. For example, a patient may be able to walk down a hall, but have considerable difficulty getting out of a chair. Walking has a large balance requirement and standing up from a chair has large muscle strength and power requirements. Also, some people may have difficulty with static standing conditions, but can easily walk a block. Knowledge of task requirements for motor control will help therapists identify motor control problems and choose appropriate interventions.

Motor control problems may include deficits in initiation of movement, termination of movement, and speed and direction control. These difficulties often are associated with abnormal movement patterns. Many factors may contribute to a patient exhibiting an abnormal movement pattern. These contributing factors may originate centrally, peripherally, or both. Central factors may include damage to the neural circuitry that generates the movement pattern, aberrant input (inhibition or facilitation) to the circuitry, or abnormal motor neuron recruitment. Peripheral factors may include muscle fiber atrophy, changes in muscle stiffness, and muscle shortening.

Producing coordinated movements requires the interaction of biomechanical and neuromuscular systems along with other body systems. Patients with upper motor neuron lesions have difficulty producing and controlling the muscle forces necessary for generating normal patterns of movement. These deficits may be related to changes in biomechanical and neuromuscular factors. For example, alterations in viscoelastic properties of muscles and tendons may increase muscle stiffness and passive restraint to movement.[49] Muscle shortening may occur from joint immobilization or an increase in muscle stiffness.[50] Stiffness also is a factor that may inhibit speed of movement.[51] These mechanical changes may affect movement patterns because mechanisms of neural control depend on the mechanical properties of the musculoskeletal apparatus. To appreciate the effects of small mechanical changes on movement patterns, consider the effect of increasing the length of your arm. Place a splint on one of your fingers and observe how often you make errors in movement and the time it takes you to adjust to the new extremity length. Although you are aware of the changes in extremity length, a period of time is necessary to adjust the movement patterns appropriately.

Factors Affecting the Initiation of Movement

Cognitive processing will affect the initiation of movement and was discussed in Chapter 10. The patient may have difficulty recognizing a command or signal to move, recalling and selecting the movement plan, or assembling and initiating the plan to move. All of this cognitive processing takes place before initial movement is observed. If patients have difficulty initiating a movement, deficits in central processing must be considered. In addition to cognitive processing, several neuromuscular factors can affect movement initiation. To move, a person must do the following:

1. Produce muscle force in a given period of time
2. Have adequate passive joint range of motion
3. Have an appropriate context and initial condition to perform the task
4. Be motivated to move

How do context and initial condition affect movement initiation? These are variables affecting the expression of a behavior. That is, a person may have the capacity to initiate a movement, but may not do so. For example, if a therapist tests the ability of a patient to reach when he is in a standing position, the patient may not perform the task. It may be because he does not have the strength in his arm muscles, or he may have the strength but will not move his arm because his balance is poor and he might fall if he lifts his arm. It also is possible that he does not have his glasses and cannot see the target, has bursitis and shoulder flexion is painful, or is nauseated and avoids any movement. The context involves factors such as balance ability and the interface between the patient and the environment.

Factors Affecting the Termination of Movement

Accuracy, target acquisition, and reversing movement direction may be affected if individuals cannot control end points of movement. Patients may have difficulty controlling the timing and magnitude of the initial agonist and antagonist muscle activation, and/or the timing and magnitude of secondary agonist and antagonist muscle bursts. This may be due to inappropriate initial scaling of muscle forces when the movement plan was generated or the inability to make modifications in force parameters. In addition to modulating magnitude of muscle activity, problems terminating movement also may be due to inappropriate timing of muscle forces. Timing difficulties with muscle activation are common in patients with neurologic problems and have been reported in patients with cerebellar, cortical, and basal ganglia disorders.[52] Sahrmann and Norton reported that patients with spastic hemiparesis had difficulty turning off agonist muscles and this was characterized by prolonged agonist activity during movement.[16]

Visual spatial deficits also may affect movement termination. If the patient does not perceive distance or location correctly, he may create erroneous parameters that will produce inaccuracies at termination or target acquisition. For specific information about sensory deficits and movement problems, refer to information presented in Chapter 9.

EXAMINATION AND EVALUATION PRINCIPLES

The purpose of an examination is to identify the problem(s). The therapist then can establish functional outcome goals with the patient and determine intervention(s). Movements that require feedback and feed-forward control and that are functional and goal directed should be used during the examination. Keep in mind that you find what you are looking for. Examinations must accurately describe the movement problem(s). Keen observational and measurement skills produce valuable objective data that assist the therapist in formulating working hypotheses about the cause of movement problems. A well-developed hypothesis should guide the goals and the selection of the interventions. At a later time, the therapist reevaluates the patient to determine the effectiveness of intervention and to make appropriate modifications in the hypothesis and the intervention. In this chapter, the examination and evaluation of spasticity, tone, and components of motor control including movement patterns, initiation, and termination of movement will be discussed.

Spasticity

Spasticity can be measured by applying quick stretch to the muscle and using simple clinical measures such as the presence of clonus, response to a tendon tap, the Ashworth Scale,[53,54] or the Modified Ashworth Scale.[11] The pendulum drop test is a clinical measure that requires equipment such as an isokinetic device or video analysis (see Chapter 8). In this test, the patient is positioned so that the extremity segment is held against gravity, and when the patient is as relaxed as possible, the examiner drops the extremity. Most commonly, this test is conducted with the patient's extremity in an isokinetic device so resistive torques can be measured, or the movement is videotaped and the velocity of the extremity segment recorded. For example, to test the quadriceps, a patient is seated, the leg is held horizontal to the ground and dropped into flexion. Measures from this test include swing excursion (arc of movement to the first resistance point), number of oscillations, and the duration of oscillations. The test is limited by the therapist's ability to position the patient for testing and is limited to the larger extremity segments. The most common physiologic measure of spasticity is the H-reflex that measures the response of the motoneuron pool to stimulation of a peripheral nerve, usually the tibial or peroneal nerve. Each of these measures has an adequate degree of reliability if the tester is well-trained in the application of the test. There may be disagreement among these measures of spasticity because not everyone agrees upon the same definitions. I am limiting my definition to that of Lance.[2]

As discussed earlier, because of the dynamic nature of muscle tone, measuring tone is more difficult and less reliable to measure than spasticity. If muscles are hypertonic, they will exhibit a resistance to movement that is not necessarily velocity dependent (as seen in Parkinson's disease). Some authors would suggest that the Ashworth Scale is a measure of tone and not spasticity, however, Ashworth's description of the examination suggests that he was interested in measuring spasticity.

Measures of muscle stiffness (ie, the length tension characteristics) are indications of muscle tone and can be measured in an active or passive muscle. Several authors are documenting stiffness measures using clinical devices[7,55,56] or EMG.[57] Malouin and her colleagues[7,55] make a good argument for differentially measuring reflexive (spasticity) and nonreflexive tone. Boiteau et al[7] compared the test-retest reliability of handheld dynamometry to isokinetic dynamometry to measure reflex and nonreflex mediated resistive forces of the plantarflexors as the extremity was moved through passive ankle dorsiflexion at low and high velocities. Both methods of measurement were reliable with ICCs between 0.79 and 0.90. The authors suggested that handheld dynamometry is a reliable and much more cost-effective method for measuring tone than using an isokinetic device. Using this measure of nonreflexive muscle tone, Malouin et al[55] measured resistive torque in patients 2 and 4 months post-CVA. Spasticity was measured with the Ashworth Scale and the Fugl-Meyer lower extremity subscore. Nonreflexive muscle tone abnormalities were present in the affected extremity at both measurements, but were not related to the level of impairment (Fugl-Meyer) or spasticity (Ashworth Scale).

Measures of muscle stiffness only measure passive resistance to movement. Tone, as discussed earlier, is dynamic, and measures of passive tone or tone at rest may have no relationship to muscle tone that is produced for voluntary movement. Hypertonus at rest is very problematic and makes personal care and positioning, such as wheelchair sitting, a challenge. Hypertonus during movement, however, poses problems with motor control. Tone at rest may be normal but when the patient attempts to move and grasp an object he may not be able to control muscle tone in the appropriate muscles for the task.

There also are devices called *tonometers* that reportedly measure muscle tone with a simple mechanical device attached over the muscle belly.[58] These may be promising instruments that will allow measurement of muscle tone in many different conditions, but there is little research published about their validity and reliability in patients with neurologic lesions or disorders.

Physical therapy that is directed at spasticity is designed to reduce muscle tone, maintain or improve ROM, and improve comfort. Intervention may include: stretching to maintain the full ROM of a joint and help prevent contracture and muscle shortening; orthoses and casts to hold a spastic extremity in a more normal position and help maintain or increase muscle length; strengthening to restore the proper level of strength to affected muscles; and positioning to improve comfort, such as seating in the wheelchair or bed positioning. Other interventions such as cold application to spastic muscles (usually for 10 minutes or longer) have limited use but may reduce muscle tone for a very short period to decrease pain. Electrical stimulation and biofeedback have little research documentation regarding their effectiveness for reducing spasticity, however, they may be useful for improving motor control.

Therapists may be interested in measuring changes in spasticity and tone to test the effects of their interventions if the goal of the intervention is to decrease spasticity and/or hypertonus. Should a therapist use measures of spasticity and tone to indicate improved motor control? As discussed earlier and is evident in the current literature, spasticity and passive measures of tone are not necessarily related to impairments or movement ability. During the evaluation process, the most important question is: What are the limiting factors for this patient to producing normal movements and improving function? If spasticity or tone is one factor, then we should direct our interventions accordingly and consult with the physician about possible alternative medical or surgical interventions. If, however, from the examination it is determined that other factors, such as force control, direction control, abnormal synergies, and/or muscle shortening, are problems, then intervention and the choice of measurements should be directed at remediating those problems and not spasticity.

Movement Patterns

When identifying movement patterns, it is important to describe the movement pattern(s), the consistency of the pattern(s), and the effect of movement speed on the pattern(s). The pattern/synergy should be described so that another therapist reading the evaluation will have a clear picture of what the patient does. Avoid describing patterns or synergies in general terms, such as "the patient has a lower extremity extensor synergy" or "the patient has severe extensor spasticity." Descriptive terms for identifying patient abilities should be used. For example, when a patient rises from a chair, does he lean forward first then push up, or is he pushing into extension with his legs before he leans his trunk forward (Figure 12-1)?

Have the patient perform a movement or task several times, if possible, without producing fatigue. Does the patient use the same movement pattern on each trial? The variability of patterns used may be just as important as the pattern itself. From a theoretical as well as a functional standpoint, variability is better than consistency in most cases, especially if the movement pattern is abnormal. If a movement pattern is consistent and abnormal, it may be more difficult to change (see Chapter 4). Observe in what other conditions/situations different patterns of movement occur. Ask the patient to perform the task or movement at different speeds, and observe the effect of speed on the pattern and the variability. Speed is a good probe for identifying difficulties we might not see if the patient moves at a self-selected speed. Changing movement speed will provide a better examination of movement control. It may also reveal problems with tone or spasticity that were not evident at slower speeds.

Remember that the patterns used for movement are specific to the task, and we cannot assume that the movement synergies used by the patient for one task will be used

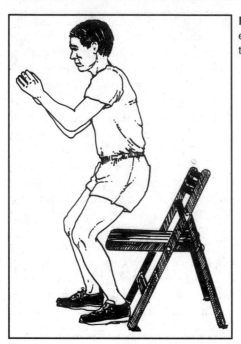

Figure 12-1. Rising from a chair to standing. If knee extension occurs before the trunk is flexed forward, the patient tends to fall backward.

for another task. Obviously, we cannot assess movement for every possible task (Figure 12-2). Selecting a few functional tasks that are meaningful and important to the patient will be most time efficient. Other tasks may be added to future examinations as time permits and the patient's abilities improve.

Initiation of Movement

Initiation of movement may be affected by numerous factors including environmental, biomechanical, neuromuscular, and central processing functions. It is an oversimplification to attribute initiation problems only to motor deficits. The first consideration is to ensure that we measure the performance that best reflects the patient's capacity for movement. This is especially important for movement initiation. The conditions and physical context of the examination affect the patient's performance.

Commands to move may also affect the patient's response. Are the commands verbal or nonverbal? Is the terminology appropriate? These factors may affect the initiation of movement more than the pattern or termination of movement. How quickly does the patient respond to a command? Measuring the length of time from the command to when the patient starts to move (reaction time) may be important for identifying movement problems. If the task requires rapid movement or a quick onset of force, we must know if the patient can meet these demands. For example, patients with Parkinson's disease may initiate movement quickly but perform movements very slowly. To examine initiation ability, we must differentiate among environmental influences, central processing deficits, and neuromuscular difficulties before determining the appropriate treatment. If the patient has a timely response to the command to move, but has difficulty producing speed and force, it is less likely to be a central processing problem. Having both processing and movement problems occurring together makes evaluation of motor function very difficult.

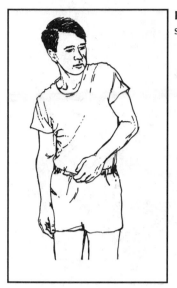

Figure 12-2. Abnormal shoulder synergy of elbow flexion and shoulder elevation when attempting to reach for an object.

Termination of Movement

For goal-directed tasks, terminating a movement is important for target accuracy. Patients who have difficulty terminating movement may overshoot or undershoot the target (Figure 12-3). Using tasks that require end point accuracy or target acquisition best examines problems with movement termination. By placing a target or object at different spatial coordinates, it can be determined if the difficulty is related to a spatial area, to specific muscle groups needed to move in different directions, or to visual spatial deficits. As with testing movement patterns or synergies, speed is a good probe. Patients may not have difficulty in accuracy when moving slowly, but when asked to move as quickly as possible, control may deteriorate. This is a well-known phenomenon for individuals with or without neurologic disorders. Whenever movement speed increases, accuracy may be compromised. Patients must be able to accomplish tasks in an adequate period of time so that they are functional and energy is conserved. Ask patients to perform unidirectional and multidirectional tasks, as well as those that require reversing movement direction. Observe when the endpoint control breaks down. Most likely, it will not be the same for all tasks or all conditions. These observations will help determine the tasks and conditions to use in treatment.

INTERVENTION STRATEGIES

Once the therapist identifies the problems, and the therapist and the patient agree on goals, an appropriate intervention strategy and specific treatment approaches can be determined. Errors in problem identification may lead to prescribing and administering a treatment that is inappropriate and ineffective, thus careful evaluation is extremely important. Practice must be specific to the ability we want to improve. If we want faster initiation and termination of movement, tasks must be structured to provide practice of these skills. Vary the practice of a particular task. Practicing movements or tasks at several different speeds is especially helpful for improving movement initiation and control.

Figure 12-3. Seated adult reaching for a glass of water. His inability to control termination of movement results in knocking over the glass.

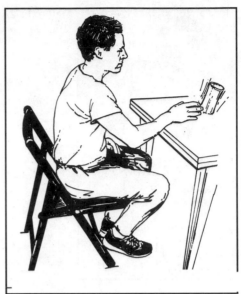

Provide feedback during practice to enhance motor learning (see Chapter 9). Feedback may be verbal, visual, or tactile. However, excessive feedback or guidance may be detrimental to the positive effects of practice. Practice provides an opportunity for the patient to learn what he is doing wrong and problem solve to correct his error. If the patient learns that feedback is always available from the therapist, he may not learn to recognize his errors and apply problem-solving skills. A patient may perform much better during treatment than when he leaves the clinic or when he returns the next day. Although the patient may look better with a therapist facilitating movement, the therapist cannot be there to provide constant correction. The type of practice and the amount of feedback given to the patient will depend on the skill(s) being developed.

Changing movement patterns in patients with neurologic disorders is difficult. Movement patterns may be changed more easily by using mechanical intervention. The use of orthotics to stabilize or restrict a joint or body segment may improve or worsen a movement pattern. Likewise, adapted seating methods may improve accuracy of reach, but, if applied incorrectly, functional ability may diminish. Therapists should emphasize goal-directed movement during practice. Asking the patient to use specific muscles or to control timing of muscle activity may be too confusing during most gross motor activities. Fine motor coordination or training after tendon transfer, however, requires this specific information and effort from the patient.

SUMMARY

Producing well-coordinated movement involving multiple extremity segments and body parts is a complex task that depends on the interaction of multiple internal and external systems. Evaluating complex movement by identifying movement patterns and problems associated with initiating and terminating movement will help therapists determine and apply effective interventions. If therapists can identify motor dysfunction using concepts of motor control and direct their interventions to the problems of motor control, they will be using a scientific approach to practice, and the time spent in intervention will be used more efficiently.

CASE STUDY #1
Jane Smith

- *Age: 74 years*
- *Medical Diagnosis: Right hemiplegia, secondary to left CVA*
- *Status: 6 months post onset*
- *Practice Pattern 5D: Impaired Motor Function and Sensory Integrity Associated with Nonprogressive Disorders of the Central Nervous System—Acquired in Adolescence or Adulthood*

EXAMINATION AND EVALUATION

Functional Limitations

Mrs. Smith has limited functional use of her right upper extremity. Her function has improved in bed mobility and gait, however, she can only walk short distances with her walker and needs standby assistance. She is not safe in transfers and is at risk for falling. She needs the assistance of at least one other adult for most transfers.

Impairments

Mrs. Smith is limited in her control of right arm movement using a flexor synergy when movement is attempted, although this has improved from an initially flaccid condition. She appears to have difficulty producing and regulating muscle activation in appropriate muscles in her upper extremity. Although she initiates movement, she has difficulty controlling movement speed. Mrs. Smith also has difficulty reciprocating joint movement. She can activate finger flexors but appears to have difficulty terminating these agonist muscles and activating the antagonist finger extensors. She has sensory loss that may contribute to difficulties with developing motor control. She has some increased stiffness (tone) in her ankle plantarflexors. Knee and ankle control are limited as indicated by a lack of knee and ankle flexion during gait. She also has slowed balance responses and an overall slowness of movement that may be due to a slowing of central processing.

PROGNOSIS/PLAN OF CARE

Goals

Treatment goals for Mrs. Smith are to:
1. Improve muscle strength throughout right upper and lower extremities
2. Improve reciprocal muscle control for hand and elbow muscles

3. Increase upper extremity coordination out of flexion synergy patterns
4. Achieve independent transfers
5. Improve balance response time
6. Improve lower extremity pattern in gait

Functional Outcomes

Following 3 months of therapy, Mrs. Smith will be able to:

1. Grasp, hold, and release objects five out of five attempts with her right hand
2. Reach to objects in various spatial locations using upper extremity coordination out of flexion synergy patterns for three out of three attempts
3. Stand from a chair independently and safely within 3 seconds on three consecutive tries
4. Climb up/down three steps (stairs) holding on to the railing
5. In 5 minutes, walk 50 feet with four direction changes using a hemi-walker without balances loss

INTERVENTION

The apparent sensory loss in Mrs. Smith's right arm and leg may be a major factor that will impede movement accuracy and learning controlled movements. All tasks should incorporate visual feedback during exercise training to help compensate for sensory loss. Active or active-assisted extension and flexion movement patterns of the entire arm, not just individual joints, should be practiced, using a goal-directed familiar task. Tasks and objects related to hobbies (eg, gardening tools or flowers) should be incorporated in the program. These activities should be performed within a ROM in which Mrs. Smith can initiate and control movement. Larger amplitudes of movement and weighted objects should be incorporated gradually and additional tasks introduced as she gains control. Tasks that promote strengthening and reciprocal movements should be used, and movement speed and direction varied. Treadmill training with a harness may help improve her gait pattern and increase her reactivity. Start at a speed she can tolerate and produce a good pattern for approximately 2-minute sessions. Gradually, increase time intervals and speed. Bicycle exercises also may be useful for improving muscle strength and facilitating timing patterns of force production for reciprocal, multisegmental movements. Mrs. Smith should practice repeated transfers from sitting to standing to improve independence and lower extremity strength. Mrs. Smith has problems with force production. Her strategy of leaning forward, stopping, and then attempting to stand reduces the momentum that assists in rising from the chair seat. Work on the movement as one continuous pattern and strengthen extensor muscles so they can produce adequate force and power to lift the body. This task also provides an opportunity for practicing movement sequencing and functional strengthening. Both rising and sitting back down should be practiced for maximum benefit in training concentric and eccentric muscle control.

CASE STUDY #2
Daniel Johnson

- *Age: 59 years*
- *Medical Diagnosis: Parkinson's disease*
- *Status: 4 years post initial diagnosis*
- *Practice Pattern 5E: Impaired Motor Function and Sensory Integrity Associated with Progressive Disorders of the Central Nervous System*

EXAMINATION AND EVALUATION

Functional Limitations

Mr. Johnson progressively is losing mobility functions with transfers and walking. His poor balance and slow responses put him at risk for falls. He has poor endurance for physical activity.

Impairments

Mr. Johnson's major problems noted during the examination include difficulty initiating and terminating movements, tremor, bradykinesia, and difficulty coordinating extremity and trunk movements. He has decreased flexibility of his trunk and pelvis, but good ROM of his extremities. He also has some memory and attention difficulties. His walking is slow and his balance is poor.

PROGNOSIS/PLAN OF CARE

Goals

Treatment goals for Mr. Johnson are to:
1. Improve initiation of movement
2. Improve trunk and pelvic flexibility
3. Increase muscle strength
4. Improve endurance for activity
5. Improve balance during gait
6. Improve speed and safety when rising from sit to stand

Functional Outcomes

Following 3 months of treatment, Mr. Johnson will:
1. Initiate upper extremity movement for reaching within 5 seconds of being requested to perform the task, and initiate walking within 5 seconds. of being requested to perform the task, 100% of the time

2. Transfer in and out of bed independently using trunk rotation, three out of three attempts
3. Demonstrate an erect posture during standing and gait 75% of the time
4. Walk 50 feet in 2 minutes
5. Maintain standing balance in response to postural perturbations

INTERVENTION

Mr. Johnson would benefit from a program for maintaining flexibility, strength, and reactivity. Goal-directed tasks of varying speed should be used. Mr. Johnson can practice adjusting speed during the movement. It is not necessary to perfect movement at one speed before changing to another. Movement patterns are sensitive to movement speed. Working with different speeds to find one that produces the best performance often is a successful strategy. Mr. Johnson can practice movement at the most effective speed for success with occasional variance of speed for maximum learning. Sometimes having a patient move to the beat of a metronome or music will improve timing. Changing directions of movements is another method for training timing. Adding direction changes to the task also increases the complexity of the task and forces the patient to repeatedly initiate and terminate movement. Mr. Johnson should practice several similar functional tasks for maximum carry over to other related tasks. Working on timed tasks may improve movement initiation. A high priority is passive and active ROM exercises for trunk axial rotation in standing and supine. This will improve and maintain joint mobility and muscle length. Improving joint movement may help improve movement speed and coordination.

CASE STUDY # 3
Shirley Teal

- *Age: 21 years*
- *Medical Diagnosis: Traumatic brain injury*
- *Status: 4 months post injury*
- *Practice Pattern 5D: Impaired Motor Function and Sensory Integrity Associated with Nonprogressive Disorders of the Central Nervous System—Acquired in Adolescence or Adulthood*

EXAMINATION AND EVALUATION

Functional Limitations

Ms. Teal has difficulty with basic mobility, requiring assistance for transfers and standing and is unable to walk. She has bilateral coordination problems that interfere with functional use of her arms. She has difficulty in grasping and manipulating objects. She is not able to cooperate fully with her rehabilitation program.

Impairments

Ms. Teal's major problems are related to decreased strength and abnormal movement patterns in the right upper extremity, trunk weakness, difficulty coordinating trunk and extremity movement, and decreased strength and coordination of the lower extremities. Her problems with controlling and coordinating extremity and trunk movements appear to be due to deficits in strength as well as timing patterns. Ms. Teal also has increased muscle tone in both upper and lower extremities and a 40 degrees plantarflexion contracture. Further examination reveals that the increased extensor tone in sitting and supine is inconsistent when she stands or when she attempts to move her extremities. The ankle plantarflexor tone has contributed to the contracture and the muscles continue to exhibit excessive tone. She has the ability to initiate selective movement of all joints in her right arm but has decreased strength and coordination.

PROGNOSIS/PLAN OF CARE

Goals

Treatment goals for Ms. Teal are to:
1. Increase strength and coordination in the right upper extremity
2. Increase strength in the trunk musculature
3. Improve coordination between trunk and lower extremities
4. Improve balance in stance
5. Increase plantarflexion ROM in the right ankle

Functional Outcomes

Following 2 months of treatment, Ms. Teal will:
1. Reach and grasp an object placed at shoulder height, using shoulder flexion and elbow extension for 15 trials while sitting in a chair
2. Roll unassisted to either the right or left side in bed
3. Rise to standing from a chair independently, 100% of the time
4. Maintain her balance in standing for 2 minutes without holding onto the parallel bars
5. Ambulate in parallel bars for 15 feet without tripping

INTERVENTION

Begin strengthening and coordination exercises for both arms using functional goal-directed tasks and resisted exercises. Use bimanual tasks to promote interextremity coordination. Upper extremity ergometry may be helpful. Emphasize simple and complex movement patterns that involve several segments and tasks that require speed and accuracy of movement. Progress the exercises with object size, weight, and repetitions to increase function. Coordination requires a variety of movement speeds and directions. Trunk flexibility and mobility tasks may improve trunk coordination patterns. Examples include mat activities requiring intersegmental coordination and changes in posture such as rolling and supine to sit (Figure 12-4). Serial casting could be administered to right plantarflexors to reduce contracture. If the muscles do not respond to casting in 2 weeks, Botox or tendon lengthening eventually may be required. As ankle muscle length increases, improved standing and gait may be possible.

CASE STUDY # 4
Shawna Wells

- *Age: 4 years*
- *Medical Diagnosis: Cerebral palsy, spastic quadriparesis, mild mental retardation*
- *Status: Onset at birth*
- *Practice Pattern 5C: Impaired Motor Function and Sensory Integrity Associated with Nonprogressive Disorders of the Central Nervous System—Congenital Origin or Acquired in Infancy or Childhood*

EXAMINATION AND EVALUATION

Functional Limitations

Shawna has difficulty with mobility and uses a bunny-hopping pattern of creeping with poor interlimb coordination. She walks on level surfaces with a posterior walker with minimal assistance from the therapist. Shawna has poor balance and does not play well with peers on movable playground equipment. She cannot walk with her walker on uneven terrain. She ambulates slowly with her walker and cannot keep up with peers. She has difficulty with reaching for objects at eye level or above.

Impairments

Shawna has tightness in ankle plantarflexors and hamstrings bilaterally. She also has reduced flexibility in her upper extremities and trunk with active shoulder flexion ROM limited to 115 degrees and abduction to 90 degrees. Her strength and endurance are impaired relative to her twin brother. She has poor sitting and standing balance.

PROGNOSIS/PLAN OF CARE

Goals

Treatment goals for Shawna are to:
1. Increase lower extremity reciprocation
2. Improve active glenohumeral movement

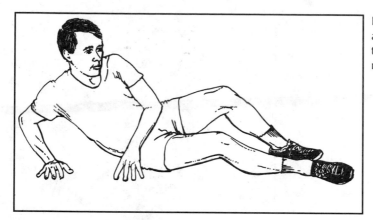

Figure 12-4. Supine to sit activities promote flexibility and segmental coordination.

3. Increase trunk flexibility
4. Increase overall strength and endurance

Functional Outcomes

Following 3 months of treatment, Shawna will:
1. Demonstrate a heel contact pattern during ambulation with a walker as measured by chalk prints on the floor
2. Reach for an object with 90 degrees of forward flexion at the glenohumeral joint without elevating the shoulder, two of three trials
3. Walk unassisted with her walker along a 50-foot obstacle course requiring multiple direction changes without losing her balance

INTERVENTION

Tricycle exercises (adapting pedals if necessary), stair climbing, and treadmill locomotion should be encouraged for reciprocal timing and increasing muscle strength (Figure 12-5). Walking can be practiced with visual cuing and verbal feedback. Walking at a speed that produces the best pattern and varying speed during the treatment session are appropriate strategies. Shawna periodically can return to the optimal walking speed for positive feedback and to decrease frustration. Arm and trunk muscles can be stretched and strengthened using wheelbarrow walking, tug of war, and resisted ball activities. To further increase ROM, Shawna should participate in practice tasks that involve stacking objects on shelves, building towers, and reaching for objects overhead. Incorporate trunk control and strengthening into the same activity for improving movement initiation. Move the support surface, for example, while sitting on a therapeutic ball, at the same time moving the upper body segments for reaching, throwing, and catching tasks. These activities encourage trunk control and automatic trunk responses. Another method of stimulating trunk activity is to practice rapid arm movements in a sitting position with no trunk support and in standing with minimal support so that Shawna has to stabilize her trunk to produce extremity movement. Using night splints or serial casts may increase ankle ROM. She has already had one tendon release which suggests that she is a high risk for muscle shortening.

Figure 12-5. Child riding a tricycle with adapted trunk and foot support.

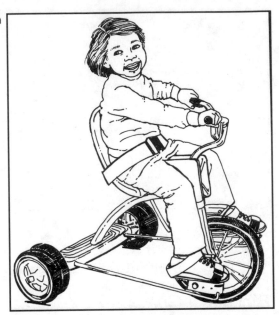

CASE STUDY # 5
Robert Anderson

- *Age: 38 years*
- *Medical Diagnosis: Incomplete T9-10 spinal cord injury with left radial nerve damage*
- *Status: 6 months post injury*
- *Practice Pattern 5H: Impaired Motor Function, Peripheral Nerve Integrity, and Sensory Integrity Associated with Nonprogressive Disorders of the Spinal Cord*

EXAMINATION AND EVALUATION

Functional Limitations

Mr. Anderson requires assistance with transfers and is unable to stand independently, but ambulates short distances wearing his knee ankle foot orthoses using crutches and a swing-through gait. He has poor endurance for standing and walking activities.

Impairments

Mr. Anderson has occasional muscle spasms in his lower extremities and increasing muscle tone from a flaccid condition in both lower extremities. He has limited active movement in his lower extremities. He has sensory loss in his lower extremities associated with his spinal cord injury.

PROGNOSIS/PLAN OF CARE

Goals

Treatment goals for Mr. Anderson are to:
1. Improve lower extremity muscle function
2. Maintain ROM in his trunk and lower extremities
3. Increase endurance during physical activities

Functional Outcomes

Following 3 months of therapy Mr. Anderson will:
1. Ambulate on the treadmill with 60% partial weight support for 10 minutes
2. Walk with his crutches and braces outside his home for 100 feet without resting

INTERVENTION

Maintain muscle length using passive ROM to lower extremities. Increase endurance and strength using upper extremity ergometry and weight lifting. To facilitate lower extremity muscle activity, use assistive exercise and proprioceptive neuromuscular facilitation techniques, electrical stimulation, and treadmill walking in a supported harness. Start with minimal weight support and assist leg movements if necessary. Increase body weight if he is able to initiate some lower extremity resistance

REFERENCES

1. Katz R, Rymer Z. Spastic hypertonia: mechanisms and measurements. *Arch Phys Med Rehabil.* 1989;70:144-153.
2. Lance J. The control of muscle tone, reflexes, and movement. *Neurol.* 1980;30:1303-1313.
3. Bobath B. *Adult Hemiplegia: Assessment and Treatment.* 2nd ed. London, England: William Heineman Medical Books Ltd; 1978.
4. Bobath K. *Neurophysiological Basis for the Treatment of Cerebral Palsy.* 2nd ed. London, England: William Heineman Medical Books Ltd; 1980.
5. Harburn KL, Vandervoort AA, Helewa A, et al. A reflex technique to measure presynaptic inhibition in cerebral stroke. *Electromyogr Clin Neurophysiol.* 1995;35:149-163.
6. Shaw J, Bially J, Deurvorst N. Clinical and physiologic measures of tone in chronic stroke. *Neurology Report.* 1999;23:19-24.
7. Boiteau M, Malouin F, Richards CL. Use of a handheld dynamometer and a Kin-Com dynamometer for evaluating spastic hypertonia in children: a reliability study. *Phys Ther.* 1995;75:796-802.
8. Boorman G, Becker WJ, Morrice BL, et al. Modulation of the soleus H-reflex during pedalling in normal humans and in patients with spinal spasticity. *J Neurol Neurosurg Psychiatry.* 1992;55:1150-1156.
9. Bajd T, Bowman B. Testing and modelling of spasticity. *J Biomed Eng.* 1982;4:90-96.
10. Bohannon RW, Larkin PA, Smith MB, et al. Relationship between static muscle strength deficits and spasticity in stroke patients with hemiparesis. *Phys Ther.* 1987;67:1068-1071.

11. Bohannon RW, Smith MB. Inter-rater reliability of a modified Ashworth scale of muscle spasticity. *Phys Ther.* 1987;67:206-207.

12. Allison SC, Abraham LD, Petersen CL. Reliability of the Modified Ashworth Scale in the assessment of plantarflexor muscle spasticity in patients with traumatic brain injury. *Int J Rehabil Res.* 1996;19:67-78.

13. Pandyan AD, Johnson GR, Price CI, et al. A review of the properties and limitations of the Ashworth and modified Ashworth Scales as measures of spasticity. *Clin Rehabil.* 1999;13:373-383.

14. Verbrugge L, Jette A. The disablement process. *Soc Sci Med.* 1994;38:1-14.

15. Bohannon RW, Andrews AW. Correlation of knee extensor muscle torque and spasticity with gait speed in patients with stroke. *Arch Phys Med Rehabil.* 1990;71:330-333.

16. Sahrmann SA, Norton BJ. The relationship of voluntary movement to spasticity in the upper motor neuron syndrome. *Ann Neurol.* 1977;2:460-465.

17. Bourbonnais D, Vanden Noven S. Weakness in patients with hemiparesis. *Am J Occup Ther.* 1989;43:313-319.

18. Gowland C, deBruin H, Basmajian JV, et al. Agonist and antagonist activity during voluntary upper-extremity movement in patients with stroke. *Phys Ther.* 1992;72:624-633.

19. Giuliani CA. Dorsal rhizotomy for children with cerebral palsy: support for concepts of motor control. *Phys Ther.* 1991;71:248-259.

20. Davidoff R. Skeletal muscle tone and the misunderstood stretch reflex. *Neurology.* 1992;42:951-963.

21. Kramer J, McPhail H. Relationship among measures of walking efficiency, gross motor ability, and isokinetic strength in adolescents with cerebral palsy. *Pediat Phys Ther.* 1994;3:3-8.

22. Landau W. Spasticity: what is it? What is it not? In: Feldman R, ed. Chicago, Ill: Year Book Publishers; 1980:17-24.

23. Landau W. Spasticity: the fable of a neurological demon and the emperor's new therapy. *Arch Neurol.* 1974;31:217-219.

24. Gordon J. Assumptions underlying physical therapy intervention: theoretical and historical perspectives. *Movement Science: Foundations for Physical Therapy in Rehabilitation.* Rockville, Md: Aspen Press; 1987:1-30.

25. Canning CG, Ada L, O'Dwyer NJ. Abnormal muscle activation characteristics associated with loss of dexterity after stroke. *J Neurol Sci.* 2000;176:45-56.

26. Peacock WJ, Staudt LA. Spasticity in cerebral palsy and the selective posterior rhizotomy procedure. *J Child Neurol.* 1990;5:179-185.

27. Engsberg JR, Ross SA, Park TS. Changes in ankle spasticity and strength following selective dorsal rhizotomy and physical therapy for spastic cerebral palsy. *J Neurosurg.* 1999;91:727-732.

28. Gul SM, Steinbok P, McLeod K. Long-term outcome after selective posterior rhizotomy in children with spastic cerebral palsy. *Pediatr Neurosurg.* 1999;31:84-95.

29. Fehlings D, Rang M, Glazier J, et al. An evaluation of botulinum-A toxin injections to improve upper extremity function in children with hemiplegic cerebral palsy. *J Pediatr.* 2000;137:331-337.

30. Hesse S, Krajnik J, Luecke D, et al. Ankle muscle activity before and after botulinum toxin therapy for lower extremity extensor spasticity in chronic hemiparetic patients. *Stroke.* 1996;27:455-460.

31. Simpson DM. Clinical trials of botulinum toxin in the treatment of spasticity. *Muscle Nerve Suppl.* 1997;6:S169-S175.

32. Wong V. Use of botulinum toxin injection in 17 children with spastic cerebral palsy. *Pediatr*

Neurol. 1998;18:124-131.

33. Cosgrove AP, Corry IS, Graham HK. Botulinum toxin in the management of the lower extremity in cerebral palsy. *Dev Med Child Neurology*. 1994;36:386-396.

34. Almeida GL, Campbell SK, Girolami GL, et al. Multidimensional assessment of motor function in a child with cerebral palsy following intrathecal administration of baclofen. *Phys Ther.* 1997;77:751-764.

35. Albright AL, Cervi A, Singletary J. Intrathecal baclofen for spasticity in cerebral palsy. *JAMA*. 1991;265:1418-1422.

36. Stempien L, Tsai T. Intrathecal baclofen pump use for spasticity: a clinical survey. *Am J Phys Med Rehabil*. 2000;79:536-541.

37. Campbell SK, Almeida GL, Penn RD, et al. The effects of intrathecally administered baclofen on function in patients with spasticity. *Phys Ther.* 1995;75:352-362.

38. Smith SJ, Ellis E, White S, et al. A double-blind placebo-controlled study of botulinum toxin in upper extremity spasticity after stroke or head injury. *Clin Rehabil*. 2000;14:5-13.

39. Hesse S, Reiter F, Konrad M, et al. Botulinum toxin type A and short-term electrical stimulation in the treatment of upper extremity flexor spasticity after stroke: a randomized, double-blind, placebo-controlled trial. *Clin Rehabil*. 1998;12:381-388.

40. Albright AL. Baclofen in the treatment of cerebral palsy. *J Child Neurol*. 1996;11:77-83.

41. Meythaler JM, Guin-Renfroe S, Hadley MN. Continuously infused intrathecal baclofen for spastic/dystonic hemiplegia: a preliminary report. *Am J Phys Med Rehabil*. 1999;78:247-254.

42. Fowler EG, Ho TW, Nwigwe A, et al. The effect of quadriceps femoris muscle strengthening exercises on spasticity in children with cerebral palsy. *Phys Ther.* 2001;81:1215-1223.

43. Brown DA, Kautz SA. Increased workload enhances force output during pedaling exercise in persons with poststroke hemiplegia. *Stroke*. 1998;29:598-606.

44. Dawes H, Bateman A, Wade D, et al. High-intensity cycling exercise after a stroke: a single case study. *Clin Rehabil*. 2000;14:570-573.

45. Weiss A, Suzuki T, Bean J, et al. High intensity strength training improves strength and functional performance after stroke. *Am J Phys Med Rehabil*. 2000;79:369-376; quiz 391-394.

46. Damiano DL, Vaughan CL, Abel MF. Muscle response to heavy resistance exercise in children with spastic cerebral palsy. *Dev Med Child Neurol*. 1995;37:731-739.

47. Damiano DL, Martellotta TL, Sullivan DJ, et al. Muscle force production and functional performance in spastic cerebral palsy: relationship of co-contraction. *Arch Phys Med Rehabil*. 2000;81:895-900.

48. Smith GV, Silver KH, Goldberg AP ,et al. "Task-oriented" exercise improves hamstring strength and spastic reflexes in chronic stroke patients. *Stroke*. 1999;30:2112-2118.

49. Dietz V, Quintern J, Barge W. Electrophysiological studies of gait in spasticity and rigidity: evidence that altered mechanical properties of muscle contribute to hypertonia. *Brain*. 1981;104:431-449.

50. Spector SA, Simard CP, Fournier M. Architectural alterations of rat hind-extremity skeletal muscle immobilized at different lengths. *Exp Neurol*. 1982;76:94-110.

51. Tang A, Rymer WZ. Abnormal force EMG relations in paretic extremities of hemiparetic humans. *J Neurol Neurosurg Psych*. 1981;44:690-698.

52. Phillips JG, Muller F, Stelmach GE. Movement disorders and the neural basis of motor control. In: Wallace SA, ed. *Perspectives on the Coordination of Movement*. Amsterdam, North Holland: Elsiever Science Publishers; 1989:361-411.

53. Ashworth B. Preliminary trial of carisorodol on minimal to moderate spasticity in multiple

sclerosis. *Practitioner*. 1964;192:540-542.

54. Gregson JM, Leathley MJ, Moore AP, et al. Reliability of measurements of muscle tone and muscle power in stroke patients. *Age Ageing*. 2000;29:223-228.

55. Malouin F, Bonneau C, Pichard L, et al. Non-reflex mediated changes in plantarflexor muscles early after stroke. *Scand J Rehabil Med*. 1997;29:147-153.

56. Worley JS, Bennett W, Miller G, et al. Reliability of three clinical measures of muscle tone in the shoulders and wrists of poststroke patients. *Am J Occup Ther*. 1991;45:50-58.

57. Pisano F, Miscio G, Colombo R, et al. Quantitative evaluation of normal muscle tone. *J Neurol Sci*. 1996;135:168-172.

58. Thiele E. Functional measuring of muscle tone. *Int J Orofacial Myology*. 1996;22:4-7.

Perspectives on Examination, Evaluation, and Intervention for Disorders of Gait

Carol A. Oatis, PhD, PT
Lisa M. Cipriany-Dacko, PT, MA

INTRODUCTION

Examination and evaluation of gait are integral components of patient management in almost every physical therapy practice pattern.[1] Physical therapists often identify achievement, restoration, or improvement of locomotion as a treatment goal. Criteria for improvement in gait typically include a more normal visual appearance in the gait pattern so parameters such as step length or joint excursions approach normal values. Such judgments usually are made using *observational gait analysis*, which is a systematic procedure in which the clinician views the behavior and compares it to normal values.[2,3] The basic premise of observational analysis is that a gait pattern is "good" if it looks *normal*, and is "not good" if it looks *abnormal*. Yet, there may be circumstances in which the underlying disability precludes a normal pattern of movement and achieving a normal visual appearance would increase the difficulty of walking. The purpose of this chapter is to provide a theoretical framework to analyze gait by considering additional factors that characterize gait besides its visual appearance.

REVIEW OF NORMAL GAIT

A clear understanding of normal gait is essential when analyzing the gait patterns of individuals with impairments. Parameters of gait generally are divided into two categories, kinematics and kinetics, each of which will be reviewed.

Kinematics

Much has been written about the kinematic parameters of locomotion. While kinematic parameters include displacement, velocity, and acceleration data, the vast majority of kinematic data is displacement data, particularly joint excursions of the lower extremities.[4-7] Most data describe motion in the sagittal plane, but some studies include all three planes.[6,8-12] A few studies include the behavior of the trunk and upper extremities.[4,13-15]

Although studies demonstrate both intra-subject and inter-subject variability in joint movement during gait, the patterns and sequencing of joint excursions are remarkably consistent across repeated trials and among different subjects.[4,16-19] However, limitations of available normative data have been presented.[20] Most of the analyses of normal locomotion are based on a limited number of unimpaired, young adult subjects, thus decreasing the applicability of the database. For example, age has been shown by most investigators to affect joint kinematics.[21-23] In addition, studies consistently demonstrate that walking velocity decreases with age.[23-26] Joint excursions generally are proportional to velocity: as walking speed decreases, joint excursions decrease; while joint excursions increase with increasing gait speed.[12,27,28] Joint excursions appear to be reduced in elderly individuals,[21,22] and consequently joint motion in an unimpaired elderly subject may be considered abnormal when compared to a younger population walking at a faster speed. The clinician is cautioned to apply appropriate standards of normalcy using relevant comparison groups in order to avoid overstating an abnormality.

Despite these limitations in the normal kinematic data, there are basic characteristics of movement that appear to be relatively constant. A grasp of these basic elements is essential to understanding gait disorders. First, consider the basic characteristics of the movement of the lower extremities in the sagittal plane. The complexity of movement increases distally, that is, beginning at ground contact the hip joint's movement is a simple single cycle oscillation from flexion to extension to flexion again (Figure 13-1). Maximum extension generally occurs at 50% of the gait cycle, so that hip joint motion is distributed evenly across the gait cycle.[4,29-31] Knee joint excursion, however, demonstrates two unequal peaks of flexion, the first appearing at about 15% of the gait cycle and the other in early swing, or at about 70% to 75% of the cycle (Figure 13-2).[4,10,29,31,32] Despite the increased complexity of the movement, there appears to be a smooth transition between flexion and extension at the knee.

The ankle demonstrates two peaks of plantarflexion (Figure 13-3).[4,29,30] The first occurs early in the stance phase as the foot descends to the floor. The second occurs early in the swing phase just after the toes leave the floor. However, the transition from plantar to dorsiflexion in midstance often is not as smooth as in the knee, as indicated by a more variable angular velocity.[20,31] Thus, the pattern of joint motions increases in complexity from the proximal to distal joints.

Another useful characteristic of joint kinematics is the apparent independence of joint movements in the lower extremity. Murray[4] noted that the ankle, knee, and hip move in

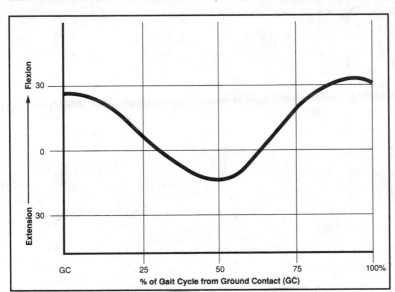

Figure 13-1. Typical kinematic pattern of hip joint movement from ground contact (GC).

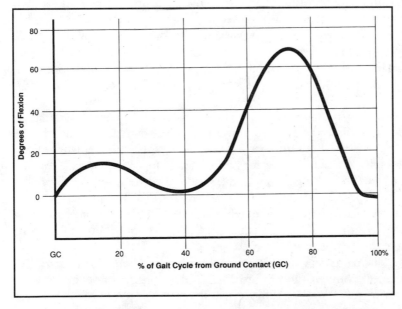

Figure 13-2. Typical kinematic pattern of knee joint movement from ground contact (GC).

the same direction only for a brief instant, in early swing, when they all move away from the ground by flexion at the hip and knee and dorsiflexion at the ankle. Throughout the rest of the gait cycle, two joints are moving toward (or away from) the ground while the other moves away from (or toward) the ground. A common impairment found in individuals following cerebral-vascular accident (CVA) is an inability to disassociate movements, compelling the individual to move the involved joints in the same direction. For example, a patient who exhibits a flexion pattern of obligatory movements flexes the knee at the same time that the hip is flexing and the ankle is dorsiflexing. Such compulsory movements interfere with the independent movements of the lower extremities found in normal gait.

Figure 13-3. Typical kinematic pattern of ankle joint movement from ground contact (GC).

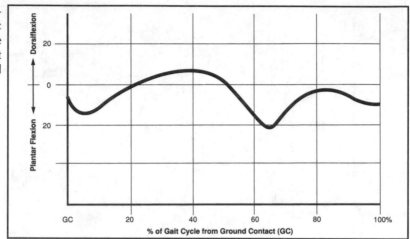

The pelvis, trunk, and upper extremities also exhibit similar patterns of smooth, cyclic movement in gait. In the sagittal plane, the pelvis moves synchronously with the two hip joints, so that the pelvis reaches a maximum anterior tilt each time one hip reaches maximum extension.[4,33-35] Therefore, the pelvis goes through two cycles of anterior rotation, but the cycles are timed evenly through the gait cycle at zero and 50%.

The trunk demonstrates only slight motion in the sagittal plane with more motion in the transverse and frontal planes. In contrast, the upper extremities exhibit almost nothing but sagittal plane motion.[4,15] Each upper extremity moves in synchrony with the opposite lower extremity. As one lower extremity swings forward the contralateral upper extremity moves forward, while the opposite lower and upper extremities extend. The trunk rotates forward with the flexing upper extremity.[4,13,35] This movement pattern constitutes a single cycle of flexion and extension of both upper extremities and the trunk. However, the trunk is rotating forward on the side opposite from the advancing lower extremity and is opposite the transverse plane rotation of the pelvis. In other words, in the transverse plane, the trunk and pelvis are 180 degrees out of phase from one another. This opposing rotation of the trunk on the pelvis contributes to the efficiency and stability of the gait pattern.

By reviewing the kinematic data, certain principles seem apparent. First, there is a progression of movement complexity from proximal to distal in the lower extremities. Second, the motions of the lower extremities require that the joints of each lower extremity move independently of each other. Next, the pelvis and trunk rotate in opposite directions, so that they are 180 degrees out of phase with each other as are the upper and lower extremities. These principles suggest that normal locomotion requires independence of the trunk and pelvis. In addition, there is a prescribed sequence of events so that the limbs and trunk move in a certain rhythm. These characteristics also are related to the kinetic parameters of locomotion. The interrelationships of kinematic and kinetic parameters hold the key to developing a more critical approach to the analysis and treatment of persons with gait disorders. Before the conceptual framework can be developed, the current level of understanding of the kinetic parameters of gait must be reviewed.

Kinetics

Kinetic parameters help describe the mechanical controls of locomotion. These parameters include joint reaction forces and muscle moments at each joint, as well as ground reaction forces. Kinetics also includes energy parameters such as mechanical energy and power, metabolic energy as in oxygen consumption, and muscle activity as indicated by electromyographical (EMG) data. Although the last is not a direct measure of muscle force, it reflects the level of muscle activity and, therefore, is a relative indicator of muscle load.

Ground reaction forces are the net forces exerted by the body onto the ground. They generally are reported as vertical force, and forward or backward, and medial or lateral shear forces. Ground reaction forces are most useful to calculate joint and muscle forces and torques rather than as unique descriptors of motion.[31,36] Joint reaction forces are the net forces applied across the joint resulting from both the inertial forces due to the acceleration of the limb segments, and the ground reaction forces.[31,37] Joint reaction forces during gait have been calculated for the hips, knees, and ankles. Peak joint reaction forces at the hip reported in men range from 2 to 6 times body weight.[38-44] Reported peak knee reaction forces range from approximately 2 to 7 times body weight.[38,39,41,42,45,46] Peak ankle forces from 1.25 to 6 times body weight also have been reported.[38,39,41,43,47,48]

Joint reaction forces in walking reportedly increase with increasing velocity.[12] Little is known of the impact of gait disorders on joint reaction forces, but data collected from nondisabled subjects remind us that walking generates large loads across joint surfaces. Techniques to minimize joint loads, such as decreasing walking speed and unloading the limbs by using an assistive device, should always be considered in the presence of joint pain or inflammation.

Gait produces large joint moments, or torques, which tend to produce joint rotations. These joint moments are generated by the external loads, such as ground reaction forces and limb weight, and by the internal forces applied by the muscles and ligaments. These joint moments are referred to as external and internal moments, respectively. Determination of internal moments during gait helps explain the role of muscles in initiating and controlling the motions of gait. The internal moments generated primarily by muscles support, propel, and control the body throughout the gait cycle.

Winter[31,49] used muscle torques to describe a support moment during the stance phase of gait in nondisabled subjects. The support moment is defined as the sum of the internal moments at the hip, knee, and ankle and is described as positive if these moments tend to push the body away from the ground. Thus, extensor moments at the hip and knee and plantarflexion moments at the ankle are considered positive. The sum of the hip, knee, and ankle moments is consistently positive throughout most of stance, indicating the muscles' role in supporting and avoiding collapse of the stance limb. Investigators note a synergistic relationship between the knee and hip extensor moments so that as one supportive component decreases another component increases to maintain a positive support moment. Elderly subjects exhibit a similar total support moment when compared to younger adults, but the support moment results from an increased hip moment with a decreased contribution from the knee and ankle.[50]

Specific muscle activity in locomotion has been studied extensively, albeit in a relatively small number of subjects.[51,52] In general, muscles are active for very short periods of time during the gait cycle (ie, 0.7 seconds or less).[52] The swing phase of gait is characterized by very little muscle activity. Winter and Yack[53] noted that distal muscles are the most active while the proximal muscles are least active during the swing phase. In stance, the plantarflexors exhibit the most prolonged activity, continuing from approximately foot-flat to almost toe-off. The quadriceps exert a brief burst of activity during loading response into midstance and the hip flexors have a brief burst of activity in late stance and early swing.

The iliacus contracts to decelerate the femur in midstance then accelerate it in late stance and early swing.[6,31,54] The gluteus maximus helps decelerate the limb in late swing. Muscle activity at the knee generally is absent throughout swing.[55-57] At the ankle, the dorsiflexor muscles are responsible for preventing foot drop or toe drag during swing.[58]

The absence of much muscle activity in swing has caused investigators to compare lower extremity motion to that of a compound or jointed pendulum[59] in which the motion of swing is dictated by gravity, given a certain initial position and velocity. Thus, muscle activity data help define three roles for muscles throughout gait. The first is that of support in the stance phase performed primarily by the hip and knee extensors (somewhat interchangeably) and by the plantarflexors. Second is propulsion performed by the plantarflexors and hip flexors, and a third is deceleration performed by the hip extensors.

Analysis of mechanical energy and joint power generated during gait provides more insight into control of locomotion and is useful in analyzing gait disorders. Mechanical energy has two forms: kinetic energy which is a function of mass and velocity, both linear and rotational; and potential energy which is a function of the distance of the body's center of mass from the ground. The principle of conservation of energy states that work must be done on an object in order to change its total energy or the sum of kinetic and potential energies (see Chapter 5). This means that if kinetic and potential energies can be changed from one form to another with no change in total energy, no work is needed in the system. In an ideal roller coaster, the car has a maximum potential energy and minimum kinetic energy at the peak of the track. At the lowest point of the track, potential energy is at a minimum, and the kinetic energy is maximized. In the ideal case, there is a complete transfer of energy so that the continued motion of the roller coaster requires no work because the total energy is unchanged.

Winter, Quanbury, and Reimer[60] investigated energy transformation within the trunk, thigh, and leg. These authors reported approximately a 50% transformation between kinetic and potential energy in the trunk and approximately a 33% exchange in the thigh, but almost no transformation in the leg. However, further analysis demonstrates energy conservation throughout the lower extremity. This conservation results from the energy transfer that can occur between body segments. For example, in the pole vault, energy is transferred from the vaulter to the pole when the athlete plants the pole after running down the runway. Energy then is transferred from the pole to the vaulter to lift the vaulter over the bar. Robertson and Winter[61] investigated the energy exchange between limb segments during locomotion, which is essentially what occurs in the game of crack-the-whip in which energy is transferred from the leader along the line of children. They found that the flow of energy between segments was significant and could account for almost all of the changes in energy in the distal limbs including the leg at the beginning and end of swing.

Mechanical power is the product of force and linear velocity or the product of moment and angular velocity. In gait, mechanical power is determined from the product of the joint's internal moment and angular velocity and helps to demonstrate the role of muscles in propelling and controlling the body.[62] Positive power indicates a shortening or concentric contraction of a muscle by which the muscle imparts energy to the system.[61] Negative power indicates a lengthening or eccentric contraction in which energy is stored in a muscle to be released later in the gait cycle. Studies of mechanical power during gait reveal that positive power is generated at the hip during limb loading, when the hip extensors are contracting concentrically. Positive power is also generated at the hip in late stance as the hip begins to flex. In contrast, slight positive power is generated only briefly at the knee. The ankle, like the hip, generates positive power late in stance when the plantarflexors are contracting concentrically. These data demonstrate that the hip flexors and extensors and the plantarflexors add energy to the lower extremity during gait. Elderly individuals and subjects with weak plantarflexors exhibit decreased power generation and increased hip flexor power.[50,63,64] The reduction in power generated by the plantarflexors may help explain the decrease in walking velocity in these individuals, as well as some of the compensatory mechanisms used.

In summary, investigations into the kinetic characteristics of locomotion provide insights into the control mechanisms which must be considered as we develop a framework for evaluating and treating abnormal locomotion. First, in normal gait, the joints of the lower extremity are exposed to significant loads that may increase under abnormal conditions and contribute to joint damage or pain. Second, muscle activity, although brief, is precisely timed, and muscle groups are activated in a coordinated way to provide support, propulsion, and deceleration. Third, mechanical power analysis reveals that muscle activity is efficient in its ability to absorb and release energy to facilitate motion. Finally, analysis of mechanical energy demonstrates that the movement of some segments allows an exchange of energy from either kinetic or potential energy to the other and that energy actually flows from one segment to another. Since mechanical energy and power are dependent on velocity and position, the motion and orientation of one limb segment or joint are, at least in part, dependent on other segments. Thus, kinetic data help identify the flaws of observational gait analysis, which only identifies the positions of limb segments or joints and compares these values with normal standards. The interdependence of limb segments and the controlling role of muscles, however, cannot be ignored. The following section develops a scheme to evaluate gait disorders, blending this kinetic information with the more conventional kinematic data.

THEORETICAL FRAMEWORK

In the preceding section, the general principles of normal locomotion were reviewed. Identification of kinematic abnormalities has limited benefit since it ignores the interrelationships of the limb segments and the energy storage capacity of muscles. The purpose of this section is to design a scheme for using these concepts to analyze and treat patients with locomotor disorders. Such a framework will provide a means to do more than merely identify deviations from normal. Rather, it should assist clinicians in evaluating the quality of gait. The *Guide to Physical Therapist Practice* describes evaluation as a dynamic process in which the therapist judges the patient's performance using data gathered during the examination.[1] Observational gait analysis is an examination procedure which yields data that allow a clinician to judge the normalcy of the kinematics of the gait pattern. By incorporating a view of gait that considers more than the kinematic appearance of the movement, a therapist can determine that a patient who exhibits abnormal movement may actually be using a "good," albeit abnormal or atypical, pattern of movement.

In order to determine the "goodness" of a locomotor pattern, basic tasks and requirements of locomotion must be considered. Das and McCollum[65] identified forward progression as the central task of bipedal ambulation and stated that this is implemented by the supporting leg. These investigators delineated the task of locomotion by considering swing and stance phases separately. They suggested that the stance phase has two implied tasks: to provide adequate upward support to avoid falling, and to provide adequate forward and backward forces for progression. These same authors offered three basic tasks for swing: safe foot clearance, placement of the swing foot onto a new and appropriate surface, and control of the transfer of angular momentum. Winter[66] also outlined three necessary (but not sufficient) tasks for safe ambulation. These included:

1. Upward support of the body
2. Maintenance of upright posture and balance during stance
3. In swing, control of foot movement for ground clearance and appropriate foot contact

Physical therapists can use these basic elements as the first criteria for judging the quality of gait. First, consider the stance phase in which support is the primary task. As detailed in the first section of this chapter, the support moment is the sum of the internal moments about the ankle, knee, and hip during the stance phase of gait.[49] Throughout most of the gait cycle, the support moment is a net positive or extensor moment (ie, the sum of ankle, knee, and hip moments tend to push the person away from the ground), providing both support and forward progression. From a clinical viewpoint, the person must generate adequate plantarflexion force and a sufficient combination of knee and hip extensor force to prevent collapse. If this combination is present, the first basic task of the stance phase is accomplished.

We can demonstrate the advantage of regarding support as a basic criterion of the quality of gait by considering a clinical example. Using support or the absence of falls as a criterion for evaluating stance could lead the clinician to the conclusion that the patient with an extension synergy has a "good" pattern of movement for the stance phase of gait because it supplies an adequate support moment to avoid collapse of the stance limb. From the kinematic perspective, an extension synergy would be a poor pattern of movement for the stance phase because it probably would lead to abnormal joint positions at ground contact and inadequate ankle plantarflexion and knee flexion following contact. Yet, an attempt to normalize the kinematic behavior might interrupt the extension synergy so that the patient would no longer have adequate support. In this case, in the stance phase, an abnormal kinematic pattern actually is a successful mechanism to accomplish one of the basic elements of stance, which is support.

The tasks of the swing phase are safe foot clearance, foot advancement, and a controlled transfer of momentum.[65,66] Safe foot clearance demands that the swinging limb is able to shorten sufficiently to allow clearance. EMG data reviewed earlier suggest that the limb shortening in swing is the result of active flexion of the hip with passive flexion of the knee. The thigh and foot transmit energy to the leg causing the knee to flex then extend. The knee's passive flexion and extension are extremely rapid and require a freely swinging knee and an adequate forward thrust of the hip to initiate the movement. The importance of a freely swinging knee is supported by investigations conducted by Olgiatti, Burgunder, and Mumenthaler.[67] These investigators reported that there was an inverse relationship between the metabolic cost of walking and the ability of subjects with multiple sclerosis to rapidly flex and extend the knee. Subjects with impaired ability to rapidly flex and extend the knee expended more energy during gait than unimpaired subjects. Inability to perform rapid knee motion was considered an indicator of increased lower extremity tone, so lower extremity "spasticity" was significantly related to a higher energy cost of ambulation.

The increased energy expenditure reported to occur with increased muscle tone reported by Olgiatti, Burgunder, and Mumenthaler[67] is consistent with Das and McCollum's second task of the swing phase of gait, transfer of momentum.[65] Joints of the lower extremity must move independently of one another, and data assessing mechanical energy transformation revealed the interdependence between limb segments and between whole limbs allowing the flow of energy between segments. Thus, some of the efficiency of the swing phase of gait depends on the coordinated movements of the adjacent limb segments.

Consider the likely effects of an extension synergy on a patient's swing phase. First, limb shortening and foot clearance are likely to be impaired since a freely swinging knee joint usually is absent in the presence of an extension synergy. Advancement of the thigh through hip flexion may be more difficult. Thus, safe foot clearance and foot placement also may be hampered. In addition, if the advancement of the thigh is diminished, there will be less energy to impart to the leg, and if flexion of the knee is limited by increased extensor tone, the entire synchronized motion of the lower extremity in swing is interrupted. Any significant beneficial energy flow through the lower extremity is unlikely. An extension synergy may seriously jeopardize the patient's safety during swing and may increase the energy expenditure to clear and advance the limb. By focusing on the general tasks embedded in stance and swing phases of gait, components of the movement pattern which are beneficial and those which are deleterious can be identified and treatment can be focused appropriately. For the patient with the extension pattern described previously, the clinician can direct intervention to ensure safety during swing and to improve the transfer of momentum through the lower extremity.

The clinician must consider the functionality of the gait pattern. Locomotion is rarely a goal in and of itself, but rather a means to an end, that is, a means of transportation to accomplish a task such as eating, shopping, working, or sleeping. Successful locomotion must be practical. Studies have shown that patients with paraplegia at the level of L1 and above generally expend less energy transporting themselves by wheelchair than by ambulating using bilateral crutches.[68] Experience has shown that many patients who are discharged from the rehabilitation facility ambulating soon abandon ambulation for the relative ease of wheelchair transportation. While this may be regarded as failure, if the efficiency of the wheelchair allows the patient to resume an active, productive lifestyle, the wheelchair should be regarded as the "better" mode of transportation. Another study suggested that one reason for the loss of independence in the aging population is an inability to cross a street within the time allotted by a standard traffic light.[69] In other words, the overall velocity is a major contributing factor to independence. Perhaps the quality of ambulation should be judged on the person's overall ability to function as a result of walking, rather than on the pattern itself. That is, despite the appearance of the gait, can the person go grocery shopping, climb stairs, or go to school? If the gait pattern is functional, the clinician must consider carefully the value of intervening. If the intervention is directed solely toward improving the appearance of the movement, it is superfluous. However, if the intervention is designed to improve the functionality of the gait, such as increasing walking speed so the individual can cross the street safely or decreasing the energy cost of walking so the individual can walk though the school corridors and still have energy to attend class, the intervention seems worth the investment.

What is the framework with which we should evaluate gait disorders? The previous discussion suggests that task evaluation can lead to a better understanding of the quality of gait. These include tasks inherent to the movements such as support, ground clearance, and transfer of momentum, as well as to the tasks that are the goals of locomotion. Examples of goals of locomotion are transportation from point A to point B within environmental constraints, such as traffic, and locomotion from point A to point B with enough residual energy to perform a desired task, such as to cook dinner or shop. Traditionally, physical therapists have considered the pattern of movement as monitored by observational gait analysis rather than considering the underlying tasks embedded within the movement. Such a narrow focus makes us susceptible to the accusation that we "cannot see the forest for the trees." As in the example of the patient with an extension synergy, it is tempting to be concerned about the absence of heel-strike or knee flexion after foot contact and to ignore the fact that the patient exhibits good, firm support in the stance phase. On the other hand, we should not be too hasty in discarding kinematic data that may help us understand the mechanisms underlying or controlling gait. Single elements within the movement of locomotion, such as joint excursions or joint moments, may influence the patient's ability to accomplish the tasks. However, single elements by themselves may not be the most useful criteria to judge the quality of the movement. Instead, gait evaluation may lead to more functionally relevant goals and more successful treatments if focused on the patient's ability to perform the basic tasks inherent in locomotion. These tasks would include support, propulsion, transfer of momentum, and the ability to use locomotion for some functional outcome. Linking standard clinical data with assessment of gait disorders can yield a judgment of the quality of the movement, possible mechanisms to explain the movement, goals of physical therapy intervention, and an intervention plan.

CLINICAL USE OF GAIT ANALYSIS

The goals of clinical gait analysis are to define a baseline pattern of behavior in order to document change, to devise a treatment plan, and ultimately to improve the behavior. To accomplish these goals, the clinician must be able to disassemble the basic tasks of gait described in the previous section and to find the relationship between those elements and the impairments that may impact the gait pattern, including impairments in strength, range of motion (ROM), and muscle tone. Identifying such relationships will allow the clinician to focus on the specific components of the movement most likely to make a difference in locomotor function.

Strength

The relationship between muscle strength and locomotion is not well-defined. Intuitively, it seems that some degree of strength is necessary, especially in the dorsiflexors for ground clearance and foot contact, in the quadriceps during weight acceptance, and in the gluteus medius for midstance. However, the level of strength required of these muscles or any others has not been determined. Investigators have attempted to define a relationship between muscle strength or weakness and gait abnormalities. Elderly subjects with weaknesses at the hip and knee exhibited decreased mechanical energy expenditure at the knee and ankle with an increased energy expenditure at the hip and low back.[63] Krebs[70] reported moderate correlations between quadriceps and hamstring muscle strength and gait function ($r = .75$ and $r = .70$, respectively) in patients with postarthrotomy femoral neuropathies in which gait function was defined by a five-point scale averaged for four activities: ambulation, stair climbing, single leg vertical jumps, and squats. Gyory, Chao, and Stauffer[71] reported a moderate correlation between quadriceps strength and knee motion during stance in patients with rheumatoid arthritis. Olgiatti, Burgunder, and Mumenthaler[67] found no significant correlation between lower extremity strength and energy cost of walking in patients with multiple sclerosis. In this latter study, strength was operationally defined as the maximum height a patient could step up. Correlations also have been reported between plantarflexion strength and joint power at the ankle during gait.[72]

The preceding studies suggest that muscle strength plays some role in gait, but how does the clinician use muscle strength data to formulate a treatment plan for patients with locomotor disorders? The basic tasks embedded in the gait cycle may provide an answer. In the stance phase, the primary task is support followed by forward progression.[65,73] According to Winter, support is provided by the plantarflexors and by the hip and knee extensors.[66,73] In addition, pelvic stability is provided by the hip abductors on the stance side. If stability during stance is the primary concern, the clinician must consider enhancing the function of the large hip and knee muscle groups. Forward progression is the role of the plantarflexors and hip flexors. The shift toward increased power generation and energy expenditure in elderly individuals and in individuals with lower extremity weakness suggests that increased focus on distal muscle activation, particularly the plantarflexors, may improve propulsion.

The primary tasks of the swing phase are foot clearance and transfer of momentum. Foot clearance, of course, requires some strength in the dorsiflexors as well as an ability to shorten the whole limb.[12] However, EMG data suggest that limb shortening occurs from an initial thrust of the hip flexors and passive flexion of the knee.[31] Threshold energy from the thigh then is transferred to the leg and foot, facilitating knee extension. Thus, the threshold strength of importance in the swing phase appears to be in the dorsiflexor and hip flexor muscles. The astute clinician will realize that many tasks in daily life require more strength than does normal walking, such as rising from a chair or stair climbing. In terms of locomotion, perhaps muscle strength should be considered as it relates to task accomplishment in stance and swing, rather than as absolute and isolated values. Further research is required to identify the level of strength throughout the lower extremities necessary for functional ambulation.

Range of Motion

Like strength, little has been written describing the relationship between flexibility of the joints of the lower extremity and a subject's walking pattern. Stauffer, Chao, and Gyory[74] reported an inverse relationship between knee flexion ROM while standing and knee motion in gait.

Krebs[70] reported a moderate correlation ($r = .74$) between percent of the patient's normal knee ROM and ambulation index based on walking, stair climbing, jumping, and squats following knee arthrotomies.

Ankle dorsiflexion ROM also is associated with ankle power during gait (r = .72) in subjects without impairment.[72] However, Salsich, Brown, and Mueller[75] suggested that individuals with decreased plantarflexion strength and decreased dorsiflexion ROM (ie, a plantarflexion contracture) may use passive tension in the plantarflexors to generate ankle joint power that contributes to propulsion. These data demonstrate the complex relationship between joint impairments and gait. Restricted ankle motion in certain individuals actually may improve function while decreased ROM in others may contribute to increased instability and inefficiency in gait.

Muscle Tone

Krebs[70] stated that only 25% to 50% of the variance in gait performance of patients after knee joint arthrotomies could be accounted for by muscle strength, motor unit activity, and knee flexibility. If strength and ROM do not completely explain locomotion performance, what other clinical factors could control locomotor behavior? As noted earlier, Olgiatti, Burgunder, and Mumenthaler[67] reported that spasticity, as measured by patients' ability to swing the knee rapidly, was significantly related to the metabolic cost of walking. Tardieu and coworkers[76] also considered the effect of spasticity on locomotion patterns in children with cerebral palsy. These authors examined the passive contribution of a plantarflexion contracture and the active contribution of normal activation or the excessive activation of the plantarflexor muscles during the push-off period of the stance phase. By analyzing the propulsive task of stance and relating this to the passive resistance to dorsiflexion measured in a separate test at rest, these investigators identified two separate mechanisms for toe-walking in children with cerebral palsy. One resulted from overactivity of the triceps surae, and the other was due to excessive passive shortening of the same muscle group. These data yield different intervention strategies for these two mechanisms of pathology. Thus, a careful analysis of muscle tone may lead to a better understanding of the mechanisms of gait disorders. This understanding may be enhanced further by relating information about muscle tone to the more standard measures of flexibility or strength.

Mechanical Parameters

In order to develop a clinical measure which reflected both the ballistic nature of the knee's movement in swing and the knee's energy storage role in stance, Oatis[77] presented a mechanical model of the knee as a damped spring linking two rigid segments, representing the leg-foot segment and the thigh, on which perched the mass of the head, arms, trunk, and opposite lower extremity (Figure 13-4). The characteristics of the damped spring, the damping and stiffness coefficients, were derived by a test in which the knee was allowed to oscillate freely after being released from an extended position. The oscillations were recorded using an electrogoniometer and the coefficients were calculated from the frequency and decay rate of the oscillations (Figure 13-5). The coefficients then were used to mathematically predict the kinematic behavior of the knee model using appropriate anthropometric data and the initial kinematic data of the thigh at heel-strike. The predicted behavior of the knee then was compared to the real kinematic data for subjects recorded by high speed cinematography.

Although the model was a very simple two-dimensional representation of the knee and required certain adjustments to describe the varied nature of the knee's role in stance and swing, the simulated data still yielded reasonable approximations of the real motion

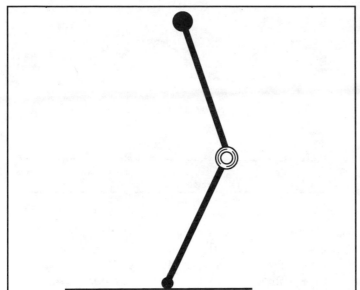

Figure 13-4. Model of the lower extremity with the head, arms, trunk, and opposite leg mounted on the thigh, which articulates with the leg-foot segment via a damped torsional spring.

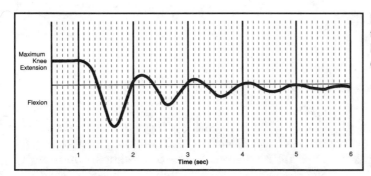

Figure 13-5. Typical electrogoniometric data of the knee joint during free oscillations.

(Figure 13-6). These results provided specific insight into the clinical behavior of the knee during gait, as well as another perspective on gait analysis. This study suggested that the knee's ability to oscillate, or swing, may be as relevant to its performance in locomotion as either strength or ROM. This study also demonstrated the usefulness of a task-oriented approach to gait analysis. The realization that the knee movement in the swing phase required very rapid flexion and extension (344 degrees per second), as well as recognition of its energy storage role in stance, led to a new measurement of knee joint function.[78]

The studies presented in this section examined relationships among functional outcome, locomotion, and some impairment variables, such as decreased strength and ROM, increased muscle tone, and the mechanical parameters of stiffness and damping. Strength and ROM influence locomotion, but impairments in these areas are insufficient to explain all gait abnormalities. Increased muscle tone appears to explain at least some of the mechanisms of gait pathology in some individuals. The stiffness and damping coefficients can be considered composite measures of joint performance perhaps comprising resting muscle tone, integrity of the articular cartilage, and joint viscosity. Each of these factors appears to have some predictive capability for the knee joint kinematics

Figure 13-6. Comparison of kinematic data of the knee from cinematography and that data simulated by the damped spring model.

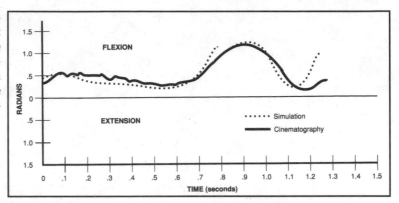

during locomotion. It is clear, however, that none of these variables can provide the full explanation for any locomotor disorder. However, these studies should emphasize to the clinician the importance of a critical approach to the application of standard clinical variables to explain and treat patients with gait pathologies. These reports also should encourage clinicians to be creative in their approach to gait analysis and intervention. A focus on the underlying tasks of locomotion and the patient's impaired ability to accomplish those tasks may lead a clinician to define a completely new measure of performance that will be more relevant to the outcome measure, locomotion, than any variables now available.

SUMMARY

The standard approach to gait analysis in the clinic is a form of observational gait analysis that documents the patient's kinematic behavior and compares it to some standard. However, this approach ignores the mechanical factors controlling the movement. Observational gait analysis enables the clinician to discriminate between normal and abnormal or atypical gait, but may not provide enough information to make a judgment about the quality of the movement. An understanding of the basic tasks inherent in locomotion, that is, support and propulsion in stance, clearance of the foot, and a transfer of momentum in swing, may provide a basis by which the clinician can assess the quality of the movement. Such understanding may lead to therapeutic interventions that are related more directly to the function of gait than treatment strategies that focus on reducing impairments. Clinicians must be critical in their review of treatment procedures to analyze their relevance to impaired task performance, and researchers must help identify and explain the mechanical and physiologic requirements of the tasks embedded in the performance of gait.

CASE STUDY #1
Jane Smith

- *Age: 74 years*
- *Medical Diagnosis: Right hemiplegia, secondary to left CVA*

- *Status: 6 months post onset*
- *Practice Pattern 5D: Impaired Motor Function and Sensory Integrity Associated with Nonprogressive Disorders of the Central Nervous System—Acquired in Adolescence or Adulthood*

EXAMINATION AND EVALUATION

Functional Limitations

Mrs. Smith is able to ambulate 30 feet with a hemi-walker and requires moderate assistance in transfers. She ambulates with slow velocity and has difficulty in advancing the right lower extremity. Her limited ability to ambulate decreases her ability to participate in functional activities within her home and in the community. During treatment, she is impulsive, is frequently frustrated, and occasionally throws things. She has difficulty expressing herself verbally.

Impairments

Examination reveals that Mrs. Smith continues to have a flexion synergy in the right upper extremity and significant weakness in the right lower extremity. There is increased muscle tone in the trunk with scapular retraction and trunk rotation to the right. The patient continues to demonstrate a pattern of increased right lower extremity muscle tone into extension and adduction at the hip. However, she is able to initiate hip flexion. One can visualize her gait pattern in the following way. She advances the walker on the left and then in swing, advances the right lower extremity by hip hiking, circumduction of the leg, or posterior rotation of the pelvis. As the right limb comes forward, the right pelvis and right shoulder simultaneously advance so the pelvis and trunk are not disassociating from one another. Mrs. Smith's stance is characterized by an initial contact as foot-flat with decreased single stance limb time on the right. Knee flexion may not be present following contact, but Mrs. Smith leans forward onto the left side during single limb support on the right so that the right hip remains flexed. Late stance is characterized by decreased or absent propulsion. She also exhibits severe verbal apraxia and moderate aphasia which make communication during therapy sessions difficult.

PROGNOSIS/PLAN OF CARE

Goals

Treatment goals are for Mrs. Smith to:
- Achieve ability to ambulate independently with her hemi-walker
- Demonstrate ability to ascend and descend stairs
- Improve the efficiency of her gait
- Preserve energy during ambulation

Functional Outcomes

Following 3 months of physical therapy, Mrs. Smith will:
- Independently ambulate 100 feet with a walker to enable her to attend a medical appointment or church

- Independently ascend and descend a flight of stairs using one rail in a one-step-at-a time pattern to enable her to enter her home, ambulate on the second floor, or attend community events
- Use pelvic advancement on the right side to equalize stride length while ambulating 10 feet within her home using a wide-based quad cane on one side and the kitchen counter on the other side
- With verbal cues, ambulate 20 feet with a walker without demonstrating genu recurvatum or forward lean
- Demonstrate active plantarflexion 50% of the time during ambulation to increase speed of gait to be more functional in community ambulation

INTERVENTION

Propulsion is an important part of the stance phase requiring active plantarflexion. Mrs. Smith has a hinged ankle foot orthosis (AFO) and continues to use the device. If the orthosis were rigid, it would preclude active contraction of the plantarflexors for propulsion. However, a hinged AFO allows the tibia to advance over the foot and allows ankle plantarflexion to occur as the strength improves in the plantarflexors. Propulsion also requires proper alignment of the trunk with the lower extremity during stance. The role of plantarflexion in the stance phase is to provide a thrust in the forward direction, which means that the trunk and pelvis must be in front of the stance foot. If Mrs. Smith has weakness of the trunk and hip, particularly the hip extensors, she may be unable to advance the trunk and pelvis over the stance limb. If the hip is flexed, she will have difficulty in advancing the pelvis over the stance foot; consequently, the ankle will not be in a position to provide propulsion, even in the presence of contracting plantarflexors. This forward lean position may contribute to genu recurvatum and a plantarflexed ankle in late stance. Therefore, emphasis on intervention should be placed on pelvic advancement during weight bearing activities and use of plantarflexion for propulsion.

Swing requires limb clearance, which means an ability to shorten the extremity adequately to avoid contacting the ground, as well as the ability to transfer momentum through the extremity. Mrs. Smith has active hip flexion, but strength of the hip muscles has not been determined. Therefore, the therapist must consider whether Mrs. Smith has adequate strength to impart a forward thrust of the thigh, which is the motive force for advancing the entire lower extremity. In addition, the knee joint must be swinging freely so that the forward momentum of the thigh can be translated into knee flexion, thus shortening the lower extremity. If this patient has increased extensor tone, then knee flexion and, consequently, limb shortening will be difficult. Intervention also must be directed toward facilitating thigh advancement with a freely swinging knee joint.

Achieving these goals requires a progressive exercise program, which first considers the general strength of the patient. Although strength by itself does not predict a gait pattern, certain threshold forces do appear necessary for functional gait. Mrs. Smith's pelvic and trunk strength must be examined, and if weakness is present, improved to promote upright posture. Mat activities in quadruped, kneeling, and half-kneeling positions will promote proximal strength, as will activities on a therapy ball. Distal strength should be facilitated and improved to enhance propulsion and improve foot clearance. Progressive standing balance activities or activities on a tilt board will help facilitate distal strength. Although progressive resistive exercises traditionally have been avoided in patients with increased muscle tone, clinical experience has demonstrated significant improvement following aggressive strengthening in patients with gait and balance disorders. Research studies also have demonstrated that strengthening programs do not increase spasticity (see Chapter 12).

To address the trunk stiffness and lack of disassociation between the trunk and pelvis, mat activities in supine, side lying, kneeling, and sitting can focus on counter rotation with the eventual progression to disassociation in standing and gait. Standing, weight-shifting, and stepping activities with manual facilitation can be performed with the focus of appropriate postural alignment in stance and pelvic advancement with adequate propulsion. This first can be performed in a supportive environment, such as within parallel bars, with the goal of a more functional environment that is outside of the bars. A long-term goal would be for Mrs. Smith to develop a two-point gait pattern with the wide-based quad cane (WBQC), which would promote upright trunk alignment during swing and stance phase.

Passive ROM should be monitored as, in the presence of increased muscle tone, inactivity, and the effects of aging, decreased ROM could become a problem over time. ROM and stretching exercises should focus on those joints that exhibit some stiffness. It will be to no avail to work on disassociation of the trunk and pelvis if the patient develops limitations due to shortening of soft tissue. ROM exercises are an integral component of home exercise programs taught to patients and their families.

Although Mrs. Smith's difficulties in communication and emotional/behavioral control may not be directly related to her locomotion problems, the approach to intervention should address these issues. We should create a quiet environment with limited distractions and build consistency in the treatment program so that the patient can discern some order in her surroundings. The exercise program should include simple exercises or task breakdown that can be followed easily with many repetitions. Creating such an environment may help decrease the patient's emotional outbursts as she begins to see and anticipate a well-ordered pattern of treatment. Simplifying the tasks will ensure greater success that may lead to greater self-esteem and less frustration. The physical therapist also must communicate with the speech therapist and occupational therapist to ensure consistency in goal setting and behavioral expectations and to avoid contradictions in approaches.

In conclusion, the emphasis of the physical therapy program should be on developing adequate strength for support, propulsion, and limb advancement and on upright trunk alignment during stance. As momentum is transferred more readily, Mrs. Smith is likely to expend less energy during each gait cycle and prolong her walking tolerance. This case demonstrates how kinematic data may be useful in developing an appropriate plan of care when the data are evaluated in light of the essential tasks of the gait cycle.

CASE STUDY #2
Daniel Johnson

- *Age: 59 years*
- *Medical Diagnosis: Parkinson's disease*
- *Status: 4 years post initial diagnosis*

- *Practice Pattern 5E: Impaired Motor Function and Sensory Integrity Associated with Progressive Disorders of the Central Nervous System*

EXAMINATION AND EVALUATION

Functional Limitations

Mr. Johnson has difficulty rising from a seated position and has a shuffling gait. He is experiencing increasing difficulty with balance, particularly with a tendency to fall during ambulation. Initiation of motion and transfers are becoming more difficult. The patient's progressive forward lean increases the danger of forward falls and inhibits his ability to impart forward propulsion. Ambulation occurs without arm swing. Mr. Johnson reports problems with remembering some things in his daily routine. His wife reports that he is often listless and uninterested in participating in social activities.

Impairments

Mr. Johnson's primary impairments include bradykinesia, akinesia, and bilateral tremors. His basic biomechanical limitations are increased rigidity and decreased isolated movements of the trunk on the pelvis and the trunk and pelvis on the lower extremities. This absence of independent movement of the trunk and limbs precludes the ability to transfer momentum along one limb or from one limb to another during locomotion. Mr. Johnson also demonstrates a mild memory loss and signs of depression.

PROGNOSIS/PLAN OF CARE

Goals

Treatment goals for Mr. Johnson are to:
1. Improve ability to ambulate independently without falling
2. Demonstrate improved speed of ambulation with festination
3. Decrease number of trips and falls during ambulation
4. Ambulate safely in a variety of environments

Functional Outcomes

Following 3 months of outpatient treatment, Mr. Johnson will:
1. Ambulate independently within the house and with standby assistance in the community without falls
2. Be able to cross the street during the time allotted by the traffic light
3. Demonstrate a heel to toe pattern during ambulation for a distance of 30 feet to prevent tripping and falls

INTERVENTION

Mr. Johnson's treatment program should be directed toward increasing extension and rotation in the thoracic and lumbar spine to enhance upright posture and facilitate independent trunk and pelvic rotations. In promoting trunk extension, the therapist must consider the strength of the trunk and hip extensors and use exercises to promote adequate strength in these muscles.

Proprioceptive neuromuscular facilitation patterns are particularly useful in promoting extensor strength throughout the trunk and limbs, and exercises such as wall squats and limb elevation in quadruped will be helpful. Trunk rotation could be facilitated in a variety of positions including supine, kneeling, and standing. Simple, slow rhythmic motions in hook-lying (supine with hips and knees flexed), sitting, and standing can be used initially, but should be progressed to larger arcs of motion with varying speeds. Facilitation of arm swing can be used to enhance trunk rotation and to disassociate trunk from pelvic rotation. For example, Mr. Johnson can be instructed in golf swing movements of both upper extremities in kneeling, which will enhance trunk control and facilitate rotation. If arm swing during ambulation is decreased because trunk rotation is limited, the trunk will be unable to impart rotational momentum to the upper extremities. Therefore, facilitation of trunk rotation may elicit more upper extremity movement. Trunk activities on a therapy ball can also be useful in promoting upright trunk responses. Postural control and balance can be facilitated through focused practice on balance strategies such as ankle, hip, and stepping strategies. Activities such as progressively decreasing the patient's base of support statically or using principal movements of tai chi to address dynamic balance are other techniques that may be helpful.

The patient's memory impairment and depression must be considered when determining goals and developing a treatment plan. Tasks should be simple and goals practical. All exercises should be written clearly so the patient has a record of his exercise regimen and does not have to depend on memory for completion of the program.

This case study reinforces the concept that concentration on joint kinematics could mask the basic problems in gait. It is undoubtedly true that this patient demonstrates decreased movements in all joint excursions, but the underlying problem is one of an absence of independent movement of trunk and limbs and decreased postural reactions. Keeping this perspective allows the therapist to concentrate on the most promising areas of treatment during the limited treatment time, that is, those areas that are most likely to produce functional benefits. Because Mr. Johnson is in the early stages of the disease, an aggressive home program should focus on all of the above areas to prevent secondary complications from a general decrease in mobility and activity.

CASE STUDY #3
Shirley Teal

- *Age: 21 years*
- *Medical Diagnosis: Traumatic brain injury*
- *Status: 4 months post injury*

- *Practice Pattern 5D: Impaired Motor Function and Sensory Integrity Associated with Nonprogressive Disorders of the Central Nervous System—Acquired in Adolescence or Adulthood*

EXAMINATION AND EVALUATION

Functional Limitations

Ms. Teal is alert but has difficulty with clear expression of speech. She has understandable speech 80% to 90% of the time if she speaks slowly. She is extremely combative during physical therapy. She is able to perform pivot transfers and stands in the parallel bars for 5 minutes with minimal assistance. She has decreased weight bearing on the right lower extremity without cues and tends to lose her balance easily if she moves quickly. She has poor endurance for standing and ambulation activities. She is unable to ascend or descend stairs without maximal assistance.

Impairments

Ms. Teal has active isolated movement of the right upper extremity with decreased strength and coordination. She has a 40 degree plantarflexion contracture at the right ankle. She also lacks 10 degrees of full right hip and knee extension. She has full active ROM of the left upper and lower extremities, but with decreased coordination.

The biomechanical problems related to her plantarflexion contracture are severe and contribute to her decreased balance and ambulation endurance. The kinematic effects of such a contracture when Ms. Teal begins to ambulate include ground contact with the toes, absence of foot-flat, inadequate knee extension in midstance, and unequal step lengths. A plantarflexion contracture results in a functional limb length discrepancy and interferes with advancement in swing as well as support and propulsion during the stance phase. The limitations in ROM at the hip and knee, although less severe, contribute to her inability to maintain the right lower extremity in a stable, weight bearing position in upright. Ms. Teal demonstrates several areas of impairment that influence her difficulties with ambulation, including behavioral, biomechanical (ie, contractures), and coordination problems.

PROGNOSIS/PLAN OF CARE

Goals

Treatment goals are for Ms. Teal to:
1. Improve available ROM in her right ankle, knee, and hip
2. Increase distance ambulated with a walker
3. Improve ability to ascend and descend stairs

Functional Outcomes

Following 2 months of physical therapy intervention, Ms. Teal will:
1. With verbal cues, ambulate 100 feet with a walker and minimal assistance so she can attend medical appointments

2. Ascend and descend 13 steps with a wide-based quad cane and one rail so she can go upstairs and downstairs at home
3. Increase passive right ankle dorsiflexion by 30 degrees and active dorsiflexion by 10 degrees to improve her balance during gait and prevent falls
4. In the walker, actively rise to tiptoe position to reach for an object on a shelf

INTERVENTION

Because the lower extremity on the involved side is functionally longer, safe clearance of the foot is a problem. To ensure safe clearance, Ms. Teal has to increase her hip and/or knee flexion in swing. This compensation disturbs the delicate timing between adjacent limb segments during swing and decreases the flow of momentum through the swing limb or between both lower extremities. The flow of momentum is disturbed even further as she moves through single limb support in stance on the involved limb. Because the limb is functionally much longer than the opposite limb, single limb support on the right is characterized by an excessive rise of Ms. Teal's center of mass. This rise interrupts the forward progression of the body over the stance limb and causes an interruption in energy flow, resulting in decreased efficiency.

In addition to the energy considerations of the lower extremity contractures, the contractures also decrease the available base of support on the involved side, which decreases stability. The base of support also is asymmetrical. Anyone who has tried to walk wearing one high heel shoe with the other foot bare can appreciate the balance difficulties that arise. If the patient's balance disturbances arise from CNS abnormalities rather than the mechanical asymmetry alone, the patient may lack the necessary compensatory mechanisms to carry out the support function of stance, and will appear quite unstable and may even fall.

Propulsion will also be the final task in gait, influenced by the plantarflexion contracture. Propulsion normally is provided by a shortening contraction of the plantarflexors pushing the ankle from 5 or 10 degrees of dorsiflexion to 20 or 30 degrees of plantarflexion. However, Ms. Teal lacks dorsiflexion ROM and does not have adequate range available to use a shortening contraction. She is incapable of imparting significant propulsive force. Therefore, an aggressive approach to resolving this contracture is required not only because of its impact on her overall function, but also because the patient is scheduled for discharge within 2 months.

Serial casting of the right ankle or surgery should be considered to provide a rapid increase in dorsiflexion ROM so she will have an enlarged base of support and symmetrical limb lengths. Ms. Teal's balance disturbances may be, in part, due to her plantarflexion contracture, but also may be the result of her brain injury. As the patient is being treated for the ankle contracture, her balance reactions can be facilitated using tall kneeling positions and a therapy ball. Ms. Teal's coordination problems appear to be the result of difficulty in sequencing activities or planning motor activities as well as the result of flawed motor output. Multiple repetitions will be useful to improve motor output, and her ability to sequence tasks will be enhanced by keeping the tasks simple and functional, using necessary cues. As the patient's ambulation ability improves, additional training using simple obstacle courses may facilitate motor planning.

This case study demonstrates the effect of a significant joint impairment in the midst of more diffuse motor pathology. Improved coordination and motor planning will be of little use if the biomechanical effects of the lower extremity contractures are not dealt with adequately. Ms. Teal's behavioral problems will be addressed through a vigorous behavioral modification program involving the entire health care team.

CASE STUDY # 4
Shawna Wells

- *Age: 4 years*
- *Medical Diagnosis: Cerebral palsy, spastic quadriparesis, mild mental retardation*
- *Status: Onset at birth*
- *Practice Pattern 5C: Impaired Motor Function and Sensory Integrity Associated with Nonprogressive Disorders of the Central Nervous System—Congenital Origin or Acquired in Infancy or Childhood*

EXAMINATION AND EVALUATION

Functional Limitations

At home and school, Shawna ambulates with a posterior control walker 50 feet with standby assistance. She has good head and trunk control, but she is most comfortable sitting in a "W" position. She rolls segmentally and creeps using a homologous pattern, but, with cues, can creep with a poorly coordinated cross diagonal pattern. She is unable to maintain her posture in any position when moved quickly. Her active movements tend to be slow and she has difficulty keeping up with her peers during motor activities. Movement through space causes autonomic distress.

Impairments

Shawna demonstrates head and trunk righting when moved in any direction. She has slow protective extension responses in her arms and legs. She is able to maintain her balance during slow tilting in prone, supine, and sitting but falls when fast tilting is attempted.

The patient's locomotor difficulties are consistent with her basic problems of diminished postural responses and inadequate isolated movements of the lower extremities. These problems limit Shawna's ability to provide adequate support and propulsion during stance. In the presence of poorly stabilized stance, swing of the contralateral leg is affected, making safe limb clearance difficult. The presence of hip weakness may contribute to poorly disassociated lower extremity movements during ambulation. The child may be using thigh contact between the limbs to provide additional stability during stance, thus compensating for gluteus maximus and gluteus medius weakness, as well as reduced pelvic stability.

PROGNOSIS/PLAN OF CARE

Goals

Treatment goals are for Shawna to:

1. Improve ability to ambulate with a posterior control walker
2. Demonstrate ability to maintain a midline posture during sitting and when standing with her walker
3. Increase lower extremity strength

Functional Outcomes

Following 3 months of physical therapy intervention, Shawna will:

1. Independently ambulate from her classroom to the cafeteria (100 feet) using the walker
2. In the walker, stand on one leg without dropping the opposite hip while kicking a ball placed in front of her foot
3. During play while standing in her walker, quickly reach and obtain a toy held out to her side one of three attempts

INTERVENTION

A complete review of Shawna's strength throughout the trunk and extremities is essential for establishing appropriate goals and developing an effective intervention program. As indicated previously, adequate support during the stance phase depends on hip and knee extensor strength as well as hip abductor strength. In their absence, Shawna may be resorting to any form of stability that is available. This may be the compensation currently available to her. However, the role of the physical therapist is to diminish the need for such compensation by increasing strength. The therapist should try to facilitate alternative synergistic patterns to provide Shawna with a broader repertoire of movements. However, isolated or varied movements may be very difficult for Shawna due to her motor control deficits (ie, cerebral palsy), as well as cognitive deficits.

A wide variety of activities to increase proximal strength are available to the physical therapist. Postural activities in prone, supine, quadruped, and kneeling can be used to facilitate activity of the trunk and pelvic girdle musculature. Decreased righting reactions and hyperactive autonomic responses to movement also limit Shawna's stability and confidence. To promote trunk control and righting reactions, Shawna can sit on an inflated wedge-shaped cushion and reach for objects that are held at various heights and distances from her body. Activities in tall kneeling and half kneeling postures also can facilitate appropriate trunk responses, as well as promote strength in the trunk and pelvis. Such activities may be used to desensitize her vestibular system and facilitate active movements. As Shawna's motor control improves, activities to promote disassociation of the lower extremities can be introduced such as reciprocal creeping, side stepping along a classroom table, kicking a ball while in her walker, and backing up while holding the walker.

Shawna demonstrates the need for proximal and isolated control to meet the requirements of the stance and swing phases of gait: support, propulsion, and transfer   of momentum. Such control depends on adequate strength because, although superior strength is not a direct requirement of functional gait, it remains an important ingredient.

CASE STUDY # 5
Robert Anderson

- *Age: 38 years*
- *Medical Diagnosis: Incomplete T9-10 spinal cord injury with left radial nerve damage*
- *Status: 6 months post injury*
- *Practice Pattern 5H: Impaired Motor Function, Peripheral Nerve Integrity, and Sensory Integrity Associated with Nonprogressive Disorders of the Spinal Cord*

EXAMINATION AND EVALUATION

Functional Limitations

Mr. Anderson has difficulty with some transfers including sit to stand with knee-ankle-foot orthoses (KAFOs). He has independent sitting balance, but cannot stand independently. He is unable to walk unless he uses a walker or forearm crutches and his orthoses. He is most efficient with a swing-through gait but does not use this method of locomotion for community ambulation due to limited endurance.

Impairments

Mr. Anderson has loss of sensation and paralysis of muscles in his lower extremities associated with his spinal cord injury. He has had increasing stiffness in his lower extremities. His balance in standing with his forearm crutches has improved, but he occasionally has difficulties, particularly on uneven terrain in the community (eg, gravel, sand).

PROGNOSIS/PLAN OF CARE

Goals

Treatment goals are for Mr. Anderson to:
1. Increase endurance for ambulation with orthoses and forearm crutches
2. Demonstrate ability to ambulate over uneven terrain with orthoses and forearm crutches
3. Improve ability to transfer from sit to stand with orthoses and forearm crutches

Functional Outcomes

Following 3 months of physical therapy, Mr. Anderson will:

1. Use his orthoses and forearm crutches for functional community activities such as attending church services or going to a movie
2. Be able to walk over a gravel driveway without loss of balance with standby assistance for safety
3. Transfer from sit to stand with his orthoses and forearm crutches independently 100% of attempts

INTERVENTION

Mr. Anderson has good cognitive skills and is highly motivated to achieve functional goals and to resume his pre-accident activities. He will be limited in his ability to ambulate by the sensory and motor loss associated with his spinal cord injury. Strengthening activities for his upper extremities are important as he will rely on his arms for transfers and ambulation with a walker or forearm crutches.

Mr. Anderson has an incomplete spinal cord lesion and has expressed interest in attempting to regain as much function as possible in his lower extremities. He has been working on a treadmill with partial weight bearing (using a harness system) and has demonstrated some ability to move his lower extremities independently, primarily at the hip joint. This activity should be continued as long as Mr. Anderson is motivated and continues to show some progress in independent movement of the lower extremities. He would need to have significant return of muscle function, however, as the limited movement he currently demonstrates will not be functional during ambulation. More realistic locomotion goals for Mr. Anderson probably are use of his orthoses and forearm crutches for household and limited community ambulation, with use of his wheelchair for prolonged community ambulation and work.

This case study demonstrates how the goals related to locomotion need to be modified in relation to pathology that limits sensory processing and motor control in the lower extremities. The assistive device (eg, wheelchair) that provides the patient with the most functional method of locomotion should be encouraged while, at the same time, activities and assistive devices (eg, orthoses and forearm crutches) are used to meet the patient's desired goal of ambulation.

REFERENCES

1. Guide to physical therapist practice. 2nd ed. *Phys Ther.* 2001;81:S31-S42.
2. Malouin F. Observational gait analysis. In: Craik RL, Oatis CA, eds. *Gait Analysis: Theory and Application.* St Louis, Mo: Mosby-Year Book, Inc; 1995:112-124.
3. Krebs DE, Edelstein JE, Fishman S. Reliability of observational gait analysis. *Phys Ther.* 1985; 65:1027-1033.
4. Murray MP. Gait as a total pattern of movement. *American Journal of Physical Medicine.* 1967;46:290-333.
5. Winter DA, Patla AE, Frank JS, et al. Biomechanical walking patterns in the fit and healthy elderly. *Phys Ther.* 1990;70:340-347.
6. Kadaba MP, Ramakrishnan HK, Wootten ME, et al. Repeatability of kinematic, kinetic, and electromyographic data in normal adult gait. *Journal of Orthopaedic Research.* 1989; 7:849-860.

7. Dujardin FH, Roussignol X, Mejjad O, et al. Interindividual variations of the hip joint motion in normal gait. *Gait and Posture*. 1997;5:246-250.

8. Sutherland DH, Kaufman KR, Moitoza JR. Kinematics of normal human walking. In: Rose J, Gamble JG, eds. *Human Walking*. Philadelphia, Pa: Willams & Wilkins; 1994: 23-44.

9. Isacson J, Gransberg L, Knutsson E. Three-dimensional electrogoniometric gait recording. *J Biomech*. 1986;19:627-635.

10. Lafortune MA, Cavanagh PR, Sommer HJ, et al. Three-dimensional kinematics of the human knee during walking. *J Biomech*. 1992;25:347-357.

11. Johnston RC, Smidt GL. Measurement of hip joint motion during walking: evaluation of an electrogoniometric method. *J Bone Joint Surg*. 1969;51A:1083

12. Inman VT, Ralston HJ, Todd F. *Human Walking*. Baltimore, Md: Williams & Wilkins; 1981.

13. Krebs DE, Wong D, Jevsevar D, et al. Trunk kinematics during locomotor activities. *Phys Ther*. 1992;72:505-514.

14. Vogt L, Banzer W. Measurement of lumbar spine kinematics in incline treadmill walking. *Gait and Posture*. 1999;9:18-23.

15. Wagenaar RC, van Emmerick REA. Resonant frequencies of arms and legs identify different walking patterns. *J Biomech*. 2000;33:853-861.

16. Eberhart HD, Inman VT, Saunders JB, et al. *Fundamental Studies of Human Locomotion and Other Information Relating to Design of Artificial Limbs*. A report to the National Research Council, Committee on Artificial Limbs, University of California, Berkeley. University of California, Berkeley; 1947.

17. Bianchi L, Angelini D, Orani GP, et al. Kinematic coordination in human gait: relation to mechanical energy cost. *The American Physiological Society*. 1998;79:2155-2170.

18. Crosbie J, Vachalathiti R, Smith R. Age, gender and speed effects on spinal kinematics during walking. *Gait and Posture*. 1997;5:13-20.

19. Crosbie J, Vachalathiti R. Synchrony of pelvic and hip joint motion during walking. **Gait and Posture**. 1997;6:237-248.

20. Wu G. A review of body segmental displacement, velocity, and acceleration in human gait. In Craik R, Oatis CA, eds. *Gait Analysis Theory and Application*. St. Louis, Mo: Mosby-Year Book, Inc, 1995:205-222.

21. Judge J, Davis RB, Ounpuu S. Step length reductions in advanced age: The role of ankle and hip kinetics. *J Geront A Biol Sci Med Sci*. 1996;51(6):M303-312.

22. Kerrigan DC. Biomechanical gait alterations independent of speed in the healthy elderly: evidence for specific limiting impairments. *Arch Phys Med Rehabil*. 1998;79:317-322.

23. Murray MP, Kory RC, Clarkson BH. Walking patterns in healthy old men. J Gerontol. 1969; 24:169.

24. Kernozek TW, LaMott EE. Comparisons of plantar pressures between the elderly and young adults. *Gait and Posture*. 1995;3:143-148.

25. Leiper CI, Craik RL. Relationships between physical activity and temporal-distance characteristics of walking in elderly women. *Phys Ther*. 1991;71:791-803.

26. Himann JE, Cunningham DA, Rechnitzer PA, et al. Age-related changes in speed of walking. *Med and Science in Sports and Exercise*. 1988;20:161-166.

27. Murray MP, Kory RC, Clarkson BH, et al. Comparison of free and fast speed walking patterns of normal men. *Am J Phys Med*. 1966;45:8-24.

28. Craik R, Cook T, D'Orazio B. Variations in healthy gait with changes in velocity. *Phys Ther*. 1980;60:575

29. Kerrigan DC. Gender differences in joint biomechanics during walking: normative study in young adults. *Am J Phys Med Rehabil.* 1998;77:2-7.

30. Kuster M, Sakurai S, Wood GA. Kinematic and kinetic comparison of downhill and level walking. *Clinical Biomechanics.* 1995;10:79-84.

31. Winter DA. *The Biomechanics and Motor Control of Human Gait: Normal, Elderly and Pathological.* Waterloo, Iowa: University of Waterloo Press; 1991.

32. Rowe PJ, Myles CM, Walker C, et al. Knee joint kinematics in gait and other functional activities measured using flexible electrogoniometry: how much knee motion is sufficient for normal daily life? *Gait and Posture.* 2000;12:143-155.

33. Murray MP, Kory RC, Sepic SB. Walking patterns of normal women. *Archives of Physical Medicine.* 1979;51:637.

34. Whittle MW, Levine DF. Sagittal plane motion of the lumbar spine during normal gait. *Gait and Posture.* 1995;3:82-82.

35. Stokes VP, Andersson C, Frossberg H. Rotational and translational movement features of the pelvis and thorax during adult human locomotion. *J Biomech.* 1989;22(1):43-50.

36. Jacobs NA, Skorecki J, Charndey J. Analysis of the vertical component of force in normal and pathological gait. *J Biomech.* 1975;5:11-35.

37. Bresler B, Frankel SP. The forces and moments in the leg during level walking. *Transactions of the ASME.* 1950;27-36.

38. Anderson FC, Pandy MG. Static and dynamic optimization solutions for gait are practically equivalent. *J Biomech.* 2001; 34: 153-161.

39. Komistek RD, Stiehl JB, Dennis DA, et al. Mathematical model of the lower extremity joint reaction forces using Kane's method of dynamics. *Biomech.* 1998;31:185-189.

40. Duda GN, Schneider E, Chao EY. Internal forces and moments in the femur during walking. *J Biomech.* 1997;30:933-941.

41. Simonsen EB, Dyhre-Poulsen P, Voigt M, et al. Bone-on-bone forces during loaded and unloaded walking. *Acta Anat (Basel)* 1995;152:133-142.

42. Paul JP. Forces transmitted by joint in the human body. *Proc Inst Mech Eng.* 1967;181:8.

43. Seireg A, Arvikar RJ. The prediction of muscular load sharing and joint forces in the lower extremities during walking. *J Biomech.* 1975;8:89-102.

44. Crowninshield RD, Brand RA, Johnston RC. The effects of walking velocity and age on hip kinematics and kinetics. *Clin Orthop.* 1978;132:140.

45. Morrison JB. Bioengineering analysis of force actions transmitted by the knee joint. *J Biomedical Engineering.* 1968;3:164-170.

46. Harrington IJ. A bioengineering analysis of force actions at the knee in normal and pathological gait. *J Biomedical Engineering.* 1976;11:107.

47. Hardt DE. Determining muscle forces in the leg during normal human walking—An application and evaluation of optimization methods. *J Biomechanical Engineering.* 1978;100: 72-78.

48. Stauffer RN, Chao EYS, Brewster RC. Force and motion analysis of the normal, diseased and prosthetic ankle joint. *Clinical Orthopaedics and Related Research.* 1977;127:189-196.

49. Winter DA. Overall principle of lower limb support during stance phase of gait. *J Biomech.* 1980;13:923-927.

50. Devita P, Hortobagyi T. Age causes a redistribution of joint torques and powers during gait. *J Appl Physiol.* 2000; 88:1804-1811.

51. Knutson LM, Soderberg GL. EMG: use and interpretation in gait. In: Craik RL, Oatis CA eds. *Gait Analysis: Theory and Application.* St Louis, Mo: Mosby; 1995:307-325.

52. Craik RL, Oatis CA. Gait assessment in the clinic: issues and approaches. In Rothstein JM ed. *Measurements in Physical Therapy.* New York, NY: Churchill Livingstone, 1985;169-205.

53. Winter DA, Yack HJ. EMG profiles during normal human walking: stride-to-stride and inter-subject variability. *Electroenceph and Clinical Neurophys*. 1987;67:402-411.

54. Shiavi R. Electromyographic patterns in adult locomotion: a comprehensive review. *Journal of Rehabilitation Research and Development*. 1985;22:85-98.

55. Milner M, Basmajian JV, Quanbury AO. Multifactorial analysis of walking by electromyography and computer. *Am J Phys Med*. 1971;50:235.

56. Dubo HIC, Peat M, Winter DA, et al. Electromyographic temporal analysis of gait: normal human locomotion. *Arch Phys Med Rehabil*. 1976;57:415-420.

57. Perry J. Functional evaluation of the pes anserinus transfer by electromyography and gait analysis. *J Bone Joint Surg Am*. 1980; 62: 973-980.

58. Hagy JL, Mann RA, Keller CW. *Normal electromyographic data gait analysis laboratory, Shriners Hospital for Crippled Children*. San Francisco, Calif: 1973.

59. Mochon S, McMahon TA. Ballistic walking. *J Biomech*. 1980;13:49.

60. Winter DA, Quanbury AO, Reimer GD. Analysis of instantaneous energy of normal gait. *J Biomech*. 1976;9:253-257.

61. Robertson DGE, Winter DA. Mechanical energy generation, absorption, and transfer amongst segments during walking. *J Biomech*. 1980;13:845-854.

62. Sadeghi H, Allard P, Duhaime M. Contributions of lower-limb muscle power in gait of people without impairments. *Phys Ther*. 2000;80:1188-1196.

63. McGibbon CA, Puniello MS, Krebs D. Mechanical energy transfer during gait in relation to strength impairment and pathology in elderly women. *Clinical Biomechanics*. 2001;16: 324-333.

64. McGibbon CA, Krebs DE. Effects of age and functional limitation on leg joint power and work during stance phase of gait. *J Rehabil Res Dev*. 1999;36:173-182.

65. Das P, McCollum G. Invariant structure in locomotion. *Neuroscience*. 1988;25:1023-1034.

66. Winter DA. Biomechanics of normal and pathological gait: implications for understanding human locomotor control. *J Motor Behav*. 1989;21:337-355.

67. Olgiatti R, Burgunder JM, Mumenthaler M. Increased energy cost of walking in multiple sclerosis: effect of spasticity, ataxia, and weakness. *Arch Phys Med Rehabil*. 1988; 69: 846-849.

68. Cerny K, Waters R, Hislop H, et al. Walking and wheelchair energetics in persons with paraplegia. *Phys Ther*. 1980; 60:1133-1139.

69. Bendersky E, Machoid P, Rorh M. *Assessment of community ambulation skill*. 1990; (UnPub Master's thesis, Beaver College, Glenside, Pennsylvania).

70. Krebs DE. Isokinetic, electrophysiologic, and clinical function relationships following tourniquet-aided knee arthrotomy. *Phys Ther*. 1989;69:803-815.

71. Gyory AN, Chao EY, Stauffer RN. Functional evaluation of normal and pathological knees during gait. *Arch Phys Med Rehabil*. 1976;57: 571-577.

72. Mueller MJ, Minor SD, Schaaf JA, et al. Relationship of plantar-flexor peak torque and dorsiflexion range of motion to kinetic variables during walking. *Phys Ther*. 1995;75:684-693.

73. Winter DA. Biomechanics of Normal and Pathological Gait: Implication for Understanding Human Locomotor Control. *J of Motor Behavior*. 1989; 21(4):337-355.

74. Stauffer RN, Chao EYS, Gyory AN. Biomechanical gait analysis of the diseased knee joint. *Clinical Orthopaedics and Related Research*. 1977;126:246-255.

75. Salsich GB, Brown M, Mueller MJ. Relationships between plantar flexor muscle stiffness, strength, and range of motion in subjects with diabetes-peripheral neuropathy compared to age-matched controls. *JOSPT*. 2000;30:473-483.

76. Tardieu C, Lespargot A, Tabary C, et al. Toe-walking in children with cerebral palsy: contributions of contracture and excessive contraction of triceps surae. *Phys Ther.* 1989;69:656-662.

77. Oatis CA. Use of a mechanical model to describe the stiffness and damping characteristics of the knee joint in healthy adults. *Phys Ther.* 1993;73:740-749.

78. Brinkman JR, Perry J. Rate and range of knee motion during ambulation in health and arthritic subjects. *Phys Ther.* 1985;65:1055-1060.

14

The Patients: Intervention and Discharge Planning

Patricia C. Montgomery, PhD, PT
Barbara H. Connolly, EdD, PT, FAPTA

INTRODUCTION

Patients with pathology of the central nervous system (CNS) seldom have isolated problems, but rather multiple problems as identified in the preceding chapters. For teaching purposes, examination and evaluation procedures and intervention strategies related to each problem area have been presented separately by the various authors. However, in the clinic, we must deal with the "whole" person, not problems in isolation. The purpose of this chapter is to summarize the primary functional limitations for each of the patients. We also hypothesize the primary impairments that are contributing to these functional limitations. Using a dynamic systems approach is essential when attempting to address the patient as a "whole" person. This ensures consideration of the multiple variables that interact on a daily basis and impact the functionality of the individual. Therefore, we have presented other areas of intervention that might be appropriate for each patient, as well as identifying future considerations for intervention and discharge.

CASE STUDY # 1
Jane Smith

- *Age: 74 years*
- *Medical Diagnosis: Right hemiplegia secondary, to left CVA*
- *Status: 6 months post onset*
- *Practice Pattern 5D: Impaired Motor Function and Sensory Integrity Associated with Nonprogressive Disorders of the Central Nervous System—Acquired in Adolescence or Adulthood*

PRIMARY FUNCTIONAL LIMITATIONS

- Requires assistance for all self-care, transfers, standing
- Sits independently, but asymmetrically
- Steers wheelchair, but bumps into objects
- Limited to walking with hemi-walker for 30 feet or with one person for assist
- Difficulty in ascending and descending stairs
- At risk for falls unless supervised
- Often unaware of visual stimuli to her right side
- Frequently sustains injuries to right arm and hand
- Does not use right hand effectively for bilateral fine motor activities
- Unaware of limitations, impulsive
- Frequently frustrated, problems expressing herself verbally

PRIMARY IMPAIRMENTS

- Sensory—right visual field cut, somatosensory deficits
- Disregard of right side of body and space
- Increased muscle tone in trunk with scapular retraction
- Increased lower extremity tone into extension and adduction
- Limited flexibility into ankle dorsiflexion, stiffness in ankle plantarflexors
- Decreased motor function/incoordination and weakness of right upper extremity
- Asymmetric weight bearing in sitting and standing
- Slowed balance responses and slowness of movement
- Impaired response selection and response programming, poor reference of correctness

PRIMARY GOALS

- Improve weight bearing symmetry in sitting, standing, and walking
- Improve attention to right side of body and space
- Improve appreciation of safety factors
- Increase flexibility of right ankle
- Increase strength of trunk and right extremities
- Improve coordinated use of right upper extremity
- Improve bed mobility and transfers
- Improve locomotion with walker (gait pattern and endurance)
- Improve ability to ascend and descend stairs
- Increase speed of response selection and accuracy in response programming
- Improve reference of correctness

PRIMARY FUNCTIONAL OUTCOMES

Self-Care

- Remove blouses and jackets independently, put on housecoat independently (with occasional assistance with buttons/zippers)
- Use both hands to assist with kitchen chores, such as drying dishes and sorting and putting away silverware
- Use her right hand as an assist during daily activities, such as holding open the refrigerator door with her right hand while obtaining an item from within with her left hand
- Transfer independently with standby supervision and verbal cues 100% of the time from bed to wheelchair, wheelchair to chair, and wheelchair to bed
- Climb up and down stairs (three steps) into her home holding onto the railing with standby assistance for safety
- Climb eight steps, with moderate assistance, in split-level home to reach bedroom level
- While supported by her walker, rise up on tiptoes to look out the kitchen window or to look for something on a high shelf
- Achieve independent bed mobility for changing positions and getting in bed (once sitting on edge of bed) and out of bed (getting into sitting at edge of bed)

Ambulation

- Transfer from her wheelchair to standing independently for 30 to 60 seconds at the kitchen or bathroom counter without assistance, then successfully transfer back to sitting in her wheelchair. This would allow her to perform functional tasks such as obtaining a drink of water, washing her hands, and putting on lipstick

- Walk 100 feet two times daily with her hemi-walker outside on level terrain. In addition, use the walker for household ambulation to move from room to room (ie, living room to kitchen, bedroom to bathroom)

Safety

- Demonstrate awareness of the right side of her body by decreasing occurrences of injury to her right arm while maneuvering around her environment in her wheelchair
- Demonstrate less impulsivity by waiting for assistance when it is needed

Additional Considerations for Intervention and Discharge

The majority and fastest rate of recovery following a cerebrovascular accident (CVA) tends to occur within the first 6 months. Mrs. Smith is now 6 months post-CVA and continues to demonstrate significant problems with communication, sensory loss, and motor function. Given her age (74 years), medical history, rate of progress for the past 6 months, and current impairments, her prognosis for improved upper extremity function and ambulation is guarded.

Two major concerns for Mrs. Smith and her family is her current living situation and her inability to effectively communicate. The team at the hospital is working with the family to obtain home care assistance for several hours each week to assist Mr. Smith with his wife's care. Mr. Smith and their two adult children are investigating an assisted living facility where there would be no stairs and Mrs. Smith could have varying levels of assistance as dictated by her long-term recovery. The family is considering placement for both Mr. and Mrs. Smith into the assisted living facility. Mr. Smith has rheumatoid arthritis and is having difficulty assisting his wife and maintaining their home. In addition, the speech language pathologist has been exploring various augmentative communication systems for Mrs. Smith. These systems would enable Mrs. Smith to communicate more effectively and thus decrease her frustration level.

Mrs. Smith has been provided with a home program of range of motion (ROM) exercises for her upper and lower extremities and trunk that is designed to maintain flexibility. Although she has attempted use of a wide-based quad cane, this has proven difficult for her. Given her limited right upper extremity function, sensory loss, and poor balance, a more realistic goal might be safe household and community ambulation with the hemi-walker.

Mrs. Smith appears to be reaching a plateau in her recovery. The team has recommended decreasing frequency of physical therapy following the current intervention period of 3 months to once per month for the next 3 months. She will be monitored during that time for progress and updating of her home program. If she continues to make progress, continued monitoring would be appropriate. Otherwise, Mrs. Smith will be discharged from physical therapy at that time.

CASE STUDY #2
Daniel Johnson

- *Age: 59 years*
- *Medical Diagnosis: Parkinson's disease*
- *Status: 4 years post initial diagnosis*
- *Practice Pattern 5E: Impaired Motor Functional and Sensory Integrity Associated with Progressive Disorders of the Central Nervous System*

PRIMARY FUNCTIONAL LIMITATIONS

- Difficulty with recreational activities (swimming and walking)
- Limits participation in physical activities because of fatigue
- Uninterested in social activities
- Requires assistance with transfers and when rising from a low chair
- Difficulty with walking: shortened stride, progressive increase in speed with festination, forward lean
- Loses balance when turning, difficulty regaining balance
- At risk for falls when walking on uneven terrain or in crowded environments
- Takes longer to complete self-care and functional household tasks
- Problems with remembering and executing multi-step activities

PRIMARY IMPAIRMENTS

- Rigidity in extremities, decreased excursions of movement
- Decreased flexibility of trunk, en bloc movements with poor trunk rotation
- Decreased isolated movements of trunk on pelvis and trunk and pelvis on lower extremities
- Center of mass displaced forward in standing and walking
- Dyskinesia, tremor, bradykinesia
- Response programming deficits, difficulty with automatic or open loop tasks
- Short-term memory problems
- Depression

PRIMARY GOALS

- Improve initiation of movement
- Improve speed and safety during transitions of movement (eg, sit to stand)
- Improve upright posture and body alignment during sitting, standing, and walking

- Increase ROM and flexibility in trunk and pelvis
- Increase speed of response to perturbations to balance in upright
- Increase stride length and balance during gait
- Increase strength, endurance, and activity level
- Improve response programming and performance of open loop tasks
- Increase short-term memory for motor tasks

PRIMARY FUNCTIONAL OUTCOMES

Transfers

- Complete sit to stand transitions from his household chairs independently
- Complete transfers, such as in and out of a car, with standby assistance for safety

Ambulation

- Stand and walk with a more erect posture so he does not have a tendency to fall forward
- Ambulate with minimal assistance (eg, holding onto another adult's arm) in the community, up and down curbs, inclines, on uneven terrain such as grass or gravel, or on slippery surfaces such as snow, ice, or wet pavement
- Ambulate independently within his home environment

Physical Activities

- Participate in community activities such as a Parkinson's disease support group and tai chi class
- Complete a home program daily to maintain extremity and trunk ROM and flexibility

Cognition

- Use cognitive strategies to complete multi-step tasks such as breaking down tasks and concentrating on doing one thing at a time in series. For example, concentrating on walking from the living room to the kitchen, then getting a can of soda from the refrigerator, then returning to the living room
- Use cognitive strategies, such as lists, for multi-step household tasks that he is having trouble remembering

Additional Considerations for Intervention and Discharge

Mr. Johnson has made progress toward achieving his goals, and it is anticipated that he will be discharged from physical therapy at the end of this 3-month intervention period. However, a major concern for Mr. Johnson's family is his increasing social isolation and depression. There is family and individual counseling available through the Parkinson's support group. Mr. Johnson and his family are being encouraged to use these services.

Additionally, the physical therapist should give the family suggestions about recreational activities in which they could participate as a family. For example, Mr. Johnson could swim with his teenage children on a regular basis at the local health club. At the local health club, the physical therapist conducts group aquatic therapy sessions that also might be beneficial for Mr. Johnson. The family should be encouraged to consider a daily walking program in which at least one member of the family walks with Mr. Johnson.

Because of the progressive nature of Parkinson's disease, Mr. Johnson will need episodic physical therapy care. As his disease progresses and he becomes unsafe with transfers and ambulation, a physical therapist will need to recommend assistive devices as necessary (eg, walker or wheelchair).

CASE STUDY #3
Shirley Teal

- *Age: 21 years*
- *Medical Diagnosis: Traumatic brain injury*
- *Status: 4 months post injury*
- *Practice Pattern 5D: Impaired Motor Function and Sensory Integrity Associated with Nonprogressive Disorders of the Central Nervous System—Acquired in Adolescence or Adulthood*

PRIMARY FUNCTIONAL LIMITATIONS

- Limits movements of head on body to reduce dizziness and vertigo
- Limits transfers/changes of position due to dizziness
- Needs minimal assist with transfers, performs pivot transfers
- Cannot stand and walk independently
- Needs maximal assistance to ascend or descend stairs
- Limited to household wheelchair mobility
- Poor coordination during bilateral upper extremity activities such as dressing, washing hands
- Inconsistent completion of two- to three-part commands and motor activities
- Difficulty with verbal communication, others unable to understand her speech
- Combative during therapy and uncooperative with therapist

PRIMARY IMPAIRMENTS

- Sensory: astereognosia, decreased proprioception and kinesthesia,
- Vertigo and dizziness (BPPN): visual dependence; stimulus identification problems

- Decreased ROM in right lower extremity joints
- Increased stiffness/muscle tone in extremities
- Generalized weakness
- Poor balance in sitting and standing
- Problems with initiation and coordination of movement
- Problems with grasping and manipulating objects
- Response selection and motor planning difficulties
- Impulsive, unsafe behavior, attention deficits (eg, maintaining and switching attention)
- Behavioral outbursts

PRIMARY GOALS

- Decrease movement-provoked symptoms of vertigo and dizziness
- Improve gaze stabilization
- Improve overall strength
- Increase ROM of right ankle dorsiflexion, hip and knee extension
- Increase symmetry and balance during sitting and standing
- Improve general coordination
- Perform independent transfers
- Increase distance ambulated with a walker
- Improve ability to ascend and descend stairs
- Improve stimulus identification ability in both hands
- Improve response selectivity and motor planning
- Increase ability to concentrate and improve attention switching ability

PRIMARY FUNCTIONAL OUTCOMES

Self-Care

- Manipulate small objects successfully, such as cosmetics, during self-care activities
- Demonstrate ability to concentrate on a self-care task for 10 minutes

Mobility

- Demonstrate ability to move her body or her head and her body through space during motor tasks without dizziness or vertigo
- Perform all transfers in and out of her wheelchair independently
- Walk with her walker sufficient distances for community ambulation
- Walk up and down 8 to 10 stairs holding on to the railing with one hand and assistance of another adult (eg, father in apartment building)
- Walk household distances with an upright posture using her hinged ankle foot orthosis and a wide-based quad cane with standby assistance for safety

Additional Considerations for Intervention and Discharge

Ms. Teal has made rapid progress since her traumatic brain injury 4 months ago. It is anticipated that she will continue to make steady progress over the next few months and will become less combative and more functional. The primary focus of her physical therapy program is to address the BPPN as she is limiting her movements due to dizziness and nausea. This issue must be resolved for her to make optimal progress in mobility skills. Because discharge to home is planned in 2 months, emphasis is being placed on independence in transfers, self-care tasks, stair climbing and descent, and assisted ambulation. When discharged, she will be living with her parents and her young child in a second-floor walk-up apartment. There is no elevator available. However, Ms. Teal's father works at home and is physically capable of providing her maximal assistance if needed.

Although Ms. Teal's attention skills are improving and her behavioral outbursts and combative behavior are decreasing, these are still areas of concern for the rehabilitation team and Ms. Teal's family. A referral has been made for a consultation with a neuropsychologist to address these issues and to develop a comprehensive program for Ms. Teal.

After discharge from the extended care facility in 2 months, she will be returning for physical therapy as an outpatient. She has expressed a desire to eventually return to work and to live alone with her young child. When the physical therapist deems Ms. Teal to be physically ready, she should be referred to vocational rehabilitation for testing and counseling. Ms. Teal will receive outpatient physical therapy as long as she continues to demonstrate measurable improvement in her functional abilities. When her skill level begins to plateau, the frequency of physical therapy services will be adjusted accordingly. It is anticipated that discharge from physical therapy will occur within 6 to 9 months.

CASE STUDY # 4
Shawna Wells

- *Age: 4 years*
- *Medical Diagnosis: Cerebral palsy, spastic quadriparesis, mild mental retardation*
- *Status: Onset at birth*
- *Practice Pattern 5C: Impaired Motor Function and Sensory Integrity Associated with Nonprogressive Disorders of the Central Nervous System—Congenital Origin or Acquired in Infancy or Childhood*

PRIMARY FUNCTIONAL LIMITATIONS

- Cannot walk independently with walker (minimal assistance) or walk on uneven terrain
- Walks too slowly to keep up with peers
- Loses her balance easily in standing in the walker

- Hesitant to play on movable toys (eg, tricycle, scooter, swing)
- Avoids object manipulation for classroom and self-care tasks
- Difficulty reaching for objects at or above eye level
- Difficulty with attending to classroom activities and changing from one activity to another
- Difficulty learning and retaining new motor skills

PRIMARY IMPAIRMENTS

- Poor respiratory function
- Sensory: tactile hypersensitivity, tactile defensiveness, somatosensory stimulus detection difficulties, postural insecurity
- Decreased ROM in ankle dorsiflexion, knee extension, upper extremities, and trunk
- Decreased strength and endurance for motor activities
- Poor sitting and standing balance
- General incoordination
- Selective attention deficits
- Mild mental retardation

PRIMARY GOALS

- Demonstrate improved discrimination of somatosensory stimuli
- Demonstrate decrease in avoidance responses to tactile stimuli
- Increase overall strength and endurance
- Demonstrate ability to maintain midline posture in sitting and standing
- Improve balance and protective reactions during play in sitting, standing, and walking with walker
- Increase flexibility of plantarflexors, hamstrings, trunk, and upper extremities
- Improve control of lower extremities during stance and swing phases of gait
- Participate in age-appropriate movement activities with her peers (eg, play-ground)
- Demonstrate improved selective attention

PRIMARY FUNCTIONAL OUTCOMES

Sensory

- Tolerate various clothing textures without complaint
- Tolerate being touched by classmates and adults without aversive reactions
- Participate in activities such as pasting and fingerpainting without complaints

Mobility

- Ride a tricycle 300 feet in 10 minutes while playing with peers
- Move into tailor sit on the floor and sit for 5 minutes during group sessions in her classroom without falling
- Demonstrate improved upper extremity ROM by being able to put on and take off a hat and to obtain toys off a high toy shelf in her classroom
- Walk with her posterior walker independently and turn it to maneuver around tables and chairs within her classroom
- Walk outside on grass with her walker for 20 feet with standby assistance for safety

Additional Considerations for Intervention and Discharge

A primary impairment that limits Shawna's ability to perform physical activity is her poor respiratory status. She has been receiving occupational therapy and speech language therapy since 4 months of age. A major focus of both of these therapies has been on improving oral motor skills and respiration. Trunk strengthening and rib cage mobility have been stressed along with functional activities such as blowing through a straw and blowing windmill type toys to increase vital capacity. However, Shawna has shown limited improvement in her respiratory function as indicated by continued breathiness during speech and lack of full inspiration and expiration. She also is susceptible to colds and respiratory infections, often missing school due to illness.

Shawna's parents continue to focus on achievement of independent ambulation for Shawna. However, from a dynamic systems perspective, all of the variables that impact Shawna's ability to achieve independent ambulate should be considered. These include: poor respiratory function resulting in increased energy expenditure, motor pathology (cerebral palsy—spastic quadriparesis), postural insecurity, mild mental retardation, and poor motivation for physical activities. In addition, Shawna has received physical therapy for the past 4 years and her gross motor skills currently are at a 6 to 10 months level. All of these factors would suggest that Shawna has a poor prognosis for independent ambulation. Shawna's physical therapist has suggested that the primary focus of Shawna's motor goals this school year should be on achieving functional classroom mobility with her walker. The physical therapist has begun to discuss with the parents that Shawna will probably need to begin using a manual or power wheelchair during the next 2 years to enable her to keep up with her peers when she reaches first grade.

It is anticipated that Shawna will continue to receive direct physical therapy services in her school program for the next 2 years. At that time, the physical therapist anticipates a change in the mode of service delivery to a consultative model with more indirect services being provided. Emphasis in the consultative model also will be on Shawna receiving adaptive physical education services in the school environment and participating in community-based recreational activities such as horseback riding, swimming, and dance classes.

CASE STUDY #5
Robert Anderson

- *Age: 38 years*
- *Medical Diagnosis: Incomplete T9-10 spinal cord injury with left radial nerve damage*
- *Status: 6 months post injury*
- *Practice Pattern 5H: Impaired Motor Function, Peripheral Nerve Integrity, and Sensory Integrity Associated with Nonprogressive Disorders of the Spinal Cord*

PRIMARY FUNCTIONAL LIMITATIONS

- Often drops items being held in his left hand
- Unable to sit for long periods of time due to susceptibility for skin breakdown
- Difficulty transferring from sit to stand with knee ankle foot orthoses (KAFOs) and crutches to bed, floor, bath, car, and wheelchair
- Cannot stand or walk independently
- Unable to walk long distances in the community with crutches and KAFOs
- Difficulty walking with his crutches and KAFOs over uneven terrain

PRIMARY IMPAIRMENTS

- Loss of sensation and motor function below T9
- Decreased sensation in left radial nerve distribution
- Increasing muscle spasms and stiffness in lower extremities
- Weakness in radial nerve innervated muscles
- Poor endurance for ambulation

PRIMARY GOALS

- Demonstrate knowledge regarding risks of skin integrity problems and maintain good skin integrity
- Manipulate small objects using left hand during activities of daily living and work-related tasks
- Maintain ROM in lower extremities
- Perform all transfers independently
- Maneuver wheelchair at mall without bumping into objects or persons
- Walk with crutches and KAFOs for short distances during community outings, such as the grocery store
- Improve ability to ambulate with crutches and KAFOs over uneven terrain

PRIMARY FUNCTIONAL OUTCOMES

Self-Care

- Become independent in all self-care activities
- Demonstrate understanding regarding skin care, ROM, and avoidance of overuse syndrome in regard to the right arm
- Use left hand without dropping objects during bilateral self-care activities (such as putting toothpaste on a toothbrush)

Mobility

- Become independent in all transfers using KAFOs and crutches
- Demonstrate ability to use KAFOs and crutches on uneven terrains, ascending and descending curbs, and movement up and down inclines without falling

Recreation

- Participate on a wheelchair basketball team to improve wheelchair skills and overall endurance
- Join a group of individuals who take outings using all-terrain vehicles (modified with hand controls)

Additional Considerations for Intervention and Discharge

Mr. Anderson is realistic about his current motor status. However, he still holds out hope for return of lower extremity motor function. He has researched the Internet and has read about the current interest in the neuroscience community regarding the benefits of treadmill ambulation. He has expressed an interest in continuing use of partial weight bearing treadmill ambulation, which has been a part of his therapy program. However, it is anticipated that he will be discharged from physical therapy at the end of this intervention period because he will have reached all of his functional outcomes. His private health insurance company will no longer pay for him to use the treadmill and receive physical therapy as he will have achieved his anticipated goals. At this point in time, no related functional outcomes can be linked to use of the treadmill, and his insurance company will most likely deny continued coverage. Mr. Anderson's physical therapist is assisting him in locating centers that are conducting clinical trials on partial weight bearing treadmill ambulation to determine if he can become a subject. If this is not feasible, Mr. Anderson's family is considering sponsorship of a series of fundraisers to raise monies so that Mr. Anderson can pay out-of-pocket to receive these services through his local hospital.

CONCLUSION

The knowledge of how contemporary theories of motor development, motor learning, and motor control can be used effectively by physical therapists will lead to greater functional outcomes in the patients we serve. The authors of the various chapters in this book have attempted to link contemporary theories to the *Guide to Physical Therapist Practice*, as well as to practical applications to patient management. Not all examination and evaluation procedures or intervention strategies were addressed in the book. However, adequate examples were provided to guide therapists as they apply concepts to overall patient management.

A variety of intervention strategies can be used to meet the same objective or several objectives simultaneously. Although repetition is important in treatment, a variety of activities makes physical therapy enjoyable and motivating for the patient and the therapist. Creativity, therefore, is the art of physical therapy.

Index

Build Your Library

Along with this title, we publish numerous products on a variety of topics. We are sure that you will find the titles below to be an essential addition to your library. Order your copies today or contact us for a copy of our latest catalog for additional product information.

CLINICAL APPLICATIONS FOR MOTOR CONTROL

Patricia Montgomery, PhD, PT and Barbara Connolly, PT, EdD, FAPTA

416 pp., Soft Cover, 2002, ISBN 1-55642-545-7, Order #45457, **$43.95**

Clinical Applications for Motor Control is a comprehensive text that will help bridge the gap between motor control/motor learning research and practical clinical applications. Written by a variety of physical therapists with a broad range of clinical expertise areas such as neurophysiology, biomechanics, and human motor control, this text is rich in a multitude of topics. The case-study format that is applied throughout the text amplifies the principles of motor control research and demonstrates the transfer of information from research studies to clinical settings.

THERAPEUTIC EXERCISE IN DEVELOPMENTAL DISABILITIES, SECOND EDITION

Barbara Connolly, PT, EdD and Patricia Montgomery, PhD, PT

240 pp., Soft Cover, 1993, ISBN 1-55642-555-4, Order #45554, **$35.95**

This innovative text is written using a problem-solving approach as opposed to specific intervention approaches. The chapters integrate case studies of four children and the application of principles discussed throughout the text as they apply to the children. An essential element to *Therapeutic Exercise in Developmental Disabilities*, Second Edition is its focus on functional limitations of the child, possibly the most important aspect of successful intervention. These factors make this text user-friendly for the beginning student and practical for the practicing clinician.

QUICK REFERENCE NEUROSCIENCE FOR REHABILITATION PROFESSIONALS: THE ESSENTIAL NEUROLOGIC PRINCIPLES UNDERLYING REHABILITATION PRACTICE

Sharon A. Gutman, PhD, OTR

288 pp., Soft Cover, 2001, ISBN 1-55642-463-9, Order #34639, **$35.95**

This text is written in a simplistic, bulleted-outlined format with accompanying full-page, color illustrations that enhance understanding of the subject matter. Clinical correlates are discussed to provide a greater understanding of the common pathological disorders that occur in response to damage to specific neuroanatomical structures. In addition to a basic understanding of neuroanatomical structures and functions, the text provides an easy-to-read discussion of the essential neuroscience information necessary for the rehabilitation professional and student.

Contact us at

SLACK Incorporated, Professional Book Division
6900 Grove Road, Thorofare, NJ 08086
1-800-257-8290/1-856-848-1000, Fax: 1-856-853-5991
E-Mail: orders@slackinc.com or www.slackbooks.com

ORDER FORM

QUANTITY	TITLE	ORDER #	PRICE
	Clinical Applications for Motor Control	45457	**$43.95**
	Therapeutic Exercise in Developmental Disabilities	45554	**$35.95**
	Quick Reference Neuroscience for Rehabilitation Professionals	34639	**$35.95**
		Subtotal	$
		Applicable state and local tax will be added to your purchase	$
		Handling	**$4.50**
		Total	$

Name: _____
Address: _____
City: _____ State:_____ Zip: _____
Phone:_____ Fax: _____
Email: _____

- Check enclosed (Payable to SLACK Incorporated):_____
- Charge my: ___ ___ VISA ___ MasterCard

Account #: _____

Exp. date: _____ Signature:_____

NOTE: Prices are subject to change without notice. Shipping charges will apply. Shipping and handling charges are non-returnable.

CODE: 328